Handbook of Food and Nutrition Security

Handbook of Food and Nutrition Security

Edited by Reagan Perry

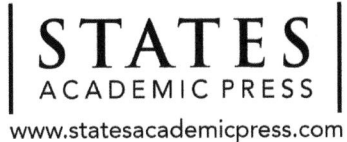

STATES
ACADEMIC PRESS
www.statesacademicpress.com

States Academic Press,
109 South 5th Street,
Brooklyn, NY 11249, USA

Visit us on the World Wide Web at:
www.statesacademicpress.com

ISBN: 978-1-63989-721-6

Cataloging-in-Publication Data

Handbook of food and nutrition security / edited by Reagan Perry.
  p. cm.
Includes bibliographical references and index.
ISBN 978-1-63989-721-6
1. Food security. 2. Food supply. 3. Nutrition policy. 4. Nutrition. 5. Food. I. Perry, Reagan.
TX357 .H36 2023
641.3--dc23

Table of Contents

Preface

It is often said that books are a boon to mankind. They document every progress and pass on the knowledge from one generation to the other. They play a crucial role in our lives. Thus I was both excited and nervous while editing this book. I was pleased by the thought of being able to make a mark but I was also nervous to do it right because the future of students depends upon it. Hence, I took a few months to research further into the discipline, revise my knowledge and also explore some more aspects. Post this process, I begun with the editing of this book.

Food and nutrition security (FNS) is attained when all individuals have physical, social and economic access to sufficient, safe and nutritious food at all times. The food should be sufficient to meet the dietary needs and food preferences of people. FNS can be ensured in an environment that promotes adequate sanitation, and health services and care. The framework of FNS is influenced by physical and temporal aspects. The physical determinant of FNS refers to the food flow in terms of availability, accessibility and utilization. The temporal aspect of FNS is concerned with stability. This book addresses the subject of food and nutrition security. It includes some of the vital pieces of works being conducted across the world, on various topics related to this topic. This book will serve as a reference to a broad spectrum of readers.

I thank my publisher with all my heart for considering me worthy of this unparalleled opportunity and for showing unwavering faith in my skills. I would also like to thank the editorial team who worked closely with me at every step and contributed immensely towards the successful completion of this book. Last but not the least, I wish to thank my friends and colleagues for their support.

Editor

Climate Change Policies in 16 West African Countries: A Systematic Review of Adaptation with a Focus on Agriculture, Food Security and Nutrition

Raissa Sorgho [1,2], Carlos A. Montenegro Quiñonez [1], Valérie R. Louis [1], Volker Winkler [1], Peter Dambach [1], Rainer Sauerborn [2] and Olaf Horstick [1,*]

[1] Heidelberg Research to Practice Group, Heidelberg Institute of Global Health (HIGH), Heidelberg University Hospital, Heidelberg University, Im Neuenheimer Feld 365, 69120 Heidelberg, Germany; raissa.sorgho@uni-heidelberg.de (R.S.); carlos.montenegro@uni-heidelberg.de (C.A.M.Q.); Valerie.Louis@uni-heidelberg.de (V.R.L.); volker.winkler@uni-heidelberg.de (V.W.); peter.dambach@uni-heidelberg.de (P.D.)

[2] Working Group on Climate Change, Nutrition & Health, Heidelberg Institute of Global Health (HIGH), Heidelberg University Hospital, Heidelberg University, Im Neuenheimer Feld 324, 69120 Heidelberg, Germany; rainer.sauerborn@uni-heidelberg.de

*   Correspondence: Olaf.Horstick@uni-heidelberg.de

Abstract: Climate change strongly impacts the agricultural sector in West Africa, threatening food security and nutrition, particularly for populations with the least adaptive capacity. Little is known about national climate change policies in the region. This systematic review identifies and analyses climate change policy documents in all 16 West African countries: (1) What are the existing climate change adaptation policies publicly available? (2) Which topics are addressed? (3) How are agriculture and food security framed and addressed? Following PRISMA guidelines, PubMed and Google scholar as key databases were searched with an extensive grey literature search. Keywords for searches were combinations of "Africa", "Climate Change", and "National Policy/Plan/Strategy/Guideline". Fifteen countries have at least one national policy document on climate change in the frame of our study. Nineteen policy documents covered seven key sectors (energy, agriculture, water resources, health, forestry, infrastructure, and education), and eight thematic areas (community resilience, disaster risk management, institutional development, industry development, research and development, policy making, economic investment, and partnerships/collaboration). At the intersection of these sectors/areas, effects of changing climate on countries/populations were evaluated and described. Climate change adaptation strategies emerged including development of local risk/disaster plans, micro-financing and insurance schemes (public or private), green energy, and development of community groups/farmers organizations. No clear trend emerged when analysing the adaptation options, however, climate change adaptation in the agriculture sector was almost always included. Analysing agriculture, nutrition, and food security, seven agricultural challenges were identified: The small scale of West African farming, information gaps, missing infrastructure, poor financing, weak farmer/community organizations, a shifting agricultural calendar, and deteriorating environmental ecology. They reflect barriers to adaptation especially for small-scale subsistence farmers with increased climate change vulnerabilities. The study has shown that most West African countries have climate change policies. Nevertheless, key questions remain unanswered, and demand for further research, e.g., on evaluating the implementation in the respective countries, persists.

Keywords: climate change; policy; adaptation; West Africa; agriculture; food security; nutrition

1. Introduction

Climate change (CC) is recognised as a threat to health, nutrition, and the livelihood of populations. Governments across the world have collectively negotiated and worked on solutions to mitigate and adapt to CC, and numerous treaties/agreements have been signed, from the Kyoto protocol in 1997 to the Paris agreement in 2015 [1–3]. Low- and middle-income countries are disproportionately affected by these impacts [4,5] and limited ability for planning, mitigation, and adaptation [6]. Hence, this study systematically determines whether West African countries have drafted and planned for adaptation through national CC policies.

CC policies are especially important for West African countries because CC is a new and amplifying risk factor for malnutrition/food security, particularly in countries with subsistence agriculture [7–9]. Preserving food security is particularly relevant for low-income countries where hunger and related productivity loss represent an enormous human and economic loss [10,11].

Between the years 2000 and 2050, CC is projected to cause additional 25.2 million chronically malnourished children <5 years, compared to a world without CC [12]. 10.5 million additional stunting cases will occur in sub-Saharan Africa, adding to the projected 41.7 malnourished children without CC occurring. This mirrors projected decreases in per capita food availability as median crop yields are expected to decrease due to CC by 0–2% per decade. At the same time, demand for crops is expected to increase by 14% per decade until 2050 [13–15].

CC policies should guide climate adaptation plans while addressing agricultural/food security. Here we focus on the West African region as a particularly vulnerable region for the effects of CC. Up to this date, no systematic analysis of existing CC policies exists for the West African region. Systematic analysis with the methods of systematic reviews have the advantage to systematically collect and analyse all relevant publications and data, ensuring that the analysis and following recommendations are not driven by expert opinion only [16].

Under this angle, this article systematically reviews the existing CC policies of 16 West African countries: Benin (BN), Burkina Faso (BF), Cape Verde (CV), Ivory Coast (IC), Gambia (GB), Ghana (GH), Guinea (GNA), Guinea-Bissau (GNB), Liberia (LB), Mali (ML), Mauritania (MR), Niger (NG), Nigeria (NGA), Senegal (SN), Sierra Leone (SL), and Togo (TG). The questions addressed are: (1) What are the existing CC adaptation policies publicly available? (2) Addressing which topics? (3) How are agriculture, food security, and nutrition framed and addressed?

2. Materials and Methods

Following the Preferred Reporting Items for Systematic Reviews and Meta-Analyses (PRISMA) [16], data were extracted by two authors until November 2020. The databases included were very broad, to reflect that CC policies may be reported or published in a wide variety of sources. The following databases were used: (1) PubMed, (2) Google Scholar, (3) Grey literature sources: United Nations databases, websites of FAO, UNDP, UNFCCC, (4) 48 West African countries' ministry governments websites (Ministry of Agriculture, Ministry of Environment, and Ministry of Health), and the (5) LSE and Grantham Research Institutes' database. The search strategy applied was the same on all databases, only on Google Scholar, the first 200 relevant hits were screened.

Search terms were combinations of "Africa" and/or country names, "Climate Change" and "National Policy/Plan/Strategy/Guideline" (Table 1).

We used adaptation as "The process of adjustment to actual or expected climate change and its effects. In human systems, adaptation seeks to moderate or avoid harm or exploit beneficial opportunities" [17]. This means that adaptation is planned for autonomous adjustments of individual groups or institutions in ecological-socio-economic systems in response to climatic stimuli, in order to reduce the society's vulnerability [18–20]. Policy documents are defined as internet-accessible plans, programmes, strategies, and guideline documents issued by national governments.

Table 1. Search phrase details for the systematic review.

Literature	Source	Search Phrases
Peer Reviewed	Google Scholar https://scholar.google.com	"Africa OR African" "Climate Change" "National Policy OR Policies" "Africa OR African" "Climate Change" "National Plan OR Plans" "Africa OR African" "Climate Change" "National Strategy OR Strategies" "Africa OR African" "Climate Change" "National Guideline OR Guidelines" "Country Name" "Climate Change" "National Policy OR Policies" "Country Name" "Climate Change" "National Plan OR Plans" "Country Name" "Climate Change" "National Strategy OR Strategies" "Country Name" "Climate Change" "National Guideline OR Guidelines"
	PubMed https://www.ncbi.nlm.nih.gov/pubmed/	(((Africa or African)) AND Climate Change) AND National Polic (((Africa or African)) AND Climate Change) AND National Plan (((Africa or African)) AND Climate Change) AND National Strateg (((Africa or African)) AND Climate Change) AND National Guideline (((Country Name)) AND Climate Change) AND National Polic (((Country Name)) AND Climate Change) AND National Plan (((Country Name)) AND Climate Change) AND National Strateg (((Country Name)) AND Climate Change) AND National Guideline
Grey	**Government Website** Ministry of Environment Ministry of Agriculture Ministry of Health Found using Google	**Ministry Webpage Information Tabs of each country:** Search each individual tab for relevant policies **Webpage Search Bar:** "National Policy" "National Plan" "National Strategy" "National Guidelines"
	Research Institute Grantham Research Institute on Climate Change and the Environment http://www.lse.ac.uk/GranthamInstitute/countries/	**Country Webpage Information Tabs:** Search each individual tab for relevant policies **Webpage Search Bar:** "Africa" "Climate Change" "National Policy" "Africa" "Climate Change" "National Plan" "Africa" "Climate Change" "National Strategie" "Africa" "Climate Change" "National Guidlines" "Country Name" "Climate Change" "National Policy" "Country Name" "Climate Change" "National Plan" "Country Name" "Climate Change" "National Stategie" "Country Name" "Climate Change" "National Guidlines"
	United Nation Organizations UNFCCC UNDP FAO https://unfccc.int http://www.adaptation-undp.org http://www.fao.org/faolex/country-profiles/en/	**UNFCCC–Main webpage Information Tabs:** Search each individual tab for relevant policies Read thought INDC, NC **UNDP–Climate Change Adaptation Portal:** Seach each individual country Read throught NAP, NAPA, NAMA **FAO–FOALEX Database** Search each individual country profile Read through policies, legislation, and international agreements

Inclusion criteria were: (1) National policy documents (2) of the 16 West African countries, (3) from any time-period, (4) publicly accessible, (5) in English, French, or Portuguese.

Publicly accessible documents are defined as document free of charge in digital or print format, accessible through internet search or by request through in-country experts at the step of identifying the full text of policies. The policy documents were often written in multiple languages (including English), contained abstracts or executive summaries in English, and were catalogued or indexed in English.

Exclusion criteria were: (1) Not written by or in collaboration with country governments, (2) no policy relevance (international reports, UN communications, scientific publications), (3) not applied nationally, (4) not specific to CC, and (5) not available in full text (Figure 1).

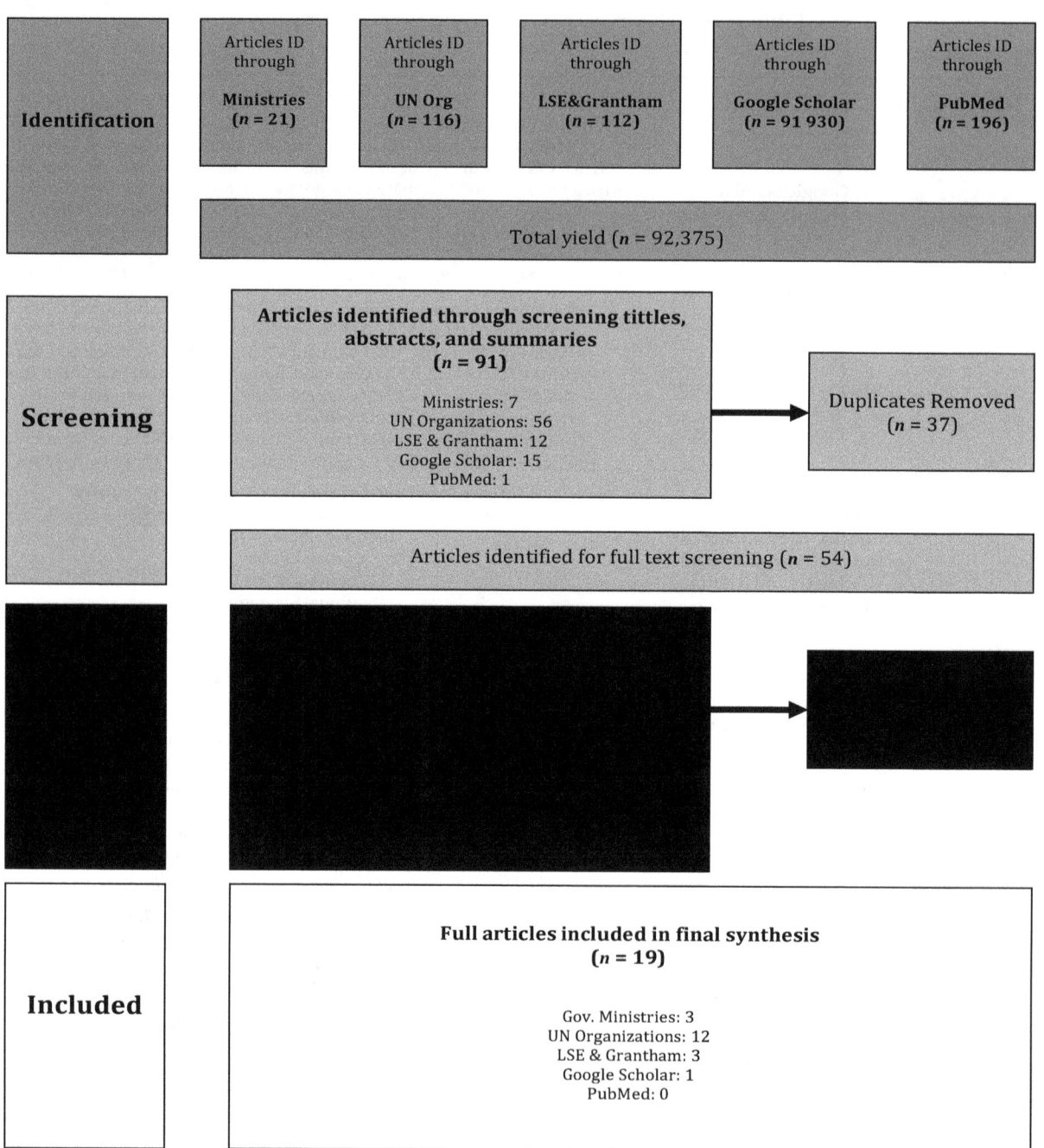

Figure 1. Flowchart of searches with the identification of policies, screening, eligibility, and inclusion.

Data were extracted from the finally included policy documents into a pre-defined data extraction sheet, covering topics as general characteristics, aims, integration into other policies, characterisation of CC and mitigation, linking of CC and agriculture including adaptation strategies, linking of CC and nutrition/food security, including adaptation strategies (Supplementary Materials Table S1).

The extracted information was analysed by country, type of document, and subject of interest. The data were then synthesised based on key points emerging from the policy documents. The content of the data was then qualitatively analysed through overarching themes developed from the documents. Next, the technical guidelines for the national adaptation plan process of the UNFCCC was used as framework for policy comparison, and lastly, a quality assessment of the policies was conducted [21].

3. Results

This section covers (Section 3) descriptive analysis with (Section 3.1) Searches and included documents (Section 3.2) key sectors, (Section 3.3) thematic areas and a (Section 3.4) comparative analysis with (Section 3.4.1) agricultural adaptation challenges, (Section 3.4.2) nutrition and food Security challenges, (Section 3.4.3) agriculture, nutrition, and food adaption solutions, and (Section 3.5) policy document comparison. Policy identification codes (PID) identify each policy document.

3.1. Searches and Document Inclusion

Searches initially retrieved 92,375 hits at the identification phase. Through screening of titles, abstracts, and summaries, 91 relevant hits were retained from all databases, then 35 duplicates were removed. Of the 47 documents identified for full text screening, 37 were eliminated based on the exclusion criteria. Eight of the 37 excluded articles were due to the inaccessibility of the full text of policies (Figure 1, Table 2, Supplementary Materials Table S2). At the end of the search, the 19 final documents were derived from following sources: Twelve United Nations organization web bases (FAO, UNDP, UNFCCC), three from LSE and Grantham, three from government ministry websites, and one from Google Scholar (Figure 1, Table 2).

Table 2. Nineteen included policies, coded by country.

	Policy Identification (PID)	Policy Document Name
1	BN1	National Strategy for Strengthening Human Resources, Learning and Skills Development to Support Green, Low Emissions and Climate Resilient Development.
2	BN2	Low Carbon and Climate Change Resilient Development Strategy 2016–2025
3	BF1	The National Strategy for implementing the Climate Change Convention
4	IC1	National Climate Change Program
5	GB1	National Climate Change Policy of The Gambia
6	GH1	Ghana National Climate Change Policy
7	GH2	Guidebook for Mainstreaming of Climate Change and Disaster Risk Reduction for MMDAs
8	GNB1	National Programme of Action of Adaptation to Climate Changes
9	LB1	Climate Change Gender Action Plan for the government of Liberia
10	LB2	National Policy and Response Strategy on Climate Change
11	ML1	National Strategy on Climate Change
12	ML2	Strategic Framework for a Green Economy Resilient to Climate Change
13	ML3	National Policy on Climate Change
14	ML4	National Climate Change Strategy: National Climate Action Plan
15	MR1	Strategy for integrating the environment and climate change in the Mauritanian education system
16	NG1	National Policy on Climate Change
17	NGA1	National Adaptation Strategy and Plan of Action of Climate Change for Nigeria
18	NGA2	National Policy on Climate Change
19	TG1	National Plan of Adaptations to Climate Change of Togo

The 19 included policy documents [22–40] originated from 14 countries. Guinea and Senegal had no relevant policy documents publicly available in the scope of this search, Benin, Ghana, Liberia, Mali, and Nigeria had more than one (Table 2). All included documents described the country, the listed agencies involved for document development, and specified aims/objectives. Seventeen of 19 documents mentioned other relevant national documents (laws, policies, reports, programmes) which were connected/relevant. Thirteen policies explained the effects of CC and elaborated on key scientific concepts as CC mitigation. Thirteen documents gave full explanations of CC mitigation, further explaining CC adaptation. Documents were often structured on key sectors and/or thematic areas. Seven common key sectors were identified across the policies: Energy, agriculture, water resources, health, forestry, infrastructure, and education (Table 3); and eight thematic areas emerged from the policy documents: Community resilience, disaster risk management, institutional development, industry development, research and development, policy making, economic investment, and partnerships/collaboration. Lastly, adaptation strategies were described for the above key sectors (Table 3).

3.2. Key Sectors

(I) Energy was discussed with a focus on electricity, petroleum, and renewable energies. More specifically, production, use, maintenance, and population need of energy and its different sources (PID: BN1, BN2, BF1, IC1, GB1, GH1, GH2, LB1, LB2, ML2, ML3, NG1, NGA1, NGA2, TG1).

(II) Agriculture was identified both as a key and vulnerable sector. Agriculture included animal husbandry, crops diversification, food granaries storage systems, and food security on a national level (PID: BN1, BN2, BF1, IC1, GB1, GH1, GH2, LB1, LB2, ML2, ML3, NG1, NGA1, NGA2, TG1).

(III) Water resource sections highlighted water use/management, desertification, fishing industry, and sometimes sanitation (PID: BN1, BN2, BF1, IC1, GB1, GH1, GH2, GNB1, LB1, LB2, ML1, ML2, ML3, ML4, MR1, NG1, NGA1, NGA2, TG1).

(IV) Health was one of the broader sectors, displaying a wide range of subtopics: Vector-borne and infectious diseases, malnutrition, heat, and human productivity, emphasising exacerbation of already existing differential social vulnerabilities (PID: BN1, BN2, BF1, IC1, GB1, GH1, GH2, GNB1, LB1, LB2, ML1, ML2, ML3, ML4, NG1, NGA1, NGA2, TG1).

(V) Forestry reiterated the importance of maintaining the environment, and the numerous ecological systems. Threats such as desertification and industrialisation were described in relation to sustainability and adaptation. (PID: BN2, BF1, IC1, GB1, GH1, GH2, GNB1, LB1, LB2, ML1, ML2, ML3, ML4, NG1, NGA1, NGA2, TG1).

(VI) Infrastructure sector centred on transport, housing, and safety. Focusing on deterioration of the above-mentioned systems, economic repercussions, and population wide effects if systems fail (PID: BN2, BF1, GB1, GH1, GH2, LB1, LB2, ML1, ML2, ML3, ML4, NGA1, NGA2, TG1).

(VII) Education mentioned three subtopics in relation to CC: (1) Education of relevant key local government members, (2) school-based education of children, (3) education of the general population (PID: BN1, BF1, GB1, GH1, GNB1, LB1, LB2, ML3, MR1, NGA1, NGA2, TG1).

Table 3. Content of the analysed policy documents in seven key sectors and eight thematic areas.

Key Sectors		BN1	BN2	BF1	IC1	GB1	GH1	GH2	GNB1	LB1	LB2	ML1	ML2	ML3	ML4	MR1	NG1	NGA1	NGA2	TG1
1	Energy	*	*	*	*	*	*	*	NMD	*	*	NMD	*	*	NMD	NMD	*	*	*	*
2	Agriculture	*	*	*	*	*	*	*	*	*	*	*	*	*	*	D	*	*	*	*
3	Water Resources	*	*	*	*	*	*	*	*	*	*	*	*	*	*	*	*	*	*	*
4	Health	*	*	*	*	*	*	*	*	*	*	*	*	*	*	D	*	*	*	*
5	Forestry	D	*	*	*	*	*	*	*	*	*	*	*	*	*	M	*	*	*	*
6	Infrastructure	NMD	*	*	M	*	*	*	D	D	*	*	*	*	*	M	M	*	D	*
7	Education	*	NMD	*	M	*	*	M	D	D	D	NMD	NMD	*	NMD	*	D	*	M	M

Thematic Areas		BN1	BN2	BF1	IC1	GB1	GH1	GH2	GNB1	LB1	LB2	ML1	ML2	ML3	ML4	MR1	NG1	NGA1	NGA2	TG1
1	Community Resilience	*	*	M	NMD	*	*	D	D	M	D	*	NMD	*	*	*	*	*	*	M
2	Disaster risk Management	M	*	NMD	*	*	*	*	NMD	NMD	D	M	*	*	M	M	M	*	*	M
3	Institutional Development	*	*	*	*	*	*	*	*	M	*	*	*	*	*	*	*	*	*	M
4	Industry Development	M	M	D	*	M	*	M	NMD	NMD	*	*	M	*	*	*	*	*	*	D
5	Research & Development	*	*	*	*	*	*	*	NMD	M	*	*	M	*	*	*	*	*	*	M
6	Policy Making	*	*	*	*	*	*	*	NMD	M	*	*	*	*	*	*	*	*	D	D
7	Economic Investment	*	*	*	NMD	*	*	*	D	M	*	*	*	*	*	*	*	*	*	M
8	Partnerships/ Collaboration	*	M	M	*	*	*	*	*	M	*	*	*	*	*	*	M	*	*	M

* (asterisk): The sector/area is highlighted as central and or key in the policy document; **D** (Discussed): The sector/area is discussed often in different ways and parts of the policy document; **M** (Mentioned): The sector/area is mentioned or briefly touched upon in the policy document; **NMD** (Not mentioned-discussed): The sector/area is not mentioned or discussed in the policy document.

3.3. Thematic Areas

Eight interconnected thematic areas were identified during the analysis of the policy documents. They were common amongst and throughout the documents, often utilised in combination with the seven key sectors (Table 3).

(i)   Partnerships and collaboration were often used in preambles. Slogans and logos of partnering country ministries and organisations were mentioned. Most frequently, the United Nations Development Program (UNDP), the United Nations Framework Convention on Climate Change (UNFCCC), German International Cooperation (GIZ), the Embassy of Norway, and the Agency for Environment and Sustainable Development (AEDD) were mentioned. Continued partnership with these organisations was encouraged, emphasising building relations with surrounding countries, regional organisations, and regional groups. Public government agencies were encouraged to stimulate, motivate, and collaborate with private businesses/private sectors (PID: BN1, IC1, GB1, GH1, GH2, GNB1, LB1, LB2, ML1, ML2, ML3, ML4, MR1, NGA1, NGA2, TG1).

(ii)   Industry development emerged with a focus on public and private sectors, involving these for growth/development. Private sector involvement in government and public initiatives such as generating renewable energy in-country was emphasised as a highly desirable outcome, as positive and sustainable development for industries. Industry development was described as a key contributor to the development of green economies, powered by growth in renewable energies and green technology (PID: BF1, IC1, GH1, LB2, ML1, ML3, ML4, MR1, NG1, NGA1, NGA2, TG1).

(iii)   Research and development focused on advancement of green technology. Policies evoked research and development for innovation, both in science on CC, and technology to cope with it. The majority of documents summarised the current climate science conducted. Documents also outlined knowledge gaps, and areas requiring further exploration through research and studies, e.g., localised weather shifts, early warning systems development (PID: BN1, BN2, BF1, IC1, GB1, GH1, GNB1, LB1, LB2, ML1, ML2, ML3, ML4, MR1, NG1, NGA1, NGA2, TG1).

(iv)   Institutional development focused on expanding the local/regional frameworks, supporting growth, for industry and research and on the local level. The rise of civil society groups centred on CC, and promotion of green employment, jobs, and careers. These opportunities should be created together with an equivalent workforce, meaning training/capacity building for promotion of climate conscious activities and lives. Educating and training members of the society strengthen the countries' institutions and communities (PID: BN1, BN2, BF1, IC1, GB1, GH1, GH2, GNB1, LB1, LB2, ML1, ML2, ML3, ML4, MR1, NG1, NGA1, NGA2, TG1).

(v)   Construction of resilient communities was a common subtopic across the documents, expressing the need for communities knowledgeable about CC effects. The first step was empowering communities to be agents of mitigation and to make use of adaptive strategies. Building resilient communities was also highlighted as essential for vulnerability reduction on a large scale: Resilient communities can stimulate more equitable social development (PID: BN1, BN2, GB1, GH1, LB1, LB2, ML1, ML3, ML4, MR1, NG1, NGA1, NGA2, TG1).

(vi)   Disaster risk management is highlighted as directly related to managing, reducing, averting, and warning against the risks faced by communities/populations. Less resilient communities would be more affected by climate related disasters, increasing the vulnerability of already vulnerable populations. Drought, heat induced wildfires, and management of important coastlines are considered to be in need of allocating funds, for adequate preparedness and response strategies (PID: BN2, IC1, GB1, GH1, GH2, LB2, ML2, ML3, NGA1, NGA2, TG1).

(vii)   Policy making revolved around promotion of all previously mentioned thematic areas on the political scene/at the policy making level. Fourteen documents state that political will makes a difference in motivating and advancing the creation of climate friendly policies (guidelines, programmes, plans, etc.). Political will and political promotion, along with governance, coordination, and integration, were also mentioned as essential at the implementation and financing stages of adopted CC policies (PID: BN1, BN2, BF1, IC1, GB1, GH1, GH2, LB1, LB2, ML1, ML2, ML3, ML4, MR1, NG1, NGA1, NGA2, TG1).

(viii) Economic investment was omnipresent. It was both an underlining factor in all key areas and cross-cutting throughout the thematic areas. This theme supports the allocation of adequate ministry budgets, which are described as increasing the possibilities of implementing proper CC adaptation measures. The implementation of adaptation measures would stimulate green industry development, nurturing green economy, and in turn fostering institutional development, partnership, and collaboration, stimulating further growth and economic revenue (PID: BN1, BN2, BF1, GB1, GH1, GH2, GNB1, LB1, LB2, ML1, ML2, ML3, ML4, MR1, NG1, NGA1, NGA2, TG1).

The key sectors and thematic areas in all policies were intertwined with discussions of the nation's development policies and aims, most often framed in the context of socioeconomic/poverty-reduction development, rural development, and sustainable development.

3.4. In Depth Analysis of Agriculture, Nutrition, and Food Security Adaptation

In addition to the key sectors/thematic areas, in depth examination of agriculture, nutrition, and food security adaptation within the general and sector-specific plans of the 19 policies yielded seven agricultural barriers.

3.4.1. Agricultural Adaptation Challenges

Agriculture was extensively discussed and interfaces with numerous thematic areas, with barriers and enabling factors. (1) Small scale farming, (2) information gaps, (3) lack of infrastructure, (4) insufficient finances, (5) weak organisation, (6) shifting agricultural calendar, and (7) ecological unsustainability were perceived as the most pressing barriers to agricultural sectors' CC adaptability.

Small scale farming is one of the largest barriers. Small farms are disproportionately affected by CC, also limiting adaptation potential. The Mali policy document (PID: ML2) states: " ... the sectors most vulnerable to climate change are, in order, agriculture, health, fishing, energy, water resources, livestock, forest-wildlife, habitat, transportation, industry and education. Smallholder farmers, along with artisans, are the most vulnerable populations ... "

Farmers lack essential information for agriculture, such as weather/precipitation data and more advanced information, as new farming strategies. Farmers also lack up-to-date information on the shifting agricultural calendar, with enormous ramifications on the entire growing season. Ivory Coast's policy document states (PID: IC1) "The mismatch between weather calendars and growing seasons poses a real problem for agricultural production ... " Lacking financial resources are also a barrier to agricultural adaptation. Policies pointed to low financial resources as a challenge at household level and on all levels of government (PID: NG1, NGA1, ML4. GB1). Farmers have limited resources to invest in adaptation, and governments have limited budgets to support farmers and essential adaptation steps such as infrastructural work (PID: GH1, ML4, GB1).

Farming communities are suffering from and contributing to deteriorating ecological structures of the land (PID ML2, NG1, GB1, GH1). Farming activities effect the lands' ecology through pollution, depletion, impoverishment of soil, water, and forest, through unsustainable, intensive, and growing exploitation (PID GH1). Mali illustrates this (PID: ML2) " ... in Mali there is a significant degradation of soils, vegetation and terrestrial ecosystems. Soil degradation results from natural phenomena (water and wind erosion) accentuated by destructive agricultural practices. These practices are linked to the strong demographic pressure that reaches 2.4% of annual growth, and to the lack of improvement in agricultural productivity ... "

Weak levels of farmer organisations were highlighted as a barrier, as their existence enables the sharing of useful data for updating. Without farmer associations/community groups, it is a challenge to foster grassroots community movements and enact larger-scale changes within communities (PID: BF1).

3.4.2. Nutrition and Food Security Challenges

Food security (availability, access, utilization, and stability) is defined by the FAO as the situation in which "all people, at all times, have physical, social, and economic access to sufficient, safe, and nutritious food that meets their dietary needs and food preferences for an active and healthy life" [41–43]. Nourishment is a key factor, as food security is related to nutrition, and conversely, food insecurity to malnutrition (undernutrition and overnutrition) [44].

Nutrition and food security were seldom addressed as independent sectors, but as sub-sectors/affiliated sectors such as human health and social protection (PID: GB1), changing agriculture landscape (PID: BN2, BF1, ML1), policy programme pillars, or collaborative NGO/IGO programmes (PID: BN1, BN2).

In Gambia's (PID: GB1), a more holistic approach entailed how CC will impact components of food security-availability, accessibility, and utilisation. CC will worsen the current food insecurity situation as quoted in (PID: GB1): "Only 18% of Gambian households are considered to be food secure while the national malnutrition prevalence rate of 9.9% verges on emergency level." This in combination with the "existing economic, environmental and health risks have translated into high levels of food and nutrition insecurity." Additionally, in Ghana's (PID: GH1), emphasis is on "Food security is a crucial issue. Ghana reduced hunger by nearly three-quarters between 1990 and 2004, but food security disparities affect the delivery of the country's development objectives." Although both documents (PID: GB1 and GH1) recognise the severity of food security, no action points were mentioned.

Guinea Bissau included a list of targeted actions, essential for adapting to the changing nutritional landscape and guaranteeing food security: "(i) Setting up of a national security stock (ii) Setting up of cereal banks (silos) by peasants to guarantee a food reserve in all regions (iii) setting up of an Early Warning System against risks (iv) Strengthening of sensitization campaigns about the importance of diversifying eating habits" (PID: GNB1).

In Guinea Bissau's (PID: GNB1), the food security concerns were not limited to rural households, but also urban/semi-urban settings: "The country has survived, at a painful cost for its populations, to cycles of chronic crises, characterized by a worsening of access to water for agricultural purposes, human and animal consumption; a marked fall in agricultural production, staple food items (rice in particular); a rise in costs of some foodstuff, particularly in urban and semi-urban centers, a deterioration in prices of cashew and cotton and an increase in food insecurity."

Several policy documents, like Nigeria's (PID: NGA1), drew attention to inequalities "Climate change will significantly affect vulnerable groups because of a variety of factors, including low adaptive capacity, limited resources, and poverty." Women and farmers are highlighted as especially vulnerable to CC, due to their dependence on natural resources for their livelihoods (PID: GH1 and LB1).

3.4.3. Agriculture, Nutrition, and Food Security Adaptation Solutions

Although the agricultural sector faces challenges due to CC, the policies illustrate that there is also adaptation potential. This sector's ability to adapt is extremely important, as agriculture is linked to both the food security and economic stability of nations, as illustrated in Burkina Faso (PID: BF1): "Burkina Faso's economy is predominantly agricultural, ... It is a subsistence agriculture based on food grains (sorghum, millet, maize) which alone occupy more than 88% of the planted area with average yields of around 850 kg/ha, dominated by small family farms of 3 to 6 ha on average." Although the rates of farming are high, production from small plots remains low related to certain non-efficient farming methods (PID: ML2). Increasing the challenges is a lack of information (environmental, weather, adaptation) (PID: IC1).

Some governments offer a two-pronged approach through reinforced promotion campaigns and the use of climate-smart agriculture (CSA).

The use of established methods under the umbrella of CSA can increase agricultural efficiency and production, as stated in Benin (PID: BN2) "The adoption of climate-smart agriculture (CSA), which relies on irrigated agriculture, the valorisation of local seeds and endemic breeds, the search for new, more adapted varieties, reliable climate information and a national policy of land tenure security" is potentially an adaption solution.

Pairing CSA with population information/promotion are suggested in Mali (PID: ML1): (1) Strengthen access to information and sensitization of the rural population regarding the agro-climatic reference calendar for the planning of agricultural activities (time of ploughing and sowing, appropriate period of agricultural interventions, timing of the appearance of certain diseases ...). (2) Promote the use of meteorological information by farmers to improve agricultural production (support, information sessions). (3) Promote and strengthen the use of seasonal forecast data in agriculture (support, information sessions).

Lack of information is coupled with lack of access to information. Upstream of the access problem, is a communication, knowledge sharing, and knowledge dissemination problem at all levels of government. Ghana plans to resolve this through training/capacity building at the local level, including the media (PID: GH1): " ... the challenge of translating complex climate science into messages that will resonate with the wider public. Here, the media has a crucial role to play in conveying "why climate change matters to me."" Although Ghana has taken steps for capacity-building at the district level, capacity-building within the local communities needs addressing.

The knowledge/information gap is mirrored by a resource gap: Few farmers and communities can make improvements to their farming and their agricultural strategies with limited financial resources or limited governmental funds. Implementation of publicly and privately-run financial mechanisms like micro-financing schemes are solutions, as in Mali (PID: ML2): "Many actions mentioned to build a green and climate change resilient economy require the population to make investments, due to their low financial capacity. It is therefore necessary to promote the development of financial services, particularly microfinance ... " These solutions, paired with saving and insurance services, could enable populations to manage CC risks.

Lack or poor infrastructure poses further challenges: There is an infrastructural gap, in areas ranging from transport, like the construction of roads, to commerce, like cash crop storage facilities (PID: BN2, BF1). Infrastructural support can improve selling agricultural products throughout the year and improve access to local and international markets, and this is precisely why the Burkina Faso government is investing in the improvement of infrastructure in their adaptation efforts. Their policy states (PID: BF1): "The Government's efforts relate to the commercial production sectors (cotton, fruit and vegetables, hides and skins, meat, etc.), the improvement of road infrastructures, etc., which are likely to favor the competitiveness of Burkinabé products in regional and international markets."

The definition of agricultural zoning is a further challenge: Some farming villages are expanding the boundaries of farmed lands with no regard to zoning rules and regulations as described in Guinea Bissau (PID: GNB1). Defining agricultural zones may minimise the multitude of problems arising from unplanned expansion, using toxic lands, plains prone to flooding, and unlawful use and occupation of pre-owned and private land.

Farmer organisations are a further solution mentioned, for example, in Gambia's (PID: GB1): "It is well recognized in Africa that secure land tenure and access rights are essential for enabling community-based adaptation, as well as harnessing any related mitigation co-benefits. The [policy] will initiate a process to identify and act upon key constraints to community-based adaptation, including land tenure and access rights."

The ecological effects/footprint of agriculture, especially in combination with livestock and animal husbandry, are outlined at the beginning of the CC policies and further elaborated on in the National Communication of each country. Enumerated solutions to reduce greenhouse gas (GHG) and adapt the agriculture methods include, for example, in Mali (PID: ML2): "Soil fertilization of soils should be organized mainly using agro-ecological solutions (improved fallow, composting, manure, organic fertilizers, bio-pesticides, agroforestry, cultural techniques such as minimum tillage or plant cover, etc.), which are generally less expensive, more easily accessible, and more effective in the long term."

3.5. Policy Document Comparison

Using the Technical Guidelines for The National Adaptation Plan Process of the UNFCCC as a framework for comparison: (1) Laying the groundwork, (2) preparatory elements, (3) implementing strategy, and (4) reporting, monitoring, and review (Supplementary Materials Table S3), the following emerges [21]:

Over a third of the documents analysed (PID: BF1, GB1, LB2, GH1, GNB1, NGA1, NGA2, TG1) followed each of the four steps, covering everything from initiating the process in multilateral collaboration to taking full stock of data gaps, information and possible hurdles of both the policy document drafting process, and of the research in their respective countries. The policy documents also analysed the weakness in adaptation to CC, and the possibilities for addressing them, and integrating further adaptation methods. Under the implementation strategy, these policy documents fulfilled all requirements, seamlessly crossing from discussion on the prioritisation of mainstreaming and integration of adaptation at the national level to promotion and coordination at regional and local levels. The last points addressed in these policy documents were elaborating, reporting, monitoring, and evaluation plans.

Policy documents from Ghana and Mali proved less developed in step 2—Preparatory elements and step 3—Implementation Strategy (PID: GH2, LB1, ML3, ML4)

In step 3, most of the policy documents successfully prioritised climate change in the national planning and developed adaptation implementation strategies, but many did not push further in addressing the last two points. They were weak in demonstrating how their national adaptation plans have been or would be updated (PID: BN2, IC1, ML1 ML2, NG1).

Furthermore, Benin (PID: BN1) specifies a strategic plan to develop and enforce knowledge of human resource personnel on the subject of green development and climate resilience. The strategy points to a missing framework and structure for growing the pool of qualified persons in the public sector, the private sector, and civil society. The document elaborates an implementation, monitoring, and evaluation plan, an institutional framework, and a 5-year action plan.

Mauritania (PID:MR1) has a strategic plan for environment and CC in their education system. In addition to discussing its environmental, geographic, and ecological situation, this strategy details the 3 levels of the education system. This provides the institutional framework for research and the overall goal of the policy document: "change in attitudes and behaviours of current and future generations vis-à-vis environmental issues and sustainable development" through integration and education at all school levels.

Liberia (PID: LB1) has an action plan specifically focused on gender and climate change. The plan's purpose is to " ... ensure that gender equality is mainstreamed into Liberia's climate change policies, programs and interventions" in order for both men and women to equally benefit from the nation's CC initiatives.

4. Discussion

4.1. Comparing Structure and Quality of the Policy Documents

Comparing the quality of the policy documents, it is important to first note the difference in the types of documents analysed. In this publication, "policy document" was used as an umbrella term covering publicly available national plans, guidelines, programmes, and policies. Although different in their development processes, aims, and outcomes, these terms are often used inconsistently and interchangeably [45]. Only the inclusive search and analysis of all these types of policy documents, as we present here, give an appropriate overview of the current state of West African CC adaptation planning [46,47].

With the expected range of policy documents, the primary aim of comparison was (1) to use a defined process of development, including a comparison to the suggested four stages by UNFCCC, and (2) to adequately review and identify the CC vulnerabilities and adaptation opportunities in the country.

(1) The majority of documents, regardless if "plan, guideline, program, or policy" followed a process similar to UNFCCC's technical guidelines for the national adaptation plan: "(1) Laying the ground work, (2) Preparatory elements, (3) Implementing strategy and (4) Reporting, monitoring and review" [21]. Except for two, the policy documents started by defining the groundwork for various subjects to be addressed throughout the document. Next, the documents also established the nation's current state and identified information and data gaps. The policy documents addressed preparatory elements by recounting the countries' previous climate related efforts and highlighting difficulties ranging from barriers in the policy drafting process itself to difficulties in acquiring and utilizing essential research for CC related activities. The policy documents analysed adaptation strength and weaknesses for which developed strategies would be implemented. After touching on implementation, most of the documents engaged discussions on the prioritisation actions and mainstreaming and integration of adaptation. They proposed various plans and methods for the reporting, monitoring, and evaluation of adaptation measure of the prioritized actions. The policy documents were thorough in discussing and covering the key aspects of the four steps. The three documents with a different development approach also had independent goals. These documents were narrow in focus and aims, each addressing only one specific aspect/sector; human resources, education, and gender. Due to this focus, they bypassed the more general analysis aspects that all other policy documents address in steps 1 and 2. Although weak in their elaboration of the entire process, they were strong in identifying vulnerabilities and barriers, then outlining the opportunities for improvements.

(2) The second quality assessment of the policy documents was performed through qualitative content analysis using structured extraction tables to review the adaptation vulnerabilities and opportunities in the policy documents. At a second stage of the content analysis, an additional focus was placed on agriculture, nutrition, and food security. The analysis illustrated that although the type of policy documents varied, the vast majority had similar content, simply under differing structures. All but two of the three divergent documents, (PID: BN1) and (PID:MR1), adequately elaborated on the country's wholistic challenges and opportunities for adaptation. From this wholistic review, seven key sectors emerged as most relevant to changing climate. These seven key sectors also illustrate a consensus in the West African countries. These are the sectors commonly deemed most vulnerable to the effects of the changing climate. Therefore, they emerge as priorities for adaptation action, which could be best implemented through actions in the eight interconnected thematic areas.

A study published in 2015 *"An overview of nationally appropriate mitigation actions (NAMAs) and national adaptation programs of action (NAPAs) in Africa"* mirrors this finding [48]. Although the review had a focus on forestry, the publication's assessment of adaptation priority areas of both East Africa and West Africa yielded a combination of the key sectors and thematic areas also highlighted in our systematic review. The Kojwang review enumerated eleven "adaptation priority areas", which overlap all seven key sectors outlined in our review with the exception of the education and energy sectors. Although energy is not on the adaptation priority list, it is first on the reviews' mitigation actions list and a focal point for NAPA projects. The education sector was not mentioned at all in the 2015 review. The eleven "adaptation priority areas" enumerated in the Kojwang review overlap some of the eight thematic areas identified in our review, except for economic investment, partnerships, and the development centred thematic areas. Research and development, institutional development, and industry development were not mentioned in the 2015 review. However, this is not surprising, as the NAMAs and NAPAs are more homogeneous than the array of policy documents our systematic review identified. This shows that outside the frame of NAPAs and NAMAs, West African countries have developed an array of policy relevant documents to address a growing variety of sectors and areas. Another difference between the two studies was the 2015 study finding that most projects within the NAPAs are for energy, early warning systems, disaster reduction, coastal protection, and food security. Food security was not found to take centre stage across the policy documents of our systematic review.

4.2. Possibilities for Integrated Adaptation

The adaption actions, solutions, and plans in the 19 national CC policy documents of this systematic review can be analysed along the lines of previously defined eight thematic areas. The proposed actions under the Disaster and Risk Management theme were focused on agriculture strategies management and water systems management. The agricultural strategies emphasised both an adaptive strategies and risk hedging methods: Diversification of crops, selection of crops based on durability, selection of crop variety based on maturation time, introduction of modified seeds based on better growth patterns, lower water requirement, and disease resistance (PID: ML2). Water system adaptation plans in the policies ranged from the creation of man-powered irrigation systems, to the use of traditional planting and bordering methods such as Zai and Half-Moon technique for increased water retention, methods supported by literature on CC and adaptation [49]. Proposed actions for water management included creating micro-dams, small dykes, and water reserves adjacent to agricultural fields. Field-adjacent water reserves have a twofold purpose, (1) as a convenient source of water in the middle of agricultural fields, and (2) serving as a drainage system in case of flooding, limiting the inundation of planted fields [50,51]. All this would preferably be performed through a participatory, integrated watershed management approach, insuring thorough analysis of the interrelation between the use of multiple methods and their impact on other sectors (PID: GB1).

The continuous development of agricultural and water management systems should be supported by industry, research, and development. Necessary research and development to better confront the changing climate and weather variables begins with the use of natural resources. The development of renewable energies, especially solar energy, not only for countries' electric grid, dominated by city use, but also for powering of equipment in rural sectors [52,53]. Development and promotion of conservative farming methods could contribute to reversing the trend of spreading and sprawling of land use for farming [54]. Ecosystem rebuilding and conservation is a subcategory of research and development, incorporating adaptive methods such as agro-forestry [55,56]. This serves to integrate agriculture and forestry, benefiting adaptation and mitigation [57,58]. This thematic area also discusses research on climate resilient ecosystems, sustainability, and energy sources. Lastly, this thematic area emphasises the inclusion of concerned community members, such as farmer's/women's groups at the centre of research and development, as they are key to the adoption and implementation of all relevant results [59,60].

Literature shows that concerned community members should also be implicated directly in the adaptation planning and activities of governing bodies [61,62]. This is necessary for building community resilience. Community resilience activities branch from integrating CC in the education system, both for teachers and students, to creating community empowerment groups [63]. These policies support strengthening social support networks, groups, and associations, since they also serve as access points for providing the population with information and tools for adaptation and protection of individuals and communities [64]. The introduction of integrated farming, alternative livelihoods systems, and income diversification are also adaptation initiatives, increasing households' and communities' resilience [50,65].

Initiation, promotion, and subsistence of the above-mentioned activities come from a new base of workers, trained in climate sciences through institutional development. These would be agents trained for capacity building purposes, at all levels of country organisation. The documents acknowledged the creation and or expansion of extension services as favourable to bridge the gap between science and research, its understanding, and application locally [63]. A trained green workforce would be essential in relaying and disseminating accurate climate related information, while simultaneously engaging in trainings and workshops with community members, making the community its own agents of change [66].

In looking at the policies, at the higher levels of government, several adaptation related actions could be mandated, grouped mainly in two areas; first, expanding governmental services, and second, strengthening government systems. For this, national policy documents need to lead to action points and implementable initiatives; followed by the development of climate actions/projects at regional and local levels. An advisory board could be set up to monitor the development of adequate and relevant guidelines, regulations, and projects. Agro-advisory boards for example could support the production of reliable weather-based crop focused information (PID: GB1). Such a board could also advise on new measures, such as establishing local weather warning systems and scaling up early warning systems for events such as floods, droughts, or famines. Lastly, these agro-advisory boards could back the promotion of agro-business both in the public and private sector (PID: ML2). Partnerships, in the private and public sectors, backing and funding green adaptation programmes are in the strategic plan of most policies [63]. Other adaptation-focused plans include the development of small-scale banking and agro-banking, primarily for implementation at local levels (PID: BN2). This is linked to a concept of weather-based insurance schemes and programmes, run either by the governments or in collaboration with international organisations (PID: BN2, GB1, GH1, ML2). The creation of national food storage facilities is another possible economic activity, including food insurance schemes.

4.3. Climate Change and Development

The relation between CC and development is both parallel and intertwined. This was evident in the policies discussion of socioeconomic/poverty-reduction development, rural development, and sustainable development. The effects of the changing climate have the potential to set the national development back in many of the West African countries, effectively undoing much of the progress across sectors from effecting meningitis epidemics in the health sector, destroying water systems in the infrastructure sectors, to pushing women, farming communities, and all other groups reliant on natural resources further into poverty [67–69]. As a result, discussions have been sparked on the interconnectivity of development and CC efforts. This intertwined connection becomes even more difficult when discussing the prioritization and funding of activities.

Though some policy documents have stated that partial funding has already been secured for their intended adaptation activities, most required significant investment to launch and upscale adaptation plans and projects. The allocation of government budget lines in West African countries are proving insufficient, therefore much funding must come from the private sector, regional, international, and non-governmental organisations and other partners [70,71]. As global funding streams expand and shift to include the allocation of funds for climate oriented, climate sensitive, and specific activities and catastrophes, there is a shift away from some previously funded development-based activities [72]. Furthermore, there is growing confusion on the differentiation of these activities, pushing the need to find a way to determine which activities are climate resilience and management, which fall under development. One of the proposed methods for differentiating development and CC activities are the use of indicators [73,74]. We would argue that although the elaboration of development and CC (mitigation and adaptation) indicators can provide a platform to sort and distinguish the two, it is more important to identify areas in which integrated approaches can be utilized and capitalized [75]. Integration would increase efficiency of results and create more efficient use of currently limited resources.

One of the next steps for West African countries will be to increase their access to adaptation funds. Such resources would allow them to address both urgent/immediate needs while continuing to monitor, evaluate, and improve current efforts and initiatives. The acquisition of funds would drive the West African region forward in its development and climate change adaptation agenda.

4.4. Limitations of the Systematic Review

The first limitation was the accessibility of CC policies. No comprehensive climate change policy data base exists for African countries. The London School of Economics and Political Science and The Grantham Research Institute on Climate Change and the Environment established a platform bridging the public to environment decrees, laws, and policies, but the database for African countries is not yet comprehensive, up-to-date, or linked to the policy texts. Searching for policy documents directly on national ministry websites proved equally limiting. Of the 48 Ministry web sites searched, only 34 were functional. The remaining 14 websites were dysfunctional in a variety of ways: From disconnected web addresses to websites indefinitely under construction. Of the functioning websites, few provided access to the policy text.

As a result, most of the policies were identified through extensive grey literature source documents, in a two-step process of (1) identifying existing policies and (2) locating a copy of the full text. Had the full text of all policy documents been accessible, the final included policies would have increased by nine, totalling 24. The search for the missing nine full text documents was extended to include the networks of three experts who were also unable to locate the policies.

The inaccessibility of policies constitutes a barrier for researchers, IGO, NGOs, and for citizens. This is an overarching difficulty in many sectors from health to economics to CC, in most low-middle income countries [76]. The public availability of policies can increase general citizen knowledge and understanding of government goals and priorities [77], encouraging public engagement, fostering transparency and stimulating accountability [78,79]. The availability and accessibility of such documents can also facilitate the monitoring of activities, not only within and between national ministries, but for all agencies interested in tracking CC adaptation progress of a country [80,81].

Lastly, this review excluded National Communications (NC), National Adaptation Plans (NAP), NAPA and NAMA for which LDCs were provided UNFCCC funding and training. Although this systematic review focused on documents drafted outside this frame, it is important to acknowledge their use as source documents in this review. All the selected West African countries have as of 2019 drafted and submitted an Initial NC and a First NC. Fourteen have submitted a Second NC, twelve a Third NC, and two have a Fourth NC. Thirteen of the sixteen countries have a NAP, four have a NAPA, four have a NAMA. A 2015 review by [48] already provides an overview of the NAMAs and NAPAs in Africa, therefore they were not re-analysed in this review. Instead, the NAP drafting guidelines were used as a framework for comparison, and the 2015 review provided for adaptation action and priority comparison. The policies in this systematic review proved more wide ranging in the scope of subjects and more diverse in the proposed areas of adaptation options, as they were not limited by a prescribed standardized format, framework, and process.

5. Conclusions

In conclusion, the systematic literature review aimed to answer the following three questions:

(1) What are the existing CC adaptation policies publicly available?

The systematic review of CC policies in West Africa identified 19 policies in 12 countries. Guinea had no policies in the frame of this review, Cape Verde, Sierra Leone, and Senegal had at least one policy in the frame of the review, but the full text was not publicly available and could not be located.

(2) Addressing which topics?

The policy documents effectively described the national situation, the agencies involved in drafting the document, and the aims/vision of the policies. The documents (17 of the 19) also strived to link and integrate other relevant national reports, laws, programmes, and policies. This is one of the initial steps in policy integration, which 13 policy documents discussed or stated as a goal.

The policy documents converged on seven key sectors: Energy, agriculture, water resources, health, forestry, infrastructure, and education. The policy documents discussed these key sectors in the context of eight thematic areas: Community resilience, disaster risk management, institutional development, industry development, research and development, policy making, economic investment, and partnerships/collaboration.

(3)   How are agriculture, food security, and nutrition framed and addressed?

Nutrition and food security challenges and adaptation were not highlighted as key points. They were seldom mentioned as an independent goal and most often under the umbrella of other sectors or areas, such as health, agriculture, and climate resilient systems.

Agriculture was a focal point of the policy documents. It was highlighted as a top three GHG emitting source in West African countries. The agricultural sector was identified as a key sector and as one of the most vulnerable sectors to CC, but it was also highlighted as a sector with immense possibilities and potential for adaptation.

The primary challenges of CC agricultural adaptation were: The small scale of farming, gap of information, lack of infrastructure, insufficient finances, weak organisation, a shifting agricultural calendar, and ecological unsustainability. The enumerated solutions ranged greatly, from solidification of farmer groups, and training of climate community agents, to the use of modified seeds, weather-based insurances, and agro-forestry.

There was also a plethora of proposed adaptation solutions for the other six key sectors, ranging from participatory integrated watershed management approaches, engagement of public–private partnerships in micro-financing and insurance schemes, construction of food-bank infrastructures, integration of CC in school curricula, training of a green human resource workforce, to serve as agents of change in communities, and also to fill a multitude of new jobs in growing renewable and green energy economies.

In addition to addressing the research questions, this systematic review compared national climate change policies using the PRISMA and UNFCCC framework, determining where on the Climate Change policy development spectrum 16 West African countries lie. This manuscript is a first in the expanding realm and intersection of climate change, policy, and health, creating a scientific bridge (between well-established methods and the newly emerging subject of climate adaptation) into new bodies of knowledge.

The results of the review can inform the policy process in the West African countries. It clearly underlines the variability of the policies, and this is probably reflected in any implementation process.

Lastly, the added value of the review is the more scientific approach for document analysis, searching and analysing in a prescribed way with the methodology of systematic reviews, making the analysis and its key conclusions stronger.

Next steps for research would be analysing the implementation of the identified CC policies. First, examining whether adaptation plans elaborated in these policies, were budgeted, developed, and implemented. Second, analysing the effect on agricultural, nutritional, and food security of the countries and their citizens.

Author Contributions: Conceptualization, R.S. (Raissa Sorgho), R.S. (Rainer Sauerborn) and O.H.; methodology, R.S. (Raissa Sorgho) and O.H.; software, R.S. (Raissa Sorgho) and C.A.M.Q.; validation, R.S. (Raissa Sorgho) and C.A.M.Q.; formal analysis, R.S. (Raissa Sorgho); investigation, R.S. (Raissa Sorgho) and C.A.M.Q.; resources, R.S. (Raissa Sorgho), V.R.L., P.D., R.S. (Rainer Sauerborn); writing—original draft preparation, R.S. (Raissa Sorgho); writing—review and editing, R.S. (Raissa Sorgho), C.A.M.Q., V.R.L., V.W., P.D., O.H. and R.S. (Rainer Sauerborn); visualization, R.S. (Raissa Sorgho) and O.H.; supervision, O.H. and R.S. (Rainer Sauerborn); project administration, R.S. (Raissa Sorgho); funding acquisition, R.S. (Raissa Sorgho) and R.S. (Rainer Sauerborn). All authors have read and agreed to the published version of the manuscript.

References

1.   UNFCCC. COP21. The Paris Agreement to the United Nations Framework Convention on Climate Change (COP21). Available online: https://unfccc.int/process-and-meetings/conferences/past-conferences/paris-climate-change-conference-november-2015/cop-21 (accessed on 3 March 2020).
2.   UNFCCC. COP8. The Delhi Declaration: Eighth session of the Conference of the Parties (COP8). Available online: https://unfccc.int/process-and-meetings/conferences/past-conferences/new-delhi-climate-change-conference-october-2002/cop-8 (accessed on 3 March 2020).
3.   UNFCCC. COP3. Kyoto Protocol to the United Nations Framework Convention on Climate Change (COP3). Available online: http://unfccc.int/essential_background/kyoto_protocol/items/2830.php (accessed on 3 March 2020).
4.   Woodward, A.; Smith, K. Chapter 11. Human Health: Impacts, Adaptation, and Co-Benefits. In *Climate Change 2014: Impacts, Adaptation, and Vulnerability. Part A: Global and Sectoral Aspects. Contribution of Working Group II to the Fifth Assessment Report of the Intergovernmental Panel on Climate Change*; IPCC: Geneva, Switzerland, 2014; p. 69.
5.   IMF. Seeking Sustainable Growth: Short-Term Recovery, Long-Term Challenges. Available online: https://www.imf.org/en/Publications/WEO/Issues/2019/08/31/World-Economic-Outlook-October-2017-Seeking-Sustainable-Growth-Short-Term-Recovery-Long-Term-45123 (accessed on 3 March 2020).
6.   Smith, J.B.; Klein, R.J.T.; Huq, S. *Climate Change, Adaptive Capacity and Development*; Imperial College Press: London, UK, 2003; p. 356.
7.   Phalkey, R.; Aranda-Jan, C.; Marx, S.; Höfle, B.; Sauerborn, R. Systematic review of current efforts to quantify the impacts of climate change on undernutrition. *Proc. Natl. Acad. Sci. USA* **2015**, *112*, E4522–E4529. [CrossRef] [PubMed]
8.   Nelson, G.; Rosegrant, M.W.; Koo, J.; Robertson, R.; Sulser, T.; Zhu, T.; Ringler, C.; Msangi, S.; Palazzo, A.; Batka, M.; et al. *Climate Change: Impact on Agriculture and Costs of Adaptation*; International Food Policy Research Institute: Washington, DC, USA, 2009.
9.   Lobell, D.B.; Burke, M.B.; Tebaldi, C.; Mastrandrea, M.D.; Falcon, W.P.; Naylor, R.L. Prioritizing Climate Change Adaptation Needs for Food Security in 2030. *Science* **2008**, *319*, 607–610. [CrossRef] [PubMed]
10. Blössner, M.; de Onis, M. *Malnutrition: Quantifying the Health Impact at National and Local Levels*; World Health Organization, Ed.; World Health Organization: Geneva, Switzerland, 2005.
11. African Union. The Cost of Hunger in Africa: The Social and Economic Impact of Child Undernutrition in Burkina Faso. In *The Cost of Hunger in Africa*; African Union Comission: Ouagadougou, Burkina Faso, 2015.
12. Nelson, G.C.; Rosegrant, M.W.; Palazzo, A.; Gray, I.; Ingersoll, C.; Robertson, R.; Tokgoz, S.; Zhu, T.; Sulser, T.B.; Ringler Msangi, S.; et al. *Food Security, Farming and Climate Change to 2050: Scenarios, Results, Policy Options*; The International Food Policy Research Institute (IFPRI): Washington, DC, USA, 2010.
13. Challinor, A.J.; Porter, J.R.; Xie, L.; Cochrane, K.; Howden, S.M.; Iqbal, M.M.; Lobell, D.B.; Travasso, M.I. Food security and food production systems. In *Climate Change 2014: Impacts, Adaptation, and Vulnerability. Part A: Global and Sectoral Aspects*; Contribution of Working Group II to the Fifth Assessment Report of the Intergovernmental Panel on Climate Change; Pramod Aggarwal, K.H., Ed.; Cambridge University Press: Cambridge, UK; New York, NY, USA, 2014; pp. 485–533.
14. Whitmee, S.; Haines, A.; Beyrer, C.; Boltz, F.; Capon, A.G.; de Souza Dias, B.F.; Ezeh, A.; Frumkin, H.; Gong, P.; Head, P.; et al. Safeguarding human health in the Anthropocene epoch: Report of The Rockefeller Foundation-Lancet Commission on planetary health. *Lancet* **2015**, *386*, 1973–2028. [CrossRef]
15. Lloyd, S.J.; Kovats, R.S.; Chalabi, Z. Climate change, crop yields, and undernutrition: Development of a model to quantify the impact of climate scenarios on child undernutrition. *Environ. Health Perspect.* **2011**, *119*, 1817–1823. [CrossRef] [PubMed]
16. Moher, D.; Liberati, A.; Tetzlaff, J.; Altman, D.G.; Prisma Group. Preferred Reporting Items for Systematic Reviews and Meta-Analyses: The PRISMA Statement. *PLOS Med.* **2009**, *6*, e1000097. [CrossRef] [PubMed]
17. IPCC. The Fifth Assessment Report of the IPCC. In *Assessment Report*; UNFCCC: New York, NY, USA, 2014.
18. Pielke, R. Rethinking the role of adaptation in climate policy. *Global Environ. Chang.* **1998**, *8*, 159–170. [CrossRef]
19. Fankhauser, S.; Smith, J.B.; Tol, R. Weathering climate change: Some simple rules to guide adaptation decisions. *Ecol. Econ.* **1999**, *30*, 67–78. [CrossRef]

20. Smit, B.; Wandel, J. Adaptation, adaptive capacity and vulnerability. *Glob. Environ. Chang.* **2006**, *16*, 282–292. [CrossRef]

21. UNFCCC NAP. *National Adaptation Plans: Technical Guidelines for the National Adaptation Plan Process*; United Nations Frameworl Convention on Climate Change: Bonn, Germany, 2012; pp. 1–152.

22. BN1. *Stratégie Nationale de Renforcement des Ressources Humaines, de L'apprentissage et du Développement des Compétences Pour Favoriser un Développement Vert, Faible en Émissions et Résilient aux Changements Climatiques*; Cotonou, Benin, 2013. Available online: https://www.uncclearn.org/wp-content/uploads/2020/10/Benin_National-Strategy_Final.pdf (accessed on 3 November 2020).

23. BN2. *Stratégie de Développement à Faible Intensité de Carbone et Résilient aux Changements Climatiques 2016–2025*; Direction General De Changement Climatique: Cotonou, Benin, 2016.

24. BF1. *Stratégie Nationale de Mise en Oeuvre de la Convention sur les Changements Climatiques*; Secrétariat Permanent du Conseil National pour la Gestion de l'Environnement, Ed.; Ministère de l'Environnement de l'Economie Verte et du Changement Climatique: Ouagadougou, Burkina Faso, 2001.

25. IC1. *Programme National Changement Climatique*; Direction Générale de l'environnement, Ed.; Bernard D. Kouakou: Abidjan, Ivory Coast, 2014.

26. GB1. National Climate Change Policy of the Gambia. Available online: https://www.google.com.hk/url?sa=t&rct=j&q=&esrc=s&source=web&cd=&cad=rja&uact=8&ved=2ahUKEwiV4K6FlantAhXCaN4KHfbRCZAQFjACegQIAxAC&url=http%3A%2F%2Fwww.lse.ac.uk%2FGranthamInstitute%2Fwp-content%2Fuploads%2Flaws%2F8109.pdf&usg=AOvVaw2tLEUby_J6bz5NQnyMmIoX (accessed on 3 November 2020).

27. GH1. *Ghana National Climate Change Policy*; National Climate Change Committee, Ed.; Ministry of Environment Science Technology and Innovation: Accra, Ghana, 2013; pp. 1–88.

28. GH2. *Integrating Climate Change and Disaster Risk Reduction into National Developement Policies and Planning in Ghana*; National Development Planning Commission (NDPC): Accra, Ghana, 2010; pp. 1–28.

29. GNB1. *National Programme of Action of Adaptation to Climate Changes*; Ministry of Natural Resources and Envronnment Government of Guinea-Bissau: Bissau, Guinea-Bissau, 2006; pp. 1–87.

30. LB1. *Climate Change and Gender Action Plan for the Government of Liberia*; Ministry of Gender and Development, Environmental Protection Agency: Monrovia, Liberia, 2012.

31. LB2. *National Policy and Response Strategy on Climate Change*; Liberia, E.P.A.o., Ed.; EPA: Monrovia, Liberia, 2018.

32. ML1. *Stratégie Nationale Changements Climatiques*; Secretariat General, Ed.; Ministere de L'environnement et de L'assainissement Republic Du Mali: Bamako, Mali, 2011; pp. 1–104.

33. ML2. *Cadre Stratégique Pour une Economie Verte et Résiliente aux Changements Climatiques*; Agence de l'Environnement et du Développement Durable: Bamako, Mali, 2011; pp. 1–32.

34. ML3. *Politique Nationale sur les Changements Climatiques*; Agence de l'Environnement et du Développement Durable, Ed.; Ministere de L'environnement et de L'assainissement: Bamako, Mali, 2011; pp. 1–45.

35. ML4. *Stratégie Nationale Changements Climatiques: Plan d'Action National Climat*; Agence de l'Environnement et du Développement Durable, Ed.; EcoSecurities Consulting: Bamako, Mali, 2011; pp. 1–104.

36. MR1. *Stratégie D'intégration de L'environnement et des Changements Climatiques Dans le Système Éducatif Mauritanien*; Ministère Delegue Aupres Du Premier Ministre Charge De L'environnement et Du developpement Durable, Ed.; Bureau NET-AUDIT: Islamique, Mauritanie, 2012; pp. 1–120.

37. NG1. *Politique Nationale en Matière de Changements Climatiques*; Le Conseil National pour l'Environnement et le Développement durable, Ed.; Programme d'Adaptation Africain: Niamey, Niger, 2012.

38. NGA1. *This National Adaptation Strategy and Plan of Action on Climate Change for Nigeria*; Building Nigeria's Response to Climate Change, Ed.; BNRCC Project: Abuja, Nigeria, 2001.

39. NGA2. *National Policy of Climate Change*; Ministry of Environment, Ed.; Department of Climate Change: Abuja, Nigeria, 2013.

40. TG1. *Plan National d'Adaption aux Changements Climatiques du Togo*; Minister de L'environnement et des Ressources Forestier: Lomé, Togo, 2016.

41. FAO. The State of Food Insecurity in the World 2001. In *Food Insecurity: When People Live with Hunger and Fear Starvation*; Food and Agriculture Organization of the United Nations: Rome, Italy, 2001; pp. 1–8.

42. FAO. *The Future of Food and Agriculture: Alternative Pathways to 2050*; Food and Agriculture Organization of The United Nations: Rome, Italy, 2018; pp. 1–228.

43. FAO. *Combining Agricultural Biodiversity, Resilient Ecosystems, Traditional Farming Practices and Cultural Identity*; Globally Important Agricultural Heritage Systems, Food and Agriculture Organization of the United Nations: Rome, Italy, 2018; pp. 1–48.

44. Cheikh Mbow, C.R. Chapter5: Food Security. In *Final Government Distribution*; Noureddine Benkeblia, A.C., Khan, A., Porter, J., Eds.; IPCC SRCCL: New York, NY, USA, 2019; p. 200.

45. WHO. *A Framework For National Health Policies, Straregies and Plans*; World Health Organization: Geneva, Switzerland, 2010; p. 10.

46. Fischer, F.; Miller, G.J. *Handbook of Public Policy Analysis: Theory, Politics, and Methods*; Taylor & Francis Group: New York, NY, USA, 2007; p. 668.

47. Pencheon, D.; Guest, C.; Melzer, D.; Gray, J.M.; Korkodilos, M.; Wright, J.; Tiplady, P.; Gelletlie, R. *Oxford Handbook Of Public Health Practice*; The First Resort For Training and Practice; Oxford University Press: New York, NY, USA, 2006.

48. Kojwang, H.O.; Larwanou, M. An overview of nationally appropriate mitigation actions (NAMAs) and national adaptation programmes of action (NAPAs) in Africa. *Int. For. Rev.* **2015**, *17*, 103–113. [CrossRef]

49. Nouhoun, Z.; Dossa, L.; Schlecht, E. Climate change and variability: Perception and adaptation strategies of pastoralists and agro-pastoralists across different zones of Burkina Faso. *Reg. Environ. Chang.* **2014**, *14*, 769–783.

50. Below, T.; Artner, A.; Siebert, R.; Sieber, S. *Micro-Level Practices to Adapt to Climate Change for African Small-Scale Farmers A Review of Selected Literature*; International Food Policy Research Institite:(IFPRI): Washington, DC, USA, 2010; pp. 1–28.

51. Mwungu, C.M.; Kizito, F.; Mwongera, C.; Koech, N.; Odhiambo, C. *Household Survey Data of Integrated Land and Water Management for Adaptation to Climate Variability and Change in West Africa*; Harvard Dataverse: Cambridge, MA, USA, 2019. [CrossRef]

52. Mohammed, Y.S.; Mustafa, M.W.; Bashir, N. Status of renewable energy consumption and developmental challenges in Sub-Sahara Africa. *Renew. Sustain. Energy Rev.* **2013**, *27*, 453–463. [CrossRef]

53. Ouedraogo, N.S. Africa energy future: Alternative scenarios and their implications for sustainable development strategies. *Energy Policy* **2017**, *106*, 457–471. [CrossRef]

54. Kimaru-Muchai, S.W.; Ngetich, F.K.; Baaru, M.; Mucheru-Muna, M.W. Adoption and utilisation of Zai pits for improved farm productivity in drier upper Eastern Kenya. *J. Agric. Rural Dev. Trop. Subtrop. (JARTS)* **2020**, *121*, 13–22.

55. Lasco, R.D.; Delfino, R.J.; Catacutan, D.C.; Simelton, E.S.; Wilson, D.M. Climate risk adaptation by smallholder farmers: The roles of trees and agroforestry. *Curr. Opin. Environ. Sustain.* **2014**, *6*, 83–88. [CrossRef]

56. Mbow, C.; Van Noordwijk, M.; Luedeling, E.; Neufeldt, H.; Minang, P.A.; Kowero, G. Agroforestry solutions to address food security and climate change challenges in Africa. *Curr. Opin. Environ. Sustain.* **2014**, *6*, 61–67. [CrossRef]

57. Mbow, C.; Smith, P.; Skole, D.; Duguma, L.; Bustamante, M. Achieving mitigation and adaptation to climate change through sustainable agroforestry practices in Africa. *Curr. Opin. Environ. Sustain.* **2014**, *6*, 8–14. [CrossRef]

58. Verchot, L.; Van Noordwijk, M.; Kandji, S.; Tomich, T.; Ong, C.; Albrecht, A.; Mackensen, J.; Bantilan, C.; Anupama, K.V.; Palm, C. Climate change: Linking adaptation and mitigation through agroforestry. *Mitig. Adapt. Strateg. Glob. Chang.* **2007**, *12*, 901–918. [CrossRef]

59. Idrissou, Y.; Assani, A.S.; Baco, M.N.; Yabi, A.J.; Traoré, I.A. Adaptation strategies of cattle farmers in the dry and sub-humid tropical zones of Benin in the context of climate change. *Heliyon* **2020**, *6*, e04373. [CrossRef]

60. Alhassan, S.I.; Kuwornu, J.K.; Osei-Asare, Y.B. Gender dimension of vulnerability to climate change and variability. *Int. J. Clim. Chang. Strateg. Manag.* **2019**. [CrossRef]

61. Few, R.; Brown, K.; Tompkins, E.L. Public participation and climate change adaptation: Avoiding the illusion of inclusion. *Clim. Policy* **2007**, *7*, 46–59. [CrossRef]

62. van Aalst, M.K.; Cannon, T.; Burton, I. Community level adaptation to climate change: The potential role of participatory community risk assessment. *Glob. Environ. Chang.* **2008**, *18*, 165–179. [CrossRef]

63. Hoff, H.; Warner, K.; Bouwer, L.M. The Role of Financial Services in Climate Adaption in Developing Countries. *Ierteljahrshefte Wirtsch.* **2005**, *74*, 196–207. [CrossRef]

64. Sorgho, R.; Mank, I.; Kagoné, M.; Souares, A.; Danquah, I.; Sauerborn, R. "We will always ask ourselves the

question of how to feed the family": Subsistence farmers' perceptions on adaptation to climate change in Burkina Faso. *Int. J. Environ. Res. Public Health* **2020**, *17*, 7200. [CrossRef] [PubMed]

65. Seo, S.N. Is an integrated farm more resilient against climate change? A micro-econometric analysis of portfolio diversification in African agriculture. *Food Policy* **2010**, *35*, 32–40. [CrossRef]

66. Gabre-Madhin, E.; Haggblade, S. Successes in African Agriculture: Results of an Expert Survey. *World Dev.* **2003**, *32*, 745–766. [CrossRef]

67. Sultan, B.; Labadi, K.; Guégan, J.F.; Janicot, S. Climate Drives the Meningitis Epidemics Onset in West Africa. *PLOS Med.* **2005**, *2*, e6. [CrossRef] [PubMed]

68. Denton, F. Climate change vulnerability, impacts, and adaptation: Why does gender matter? *Gend. Dev.* **2002**, *10*, 10–20. [CrossRef]

69. Beg, N.; Morlot, J.C.; Davidson, O.; Afrane-Okesse, Y.; Tyani, L.; Denton, F.; Sokona, Y.; Thomas, J.P.; La Rovere, E.L.; Parikh, J.K.; et al. Linkages between climate change and sustainable development. *Clim. Policy* **2002**, *2*, 129–144. [CrossRef]

70. Fonta, W.M.; Ayuk, E.T.; van Huysen, T. Africa and the Green Climate Fund: Current challenges and future opportunities. *Clim. Policy* **2018**, *18*, 1210–1225. [CrossRef]

71. Nakhooda, S.; Caravani, A.; Bird, N. *Climate Finance in Sub-Saharan Africa*; Overseas Development Institute: Berlin, Germany, 2011; pp. 1–8.

72. Smith, J.B.; Dickinson, T.; Donahue, J.D.; Burton, I.; Haites, E.; Klein, R.J.; Patwardhan, A. Development and climate change adaptation funding: Coordination and integration. *Clim. Policy* **2011**, *11*, 987–1000. [CrossRef]

73. Ford, J.D.; Berrang-Ford, L.; Lesnikowski, A.; Barrera, M.; Heymann, S.J. How to Track Adaptation to Climate Change: A Typology of Approaches for National-Level Application. *Ecol. Soc.* **2013**, *18*, 1–14. [CrossRef]

74. Austin, S.E.; Biesbroek, R.; Berrang-Ford, L.; Ford, J.D.; Parker, S.; Fleury, M.D. Public Health Adaptation to Climate Change in OECD Countries. *Int. J. Environ. Res. Public Health* **2016**, *13*, 889. [CrossRef] [PubMed]

75. Syrovátka, M. *Financing Adaptation to Climate Change in Developing Countries*; Department of Development Studies; Palacky University: Olomouc, Czech Republic, 2009; pp. 59–74.

76. Kim, P.S. A Daunting Task in Asia. *Public Manag. Rev.* **2008**, *10*, 527–537. [CrossRef]

77. Wooden, R. The Principles of Public Engagement: At the Nexus of Science, Public Policy Influence, and Citizen Education. *Soc. Res. Int. Q.* **2006**, *73*, 1057–1063.

78. Finkelstein, N.D. (Ed.) Introduction: Transparency in Public Policy. In *Transparency in Public Policy: Great Britain and the United States*; Palgrave Macmillan: London, UK, 2000; pp. 1–9.

79. Whitmarsh, L.; O'Neill, S.; Lorenzoni, I. *Engaging the Public with Climate Change: Communication and Behaviour Change*; Earthscan: London, UK, 2011.

80. Lesnikowski, A.C.; Ford, J.D.; Berrang-Ford, L.; Barrera, M.; Heymann, J. How are we adapting to climate change? A global assessment. *Mitig. Adapt. Strateg. Glob. Chang.* **2015**, *20*, 277–293. [CrossRef]

81. Lesnikowski, A.; Ford, J.; Biesbroek, R.; Berrang-Ford, L.; Heymann, S.J. National-level progress on adaptation. *Nat. Clim. Chang.* **2015**, *6*, 261. [CrossRef]

2

Green Food Development in China: Experiences and Challenges

Jiuliang Xu [1,2,3], Zhihua Zhang [4], Xian Zhang [4], Muhammad Ishfaq [1], Jiahui Zhong [1], Wei Li [5], Fusuo Zhang [1,2,3] and Xuexian Li [1,2,3,*]

[1] Department of Plant Nutrition, The Key Plant-Soil Interaction Laboratory, Ministry of Education, China Agricultural University, Beijing 100193, China; jlxu9@cau.edu.cn (J.X.); ishfaq@cau.edu.cn (M.I.); zhongjiahuicau@126.com (J.Z.); zhangfs@cau.edu.cn (F.Z.)
[2] National Academy of Agriculture Green Development, China Agricultural University, Beijing 100193, China
[3] Chinese Academy of Green Food Development, Beijing 100193, China
[4] China Green Food Development Center, Beijing 100081, China; 13911389022@163.com (Z.Z.); zx695641084@163.com (X.Z.)
[5] Fujian Key Laboratory of Agro-Product Quality and Safety, Fuzhou 350003, China; liwei6055@126.com
* Correspondence: steve@cau.edu.cn.

Abstract: China feeds approximately 22% of the global population with only 7% of the global arable land because of its surprising success in intensive agriculture. This outstanding achievement is partially overshadowed by agriculture-related large-scale environmental pollution across the nation. To ensure nutrition security and environmental sustainability, China proposed the Green Food Strategy in the 1990s and set up a specialized management agency, the China Green Food Development Center, with a monitoring network for policy and standard creation, brand authorization, and product inspection. Following these 140 environmental and operational standards, 15,984 green food companies provided 36,345 kinds of products in 2019. The cultivation area and annual domestic sales (CNY 465.7 billion) of green food accounted for 8.2% of the total farmland area and 9.7% of the gross domestic product (GDP) from agriculture in China. Herein, we systemically reviewed the regulation, standards, and authorization system of green food and its current advances in China, and then outlined its environmental benefits, challenges, and probable strategies for future optimization and upscaling. The rapid development of the green food industry in China suggests an applicable triple-win strategy for protecting the environment, promoting agroeconomic development, and improving human nutrition and health in other developing countries or regions.

Keywords: green food; authorization; standard; food quality; environment; sustainable development

1. Introduction

A leading challenge of the 21st century is to ensure global food security on a socioeconomically sustainable basis; annual grain production needs to increase by approximately 580 million tons (MT) by 2030—a 2% increase per year—in order to meet the grain demands of the rapidly growing population [1]. With 22% of the world's population depending on only 7% of the cultivated land [2], the total annual grain production in China has increased from 280 to 617 million tons (~120%), and the average grain yield has increased from 2949 to 6081 kg ha^{-1} (~106%) over the last four decades (1980–2018) [3,4]. Such achievements in grain production rely heavily on high levels of resource inputs. The increase in the application of chemical nitrogen (N) fertilizers, from 9.34 to 20.65 million tons (National Bureau of Statistics of China), has resulted in a lower overall N use efficiency of 0.25, compared with 0.42 in developed countries [5]. If an excessive amount of synthetic N enters the surrounding environment, it causes soil acidification and the intensification of greenhouse gas emissions, N deposition, and the eutrophication of surface water [5–7]. Soil acidification in southern China significantly stimulates the bioavailability of heavy metals, i.e., Cd and Mn, and certain levels of heavy metals are unintentionally included in composts and phosphate fertilizers [8]. Almost 20% of the farmland in China has been polluted by heavy metals, especially cadmium (Cd), nickel (Ni), and arsenic (As) [9], and the related food contamination has become an increasingly serious agricultural and social issue [10]. The overuse of pesticides is another challenge for improving food quality; the intensity of pesticide use increased from 5.83 kg/ha in 1990 to 13.07 kg/ha in 2018, with an average annual growth of 4.28% [3]. The public policy "zero growth of chemical fertilizer and pesticide use by 2020" was therefore initiated in 2015 in order to sustain agriculture development in China.

Green food was first introduced in China by the Ministry of Agriculture (MOA) in 1990, and it primarily refers to a full range of edible plants, animals, fungal raw materials, value-added processed products, and condiments. According to the principle of sustainable development, standard operational protocols apply to the full industry chain, including the production, processing, packing, storage, and transportation of green foods for farm-to-fork quality control and the efficient utilization of resources, as designed by the China Green Food Development Center (CGFDC). With strict regulations and regular inspection, green food dramatically reduces resource inputs, i.e., chemical fertilizers, pesticides, and related additives; disseminates new technologies; improves environmental and food quality; increases farmers' earnings [11]. Over the past three decades, green food has undergone exponential development in terms of the cultivation area, number of products and companies, and domestic and international markets and sales. Herein, we systematically summarize the regulation and development of the green food industry, as well as its broad significance and challenges.

2. Classification, Standardization, and Development of Green Food in China

China adopted three food categories in order to ensure food safety and quality, namely, organic food, green food and safe food (pollution-free food), officially introduced in 1989, 1990, 2001 respectively. The standards and logos of each category are shown in Figure 1. One of the most obvious features of such a classification system is the limitations regarding the type and amount of chemical inputs for the three levels. Organic food allows only organic fertilizers, encourages biological pathogen control, and minimizes other chemical inputs. However, the high standard and price of organic food makes it available to a small percentage of customers [12]. Rather than eliminating chemical fertilizers, pesticides, and additives, the green food category reduces chemical N fertilizers by 50% compared with local farmers' fertilization levels, and excludes nearly 72% of commercially available pesticides in China, which is more acceptable for Chinese farmers and is better for meeting the quality and safety demands of customers. As a "middle ground" between organic and safe food, green food has the highest consumer awareness [13] and improves the competitiveness of the food industry and farmers' income, as well as protecting the environment and ensuring the sustainability of agricultural development [14]. Certification of safe food was stopped in 2018 because its standard had been adopted by most farmers and producers.

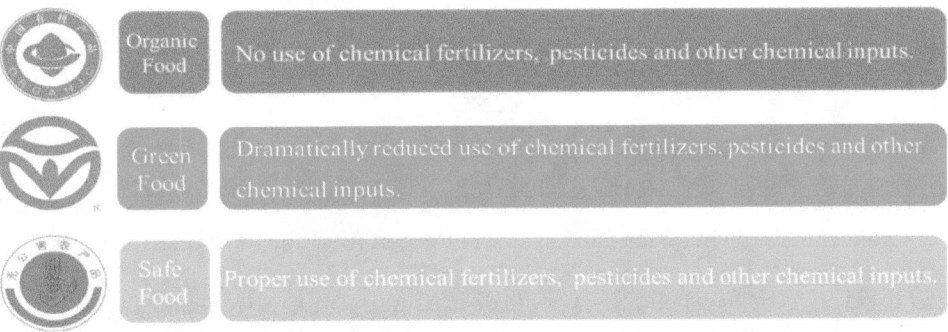

Figure 1. The three levels of food classification in China.

2.1. Administration, Standards, and Authorization of Green Food

CGFDC, founded by the Ministry of Agriculture in 1992, is a specialized agency in charge of national green food regulation and development. It has a general office and six divisions of trademark management, namely, authentication, science–technology and standards, quality inspection, planning and finance, market, and information. Since its establishment, CGFDC has functioned extremely successfully and efficiently in policy formulation, standard upgrading, authentication, accreditation, and quality control. A nationwide monitoring network led by CGFDC ensures policy and standard implementation, including 36 local green good management departments, as well as 96 monitoring organizations.

Green food regulations and standards were developed and established following the Codex Alimentarius programmed by the Codex Alimentarius Commission (CAC) which is the central managing body of the Food and Agriculture Organization (FAO)/World Health Organization (WHO) Food Standards Program to ensure food safety, promote consumer health, and facilitate global food trade. As shown in Figure 2, CGFDC has put 140 standards into effect for food quality control, from the farmland to the dining table. The standard system covers essential requirements for the environment, production technology, product quality, packaging, storage and transportation along the industry chain, and other production material standards, such as fertilizer standards, pesticide standards, food additive standards, and feed additives.

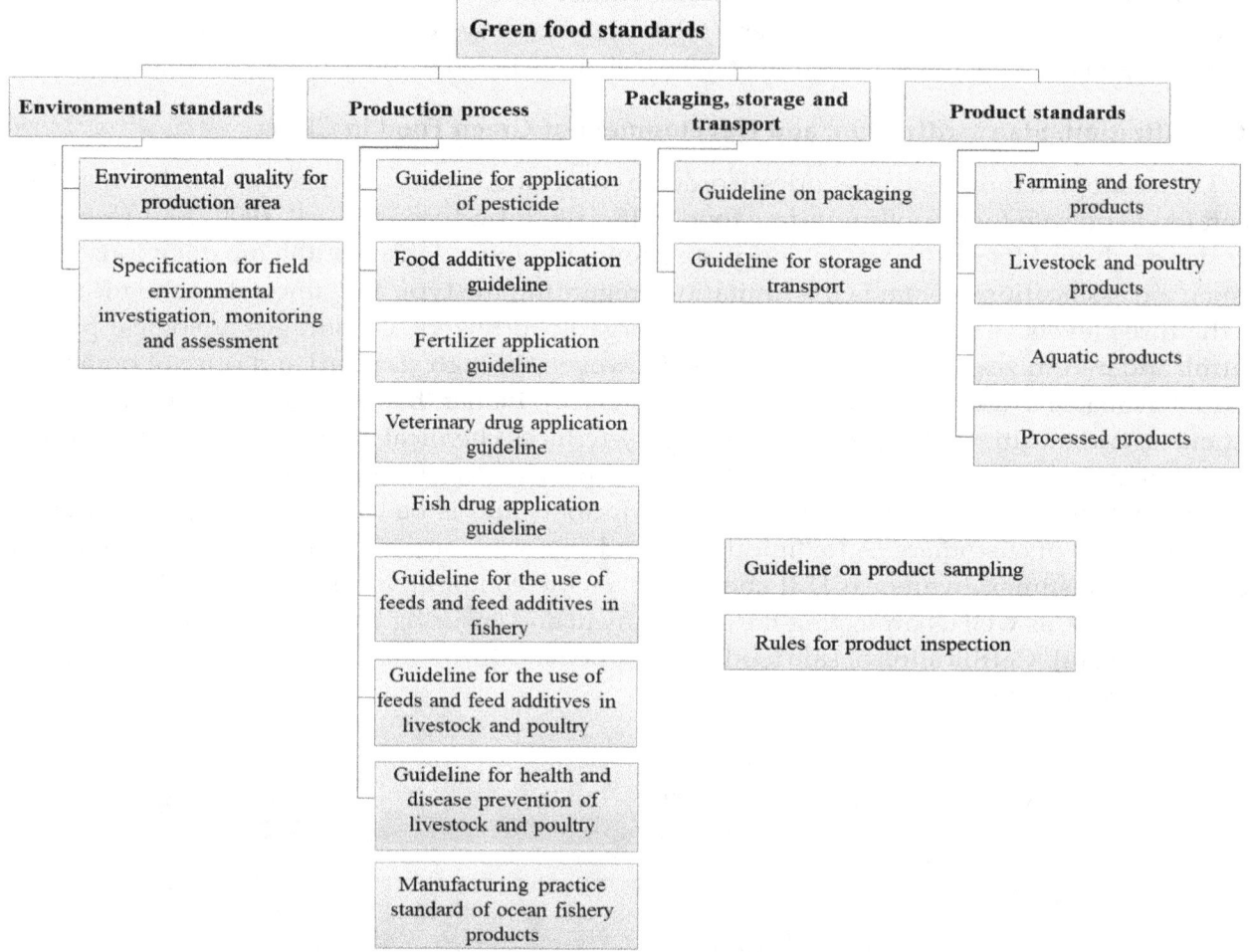

Figure 2. The well-established standard system of green food for food quality control in China.

Unlike safe food, green food places special emphasis on environmental control by specifying the field investigation, monitoring, and assessment. The soil, water, and air quality indexes in the production area are that of the highest national level, and are free of heavy metals or other contaminants. To maintain a superior environment, chemical inputs, including fertilizers and pesticides, are dramatically reduced, therefore, as listed in Table 1, the threshold level of heavy metals, biohazards, and pesticide residues in rice grains of green food is comparable or lower than that of CAC standards. Green food encourages the increased application of organic fertilizer, including animal manure, compost, crop straw fertilizer, and some other commercial fertilizers. The green food fertilizer standards require the use of a fertilizer that meets the crop nutrient requirement of returning a sufficient amount of organic matter to the soil in order to maintain or increase soil fertility and soil biological activity. In China, 527 kinds of pesticides are available for general agricultural producers according to the national food safety standard; however, only 131 kinds of much safer pesticides are listed in the green food guide. Green food has successfully registered in more than 10 foreign countries including USA, UK, France and Japan, and a series of products have been certified. Lastly, green food follows a "from farm to fork" control principle similar to the Hazard Analysis Critical Control Point (HACCP) system.

Table 1. Comparative safety standards of "green food", "safety food" and "CAC" in terms of heavy metals, biohazards and pesticide residues (mg/kg) in rice grains.

	Green Food [1]	Safety Food [2]	CAC [3]
Pb	≤0.2	≤0.2	≤0.2
Cd	≤0.2	≤0.2	≤0.4
Aflatoxin B1	≤0.005	≤0.01	≤0.005
Fenitrothion	≤0.01	≤1.0	≤0.01
Triazoophos	≤0.01	≤0.05	≤0.02
Dimethoate	≤0.01	≤0.05	≤0.01
Bisultap	≤0.01	≤0.2	-
Butachlor	≤0.01	≤0.5	≤0.5
Buprofezin	≤0.3	≤0.3	-

[1] Green Food Standard for Rice, NY/T419-2014; [2] Agricultural Trade Standard of Safe Food for Rice of China, NY 5115-2008; [3] CAC: Codex Alimentarius Commission for rice.

The applicant initially submits their application to the Provincial Green Food Office for primary screening and for examination of the environment and products. Suitable candidates are then transferred to the CGFDC and the Green Food Authentication Review Committee for systematic evaluation. Certified applicants are then authorized to use the "Green food" logo from the CGFDC for production and marketing (Figure 3). Authorization takes effect immediately, is applicable for the following three years, and requires renewal before expiration. Monitoring staff annually inspect the operational procedures and product quality of the green food logo-users. The permit of "Green food" logo users is canceled under following conditions: (1) production environment fails to reach the green food level; (2) products are not up to the quality standard of green food; (3) industries fail to fulfil the contract of green food logo; (4) industries use unregulated raw materials; (5) industries refuse sampling inspection. Accordingly, for example, 52 products out of 8896 were screened out and ceased when 28.8% randomly selected green food products were sampled in 2018.

2.2. Rapid and Steady Growth of the Green Food Industry

Certified products and companies have undergone historic increases since the 1990s (Figure 4 and Table 2). In 2019, a total of 15,984 green food companies provided 36,345 (127 in 1990s) products. The cultivation area expanded from 0.82 million ha in the 1990s to 11.1 million ha in 2019, accounting for 8.20% of the total farmland area in China. In recent years, small-holder farmers have been encouraged to shift from conventional agriculture to the green food mode, resulting in the growing number of companies without obvious expansion of the cultivated area. Additionally, more newly certified companies prefer food processing for higher added value rather than primary products, which contributes more to industry upgrading than area expansion. The annual domestic sales in 2019 reached CNY 465.7 billion, and approximately 9.7% of the GDP was from agriculture (National Bureau of Statistics of China). A huge leap in international sales, from USD 0.04 to 4.13 billion, over the period of 2001–2019, suggests robust growth in the green food market outside of China. The steady development of the green food industry has attracted many farmers and has promoted industrial standardization.

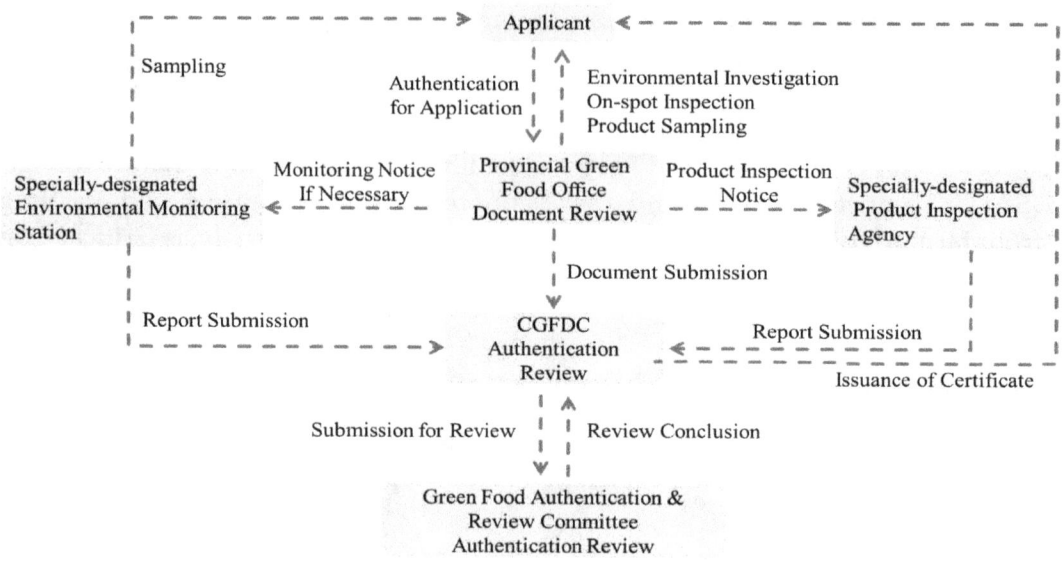

Figure 3. Schematic illustration of green food authorization in China. CGFDC, China Green Food Development Center.

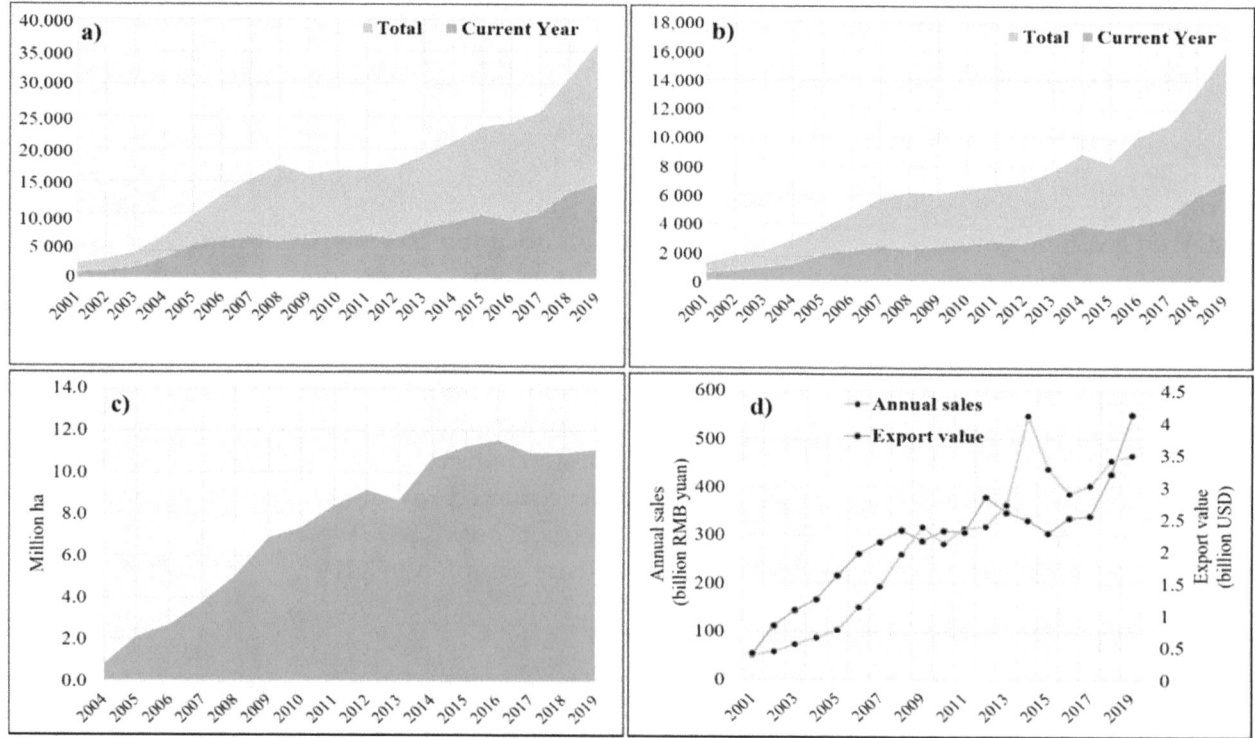

Figure 4. Green food development in China over the last two decades (2001–2019): (**a**) Number of certified products, (**b**) number of certified companies, (**c**) cultivated area, and (**d**) annual sales and export value. "Total" in (**a,b**) indicates cumulative number to date, and "Current year" refers to the number of newly certified products or companies in a particular year.

Table 2. Current status of the green food industry in China in 2019 (Source: CGFDC).

Item	Number
Product	36,345
Company	15,984
Farm	721
Farmer (million)	21.7
Cultivation area (million ha)	11.1
Domestic sales (billion CNY)	465.7
Export value (billion USD)	4.1
Technical standards	15
Product standards	125

2.3. Categories and Proportions of Green Food Products

Green food is generally classified into five categories, namely, primary and processed products of agriculture/forestry, beverage, livestock and poultry, aquaculture, and others (Figure 5 and Table S1). There are 23,986 agricultural and forest products (73.5 million tons), accounting for 77.5% of the overall green food. Subgroups of vegetables, fruits, and rice amount to 60.6% of the total amount of green food. The other agricultural and forest subgroups include soybean, maize, coarse cereals, wheat flour, edible forestry products, and vegetable oil, among others.

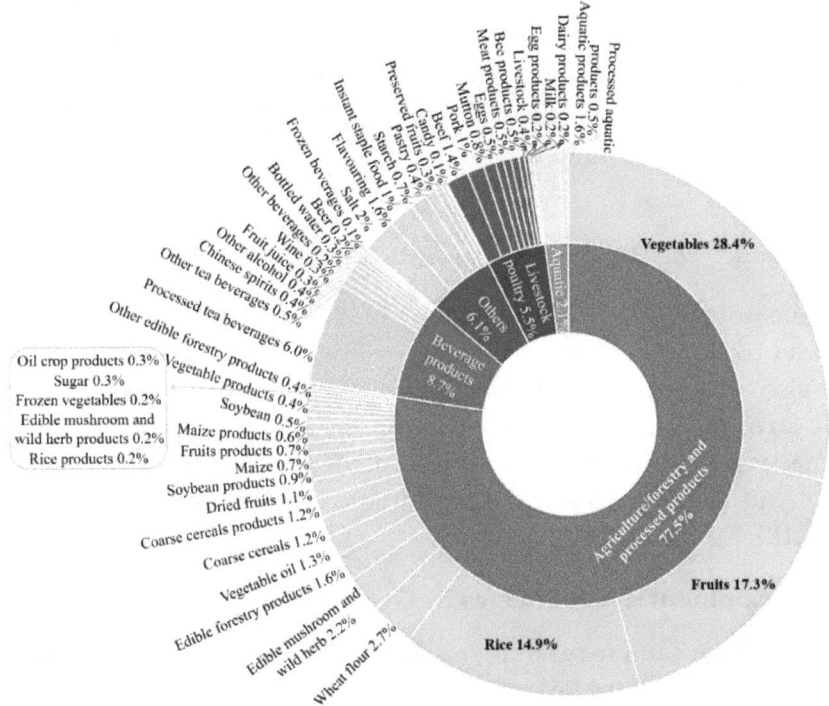

Figure 5. Green food categories and their corresponding proportions on the basis of the amount of product in China.

The second largest category (8.7%) is beverages, with a lower cost and higher profit; processed tea (nearly 6%) dominates this category. The third category (5.5%) is livestock and poultry products, including beef (1.4%), pork (1%), mutton (0.8%), and eggs (0.5%), as well as their products. Aquatic products rank fourth (2.1%). Notably, compared with agricultural/forestry or livestock products, the proportion of poultry and aquatic products is fairly low because of the strict prohibition of genetically modified (GM) ingredients according to the standard of "Green Food: Guideline for the Use of Feeds and Feed Additives in Animals." Most Chinese customers dislike GM food [15,16], and therefore, green food excludes direct GM feed or additives, which considerably hinders the application and authorization for livestock, poultry, and aquatic producers.

2.4. Distribution Patterns of Green Food Production

By the end of 2019, green food had spread across all province-level administrative regions in the mainland (Figure 6), with the highest density in the eastern coastal area and Heilongjiang. More than 40% of green food companies are concentrated in five provinces—Shandong, Anhui, Jiangsu, Heilongjiang, and Zhejiang—with Shandong being the province with the greatest number of green food companies (1625; 10.2%) and products (3898; 10.7%). By contrast, 5.9% of the green food companies are scattered in Xinjiang, Tibet, Qinghai, Shanxi, Shaanxi, and Ningxia. Tibet has the least companies (17) and products (42). Such an asymmetric distribution suggests good development of green food in eastern and northeastern China and underdevelopment in Western China. Given the high-grade environmental conditions in the west, western China possesses a great advantage for accelerating green food growth for local rural and economic development.

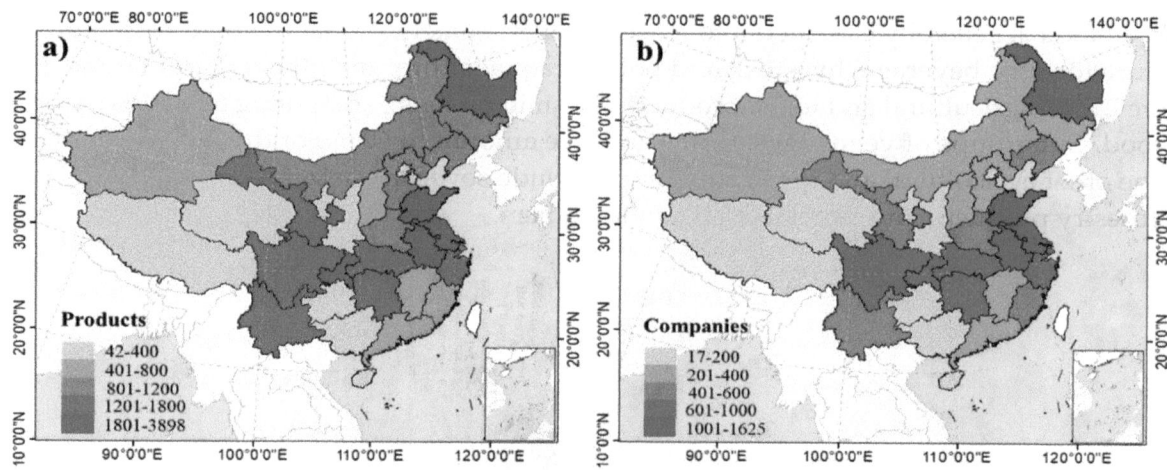

Figure 6. (a) Product- and (b) company-based distribution of green food in China in 2019.

Green food is a quite unique system well developed in China to ensure food quality on a sustainable basis. However, in order to ensure sustainable farming, environmental protection, and human health, other approaches are also adopted across the world with different principles from those of green food. In particular, organic farming and integrated farm management practices can be observed in USA, Germany, France, Canada, UK, Italy, etc. For example, a UK-based leading organization namely LEAF (Linking Environment And Farming) is actively working to deliver more sustainable and resilient food and farming chain [17,18].

3. Agricultural and Environmental Advantages of Green Food

Green food has brought about far-reaching environmental, economic, and social impacts with its rapid development across the mainland over the past three decades. Here, we consider how a 50% cut of chemical nitrogen fertilizers and the supplementation of organic fertilizers (N fertilization guide for green food) affect crop production and environmental protection (Table S2).

3.1. Crop Yield and Quality

Numerous studies have suggested that less than 50% of the N fertilizers that are applied are absorbed by crops, and a large percentage of the remaining active N goes into the soil, water, or air, causing severe environmental damage [19]. In the North China Plain and the Taihu Region, a 30–60% decrease in chemical N fertilizers does not affect the yields of rice, wheat, or maize [20]. A more recent meta-analysis has revealed that the substitution of 50–75% of chemical N fertilizers with livestock manure improves the crop yield by 12.7% [21]. In a 19-year long-term field experiment in China, using a similar 50% replacement strategy, the crop yield was improved and yield variability was reduced; these results are also supported by experiments with other crops [22]. Beyond annual crops, apple yields can increase from 31.5 to 42.1 t/ha when supplied with mixed N (50% chemical N and 50% swine manure); more importantly, a combinatorial N supply significantly improves the fruit quality, as indicated by the higher values for the sugar/acid ratio, concentrations of vitamin C and soluble solids, and firmness [23]. Green cucumber grown in this manner is free from environmental contamination and is safer for human consumption compared with local farmers' cucumber [24].

3.2. Environmental Consequences

The application of organic fertilizers improves the organic matter content, soil microbial activities, and water and nutrient holding capacities, while reducing water contamination [25–28]. Green food favors organic fertilizers because of its greater nutrient-use efficiency, less nutrient leaching and volatilization, and lower environmental costs in different agroecosystems, as supported by numerous studies with a comparable N regime [28–33]. The mixed and balanced organic and inorganic N supply promotes soil carbon sequestration in the rice–wheat rotation system [34], and considerably reduces N_2O emissions compared with inorganic N dominant treatment [35]. Therefore, the green food model may serve as a win–win strategy for sustainable environmental and economic development.

4. Major Challenges of the Green Food Industry

In spite of the considerable progress and environmental benefits, the cultivation area of green food has maintained a relatively low level (8.20% of the total arable land in China). More livestock, poultry, aquatic, and processed products are needed in order to meet the market demand. Making green food a stronger public brand is another challenge in the long run.

4.1. Unbalanced Development of Green Food

The green food industry needs to be well-structured in terms of food processing, food categories, and regional distribution. (i) As described in Section 2.3, primary agricultural products dominate green food production, and primarily processed and further-processed products account for only 25.5% of the overall green food products, which makes green food less value-added and favorable for producers. (ii) Crop products make up a particularly large proportion of green food, while products of an animal origin hold a proportion of only 7.6%, which weakens the competitiveness and profitability of the industry. Such a product structure cannot meet the food consumption pattern or nutrient requirements. (iii) Green food is more preferentially distributed in eastern China, although western China, rich in natural resources and ideal for green food production, is still relatively less developed. For instance, Xinjiang and Ningxia are major grape production regions in China both for fresh and wine-brewing grape under favorable environmental conditions. If production is properly upscaled with sequential processing and optimized logistic organization, green food boosts local economic development, improves employment and farmers' earnings.

4.2. Insufficient Technological Innovations

Technology plays a critical role in improving production efficiency and product values, reducing food waste, and promoting industry upgradation. Green food calls for new techniques for nutrient management, crop and animal management, disease control, food processing, cold storage, and waste recycling along the industry chain. Technological innovation also ensures food quality, helps nurture leading companies, and enables better marketing and advertising strategies, and also improves export competitiveness. To date, more than 60% of green food companies are small-sized producers with limited capabilities in terms of scientific and technical innovations. Underdevelopment of farmer training programs and a lack of awareness regarding the essence of green food production technology is one of the reasons for its low popularity among local growers.

4.3. Weak International Competitiveness

The overall competitiveness of the green food industry is still very weak and the trade levels are relatively low. The green food industry in China has achieved remarkable development; however, the total output of green food is still relatively low compared to the demand for safe agricultural products in both the international and domestic markets. The global consumption expenses for organic food in 2017 exceeded USD 69.8 billion [36], so it has a big sale potential in the international market. However, the export value of Chinese green food was only approximately USD 2.5 billion in 2017. Green food allows the use of chemical compositions in production and does not meet certain international standards. Insufficient product diversification and lack of processed products also are significant barriers facing green food exportation.

4.4. Consumer Mistrust, Awareness, and Higher Prices of Green Food Products

The demand for green food or organically produced food plays a central role in the successful proliferation of these industries. Apart from the abovementioned strict certification and quality maintenance standards (see Section 2.1. Administration, Standards, and Authorization of Green Food), Chinese and international consumers are very much concerned about food safety. There is a lot of consumer mistrust about the quality of labeled food and there is not enough awareness about the quality standards of the current green food; therefore, there are not many consumers who demand green food. The second, and one of the most important reasons, for the limited demand for green good is the price difference, as the price of green food-labeled products is comparatively higher than conventionally produced food. Therefore, developing domestic market and awareness programs regarding product quality standards is needed in order to build solid trust among consumers.

4.5. Inadequate Policy Support

Proper policies accelerate industry development, and the challenges facing green food indicate inadequate policies for further expansion of the industry. Less support from government and enterprises is another constraint for farmers, preventing them from shifting from intensive agriculture toward green food production technology. Often, policymakers find it difficult to encourage the development of the green food industry. Considerably less funding has been put toward the research and development of the green food industry, and this has resulted in a lack of dearth knowledge regarding this industry.

5. Way Forward

In order to tackle the above challenges, we propose the following strategies to boost the development of the green food industry.

5.1. Optimize the Industry Structure

Better regulations in order to optimize the industry structure are conductive to green food development. This could be achieved by optimizing the industry structure through strengthening the provision of livestock, poultry, and value-added products so as to meet the demands of different customer populations in domestic and international markets. Furthermore, attention should be paid to insects and aquatic organisms as green food which provide quality products with low impact on environment. Insects have promising potential to provide sustainable alternative source of proteins for humans and livestock. They utilize water and food more efficiently, with higher feed conversion rates and better growth efficiencies, compared to conventional livestock [37–39]. Additionally, insect-based diets aid in maintaining diversity of habitats for other beneficial organisms by reducing pesticide use. Similarly, seafood such as jellyfish can be further developed as another alternative source of protein having less carbohydrates and fats with lower environmental impacts [40–43]. In brief, to develop a regional industry with specific products and an industrial structure and to exert the superiority of resources are key for regional green food development.

5.2. Update Standards and Strengthen Technological Innovation

The standard system and related techniques need to be updated by: fostering cooperation with universities and research institutions, training farmers for knowledge and technology transfer, such as through farmer field schools and communication technologies, integrating industry expansion with quality improvement and attaching more technology to the development of green food, supporting leading enterprises so as to enhance the formation of green food industry groups, green food industry and government should be clearer about understanding the international quality standards, and should improve the output quality and export competitiveness.

5.3. Optimize Supply Chain Management

Creative management of a supply chain can be achieved in the context of green food development, which not only increases farmer and industry profits, but also creates environmental benefits. This can help to explore demand-related information sharing among supply chain actors, including farmers, enterprises, suppliers, and consumers to strengthen both the forward and backward supply chains from the industry, to characterize the food supply chains in connection with sustainable consumption and production, to strengthen integration of a dominant industrial chain, balance the development of primary, secondary, and tertiary industries and to ensure the efficient use of byproducts and rural waste.

5.4. Exploit the Brand Effect

Green food brand advantage is a major element in marking strategies. In order to improve competitiveness in domestic and international markets, the green food industry should carry out a prominent brand strategy to further exploit the brand effect by incubating leading companies, improving food quality, increasing public awareness, and establishing the trace system so as to enhance the brand value in a favorable social environment; distinguish the products' value of being "green, safe, and environmentally friendly" so as to improve consumers' quality trust, establish more marketing channels in order to cut down customers' perceived costs and strengthen the control of advertisements through the media.

5.5. Make More Supportive Policies

The success of encouraging green food industry initiatives profoundly depends on governmental policies. The Chinese government should make more favorable supportive policies, i.e., subsidies, tax deductions, reduced certification costs, and low-interest loans, so as to encourage more farmers and companies to produce environmentally friendly organic fertilizers, pesticides, and processed green foods. Special ecological subsidies may apply to green crop production for a reduction in chemical fertilizers and for increases in carbon sequestration. Significant tax deductions would encourage livestock, poultry, and aquatic production, food processing, and the full provision of organic fertilizers. Other supportive policies may enhance farmers' motivation to shift from conventional intensive agriculture to green food mode.

6. Potential and Large-Scale Impact of Green Food Farming Scenario

The potential larger-scale impact of the green food industry in China has been projected through a scenario analysis. For instance, the large-scale adaptation of the "Green Food Fertilizer Application Guideline," namely, reducing chemical N fertilizers by 50% so that the proportion of green food in China increases to 20%, would determine the potential N fertilizer and emission reduction. In this simulation, the chemical N fertilizer (N fer) input of conventional farming was based on a previous study—a database constructed by Zhang et al. from a national survey of 6.6 million producers covering 54 crops in China, representing >95% of the cropland of China, which were categorized into cereals (133 kg N/ha), fruits (429 kg N/ha), vegetables (275 kg N/ha), and others (132 kg N/ha) [44]. The reduction of N consumption was estimated based on reducing chemical N fertilizers by 50%

compared with conventional farming on the same cultivated area. The emission factors/models of nitrate (NO_3^-–N) leaching, ammonia (NH_3–N) volatilization, and nitrous oxide (N_2O–N) emissions were calculated using exponential or linear models developed by Wang et al. for wheat and maize [45], by Cui et al. for rice [46], and by Wang et al. for vegetables [47]. For fruits, it was assumed that they have similar N losses as vegetables.

Based on the scenario analysis, with the green food standard, chemical N fertilizer use would be reduced by 2.2. MT (1.33 MT for cereals, 0.24 MT for vegetables, 0.25 MT for fruits, and 0.34 MT for other crops; Figure 7). The estimated NH_3 emissions would be reduced by 0.17 MT, the N_2O emissions would be reduced by 0.01 MT, and NO_3^-–N leaching would be reduced by 0.14 MT. If the proposition of the green food industry reached the predicted 20%, chemical N fertilizer use would be reduced by 5.53 MT; the emissions of NH_3 and N_2O would be reduced by 0.40 MT and 0.03 MT, respectively; NO_3^-–N leaching would be reduced by 0.33 MT. The green food industry has the ability of achieving remarkable reductions in terms of chemical N use, and developing green food is an effective way to reduce the fertilizer N input and to decrease environmental pollution. Nevertheless, because nitrogen loss is only calculated by chemical N reduction, it is currently quite difficult to obtain the organic fertilizer information, which is also a major source of emissions, and needs greater investigation in order to support further analysis. In addition, future research needs to recognize the effects across the full food system in order to investigate green food industry effects, such as health, environmental, social, and economic effects.

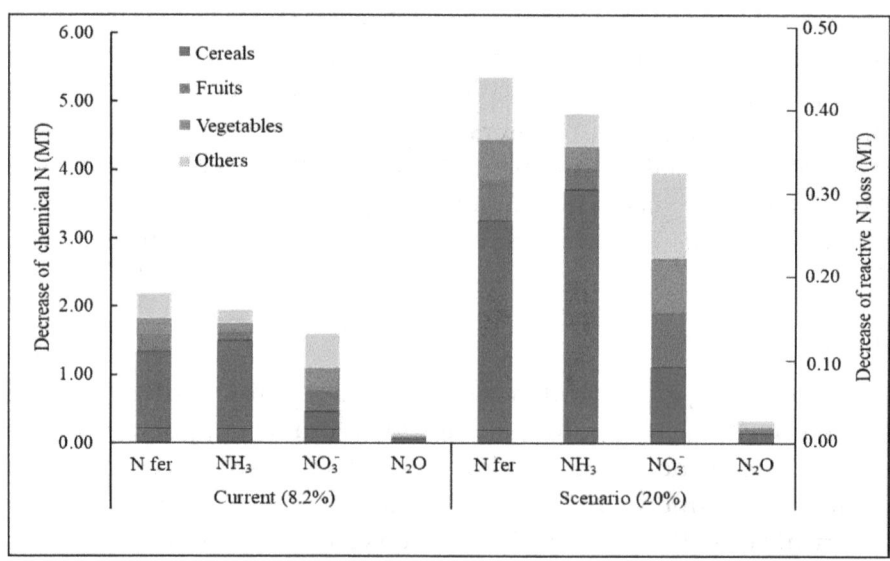

Figure 7. Achievable reduction in chemical N input (N fer), ammonia volatilization (NH_3), nitrate leaching (NO_3^-), and nitrous oxide emission (N_2O) if the proportion of green food in China increases to 20%.

While N fertilizer is excessively overused in China, sustainable agriculture has become a priority for China. China released the "action to achieve zero growth of chemical fertilizer use by 2020" policy in order to achieve zero growth for chemical fertilizer use for principal crops by 2020 [44]. By 2019, 83% of the provinces reached a negative three-year average annual growth of fertilizer use, showing the potential for successfully achieving this policy [48]. Nevertheless, China's agriculture still has a long way to go in facing the challenges of further enhancing agricultural productivity while minimizing environmental impacts. Green food is a sustainable and environmentally friendly approach, as its limited use of chemical inputs can considerably reduce environment-related concerns. Therefore, shifting from intensive conventional agriculture toward green food farming at a large scale is an effective way to realize sustainable development in China.

In addition to mitigation of environmental pollution, shifting from conventional to green food-like farming system has the potential to improve soil health by improving its physical, chemical and biological properties [49–52]. Sustainable soil health depends on the application of carbon-rich amendments that support the biological processes, which are the central foundations of healthy soil. Additionally, systemic reduction of chemical nitrogen, according to the green food rule, prevents its overuse by small-hold farmers and better balances crop nutrition, improving the quality of agricultural commodities, i.e., increasing the sugar/acid ratio of apple and grape [23,53]. It helps prepare farms and people to be more resilient to climate change; primarily, the addition of organic fertilizers improves water use efficiency, consequently, resistance to risky weather, and ultimately lowers the chances of crop failure. Pesticides and heavy metals are also critical substances under regulation of green food, however, more data and field experiments are required for in-depth quantitative analysis in the future. In brief, large-scale expansion of green food farming has promising potential to produce safe and nutritious food, improve soil fertility and quality, and eventually uplift the living standard of people on a sustainable basis.

7. Conclusions

In sharp contrast to long-standing yield-centered production systems, green food, as a national program, has historically put a high priority on environment and food quality since early 1990s by stringent selection of arable land, dramatic cuts in chemical inputs, and a wide array of gradually-established detailed regulations of postharvest processes. After nearly 30 years' steady and rapid development, green food accounts for 8.2% of the total farmland area and 9.7% of the GDP from agriculture in China, signifying high efficiencies of existing regulations and broader practical applicability of current standards in the future. Here, for the first time, we systematically summarized its regulation, standards, achievements, environmental benefits, challenges, and future strategies.

Economic growth in China has averaged 9.5% over the past two decades and the country is currently experiencing rapid urbanization. More and more attention is being focused on environment- and health-related problems, and a healthy diet has become a new consumption trend, which conditions a much more favorable socioeconomic environment for green food. Increasingly strict environment protection policies further favors the implementation of green food standards. To meet the environment requirements and increase the food value, more non-green food farmers are willing to reduce chemical nitrogen fertilizers by 50% and properly utilize 131 kinds of pesticides out of 527 market available products. In the long run, green food represents a sustainable agricultural developmental model that can drastically reduce environmental costs, while increasing product value and producer profit. Optimizing the industry structure, upgrading standards and technologies, strengthening brand impact, and establishing supportive policies will boost green food growth in the future.

Author Contributions: Conceptualization, J.X. and X.L.; writing—original draft preparation, J.X.; writing—reviewing and editing, J.X., Z.Z., X.Z., M.I., J.Z., W.L., F.Z., and X.L. All authors have read and agreed to the published version of the manuscript.

Acknowledgments: This work was supported by the China Green Food Development Center (GXTC-C-19050052).

References

1. Fan, M.S.; Shen, J.B.; Yuan, L.X.; Jiang, R.F.; Zhang, F.S. Improving crop productivity and resource use efficiency to ensure food security and environmental quality in China. *J. Exp. Bot.* **2011**, *63*, 13–24. [CrossRef] [PubMed]

2. Yu, X.; Sun, J.X.; Sun, S.K.; Yang, F.; Lu, Y.J.; Wang, Y.B.; Wu, F.J.; Liu, P. A comprehensive analysis of regional grain production characteristics in China from the scale and efficiency perspectives. *J. Clean. Prod.* **2019**, *212*, 610–621. [CrossRef]

3.   FAO. Statistics Division of the Food and Agriculture Organization of the United Nations. Agriculture Database. FAOSTAT. 2018. Available online: http://www.fao.org/faostat/en/#data/QC/ (accessed on 1 December 2018).

4.   Ying, H.; Yin, Y.L.; Zheng, H.F.; Wang, C.Y.; Zhang, Q.S.; Xue, Y.F.; Stefanovski, D.; Cui, Z.L.; Dou, Z.X. Newer and select maize, wheat, and rice varieties can help mitigate N footprint while producing more grain. *Glob. Chang. Biol.* **2019**, *25*, 4273–4281. [CrossRef] [PubMed]

5.   Cui, Z.L.; Zhang, H.Y.; Chen, X.P.; Zhang, C.C.; Ma, W.Q.; Huang, C.D.; Zhang, W.F.; Mi, G.H.; Miao, Y.X.; Li, X.L.; et al. Pursuing sustainable productivity with millions of smallholder farmers. *Nature* **2018**, *555*, 363–366. [CrossRef] [PubMed]

6.   Guo, J.H.; Liu, X.J.; Zhang, Y.; Shen, J.L.; Han, W.X.; Zhang, W.F.; Christie, P.; Goulding, K.W.; Vitousek, P.M.; Zhang, F.S. Significant acidification in major Chinese croplands. *Science* **2010**, *327*, 1008–1010. [CrossRef] [PubMed]

7.   Liu, X.J.; Duan, L.; Mo, J.M.; Du, E.Z.; Shen, J.B.; Lu, X.K.; Zhang, Y.; Zhou, X.B.; He, C.N.; Zhang, F.S. Nitrogen deposition and its ecological impact in China: An overview. *Environ. Pollut.* **2011**, *159*, 2251–2264. [CrossRef]

8.   Zhu, Q.C.; Liu, X.J.; Hao, T.X.; Zeng, N.F.; Zhang, F.S.; Wim, D.V. Modeling soil acidification in typical Chinese cropping systems. *Sci. Total Environ.* **2018**, *613*, 1339–1348. [CrossRef]

9.   Shang, E.P.; Xu, E.Q.; Zhang, H.Q.; Huang, C.H. Temporal-spatial trends in potentially toxic trace element pollution in farmland soil in the major grain-producing regions of China. *Sci. Rep. UK* **2019**, *9*, 19463. [CrossRef]

10. Yang, S.Y.; Zhao, J.; Chang, S.X.; Collins, C.; Xu, J.M.; Liu, X.M. Status assessment and probabilistic health risk modeling of metals accumulation in agriculture soils across China: A synthesis. *Environ. Int.* **2019**, *128*, 165–174. [CrossRef]

11. Hassan, M.U.; Wen, X.; Xu, J.L.; Zhong, J.H.; Li, X.X. Development and challenges of green food in China. *Front. Agric. Sci. Eng.* **2020**, *7*, 56–66. [CrossRef]

12. Yin, S.J.; Wu, L.H.; Du, L.; Chen, M. Consumers' purchase intention of organic food in China. *J. Sci. Food Agric.* **2010**, *90*, 1361–1367. [CrossRef]

13. Liu, L.Q.; Liu, C.X.; Wang, J.S. Deliberating on renewable and sustainable energy policies in China. *Renew. Sustain. Energy Rev.* **2013**, *17*, 191–198. [CrossRef]

14. Liu, R.D.; Pieniak, Z.; Verbeke, W. Consumers' attitudes and behaviour towards safe food in China: A review. *Food Control.* **2013**, *33*, 93–104. [CrossRef]

15. Cui, K.; Shoemaker, S.P. Public perception of genetically-modified (GM) food: A Nationwide Chinese Consumer Study. *NPJ Sci. Food.* **2018**, *2*, 10. [CrossRef] [PubMed]

16. Prakash, C.S. GM crops in the media. *GM Crop. Food.* **2015**, *6*, 63–68. [CrossRef]

17. Drummond, C. Environmental management systems in practice: The experiences of LEAF (Linking Environment and Farming) in meeting the needs of farmers, consumers and environmentalists. *Asp. Appl. Biol.* **2000**, *62*, 165–172.

18. Drummond, C.; Harris, C. Linking Environment and Farming: Integrated Systems for Sustainable Farmland Management. In *Sustainable Farmland Management: Transdisciplinary Approaches*; CABI: Wallingford, UK, 2008; p. 169.

19. Zhang, F.S.; Chen, X.P.; Vitousek, P. An experiment for the world. *Nature* **2013**, *497*, 33–35. [CrossRef]

20. Ju, X.T.; Xing, G.X.; Chen, X.P.; Zhang, S.L.; Zhang, L.J.; Liu, X.J.; Cui, Z.L.; Yin, B.; Christie, P.; Zhu, Z.L. Reducing environmental risk by improving N management in intensive Chinese Agricultural Systems. *Proc. Natl. Acad. Sci. USA* **2009**, *106*, 3041–3046. [CrossRef]

21. Xia, L.L.; Lam, S.K.; Yan, X.Y.; Chen, D.L. How does recycling of livestock manure in agroecosystems affect crop productivity, reactive nitrogen losses, and soil carbon balance? *Environ. Sci. Technol.* **2017**, *51*, 7450–7457. [CrossRef]

22. Li, Y.Y.; Shao, X.H.; Guan, W.H.; Ren, L.; Liu, J.; Wang, J.L.; Wu, Q.J. Nitrogen-decreasing and yield-increasing effects of combined applications of organic and inorganic fertilizers under controlled irrigation in a paddy field. *Pol. J. Environ. Stud.* **2016**, *25*, 673–680. [CrossRef]

23. Zhao, Z.P.; Yan, S.; Liu, F.; Ji, P.H.; Wang, X.Y.; Tong, Y.A. Effects of chemical fertilizer combined with organic manure on Fuji apple quality, yield and soil fertility in apple orchard on the Loess Plateau of China. *Int. J. Agric. Biol. Eng.* **2014**, *7*, 45–55. [CrossRef]

24. Wang, F.; Liu, Y.X.; Ouyang, X.H.; Hao, J.Q.; Yang, X.S. Comparative environmental impact assessments of green food certified cucumber and conventional cucumber cultivation in China. *Renew. Agric. Food Syst.* **2018**, *33*, 432–442. [CrossRef]

25. Bedada, W.; Karltun, E.; Lemenih, M.; Tolera, M. Long-term addition of compost and NP fertilizer increases crop yield and improves soil quality in experiments on smallholder farms. *Agric. Ecosyst. Environ.* **2014**, *195*, 193–201. [CrossRef]

26. Gogoi, B.; Kalita, B.; Deori, B.; Paul, S. Soil properties under rainfed rice (*Oryza sativa* L.) crop as affected by integrated supply of nutrients. *Int. J. Agric. Innov. Res.* **2015**, *3*, 1720–1725.

27. Li, R.; Tao, R.; Ling, N.; Chu, G.X. Chemical, organic and bio-fertilizer management practices effect on soil physicochemical property and antagonistic bacteria abundance of a cotton field: Implications for soil biological quality. *Soil Tillage Res.* **2017**, *167*, 30–38. [CrossRef]

28. Wang, Z.T.; Geng, Y.B.; Liang, T. Optimization of reduced chemical fertilizer use in tea gardens based on the assessment of related environmental and economic benefits. *Sci. Total Environ.* **2020**, *713*, 136439. [CrossRef]

29. Banger, K.; Kukal, S.S.; Toor, G.; Sudhir, K.; Hanumanthraju, T.H. Impact of long-term additions of chemical fertilizers and farm yard manure on carbon and nitrogen sequestration under rice-cowpea cropping system in semi-arid tropics. *Plant Soil* **2009**, *318*, 27–35. [CrossRef]

30. Huang, Y.; Tang, Y.H. An estimate of greenhouse gas (N_2O and CO_2) mitigation potential under various scenarios of nitrogen use efficiency in Chinese croplands. *Glob. Chang. Biol.* **2010**, *16*, 2958–2970. [CrossRef]

31. Zhang, X.; Zhang, J.; Zheng, C.Y.; Guan, D.H.; Li, S.M.; Xie, F.L.; Chen, J.F.; Hang, X.N.; Jiang, Y.; Deng, A.X.; et al. Significant residual effects of wheat fertilization on greenhouse gas emissions in succeeding soybean growing season. *Soil Tillage Res.* **2017**, *169*, 7–15. [CrossRef]

32. Chen, J.; Lu, S.Y.; Zhang, Z.; Zhao, X.X.; Li, X.M.; Ning, P.; Liu, M.Z. Environmentally friendly fertilizers: A review of materials used and their effects on the environment. *Sci. Total Environ.* **2018**, *613*, 829–839. [CrossRef]

33. Zhang, Y.T.; Wang, H.Y.; Lei, Q.L.; Luo, J.F.; Lindsey, S.; Zhang, J.Z.; Zhai, L.M.; Wu, S.X.; Zhang, J.S.; Liu, X.X.; et al. Optimizing the nitrogen application rate for maize and wheat based on yield and environment on the Northern China Plain. *Sci. Total Environ.* **2018**, *618*, 1173–1183. [CrossRef]

34. Yang, B.; Xiong, Z.Q.; Wang, J.Y.; Xu, X.; Huang, Q.W.; Shen, Q.R. Mitigating net global warming potential and greenhouse gas intensities by substituting chemical nitrogen fertilizers with organic fertilization strategies in rice-wheat annual rotation systems in China: A 3-year field experiment. *Ecol. Eng.* **2015**, *81*, 289–297. [CrossRef]

35. Cai, Y.J.; Ding, W.X.; Luo, J.F. Nitrous oxide emissions from Chinese maize-wheat rotation systems: A 3-year field measurement. *Atmos. Environ.* **2013**, *65*, 112–122. [CrossRef]

36. Bazaluk, O.; Yatsenko, O.; Zakharchuk, O.; Ovcharenko, A.; Khrystenko, O.; Nitsenko, V. Dynamic Development of the global organic food market and opportunities for Ukraine. *Sustainability* **2020**, *12*, 6963. [CrossRef]

37. Christina, H.; Jing, S.; Alice, G.; Michael, S. The psychology of eating insects: A cross-cultural comparison between Germany and China. *Food Qual. Prefer.* **2015**, *44*, 148–156. [CrossRef]

38. Oonincx, D.G.A.B.; Van Broekhoven, S.; Van Huis, A.; van Loon, J.J.A. Feed conversion, survival and development, and composition of four insect species on diets composed of food by-products. *PLoS ONE* **2015**, *10*, e0144601. [CrossRef]

39. Raheem, D.; Carrascosa, C.; Oluwole, O.B.; Nieuwland, M.; Saraiva, A.; Millán, R.; Raposo, A. Traditional consumption of and rearing edible insects in Africa, Asia and Europe. *Crit. Rev. Food Sci. Nutr.* **2019**, *59*, 2169–2188. [CrossRef]

40. Raposo, A.; Coimbra, A.; Amaral, L.; Gonçalves, A.; Morais, Z. Eating jellyfish: Safety, chemical and sensory properties. *J. Sci. Food Agric.* **2018**, *98*, 3973–3981. [CrossRef]

41. Bonaccorsi, G.; Garamella, G.; Cavallo, G.; Lorini, C. A systematic review of risk assessment associated with jellyfish consumption as a potential novel food. *Foods* **2020**, *9*, 935. [CrossRef]

42. Khong, N.M.; Yusoff, F.M.; Jamilah, B.; Basri, M.; Maznah, I.; Chan, K.W.; Nishikawa, J. Nutritional composition and total collagen content of three commercially important edible jellyfish. *Food Chem.* **2016**, *196*, 953–960. [CrossRef]

43. Bleve, G.; Ramires, A.; Gallo, A. Leone Identification of safety and quality parameters for preparation of jellyfish based novel food products. *Foods* **2019**, *8*, 263. [CrossRef]

44. Zhang, Q.; Chu, Y.; Xue, Y.; Ying, H.; Chen, X.; Zhao, Y.; Ma, W.; Ma, L.; Zhang, J.; Yin, Y.; et al. Outlook of China's agriculture transforming from smallholder operation to sustainable production. *Glob. Food Sec.* **2020**, *26*, 100444. [CrossRef]

45. Wang, G.L. Quantitative Analysis of Reactive Nitrogen Losses and Nitrogen Use Efficiency of Three Major Grain Crops in China. Ph.D. Thesis, China Agricultural University, Beijing, China, May 2014. (In Chinese).

46. Cui, Z.; Wang, G.; Yue, S.; Wu, L.; Zhang, W.; Zhang, F.; Chen, X. Closing the N-use efficiency gap to achieve food and environmental security. *Environ. Sci. Technol.* **2014**, *48*, 5780–5787. [CrossRef]

47. Wang, X.Z. Environmental Impacts, Mitigation Potentials and Management Approaches in Chinese Vegetable Production System—Pepper as a Case. Ph.D. Thesis, China Agricultural University, Beijing, China, May 2018. (In Chinese).

48. Jin, S.; Zhou, F. Zero Growth of Chemical Fertilizer and Pesticide Use: China's Objectives, Progress and Challenges. *BioOne Complet.* **2018**, *9*, 50–58. [CrossRef]

49. Guo, L.Y.; Wu, G.L.; Li, Y.; Li, C.H.; Liu, W.J.; Meng, J.; Liu, H.T.; Yu, X.F.; Jiang, G.M. Effects of cattle manure compost combined with chemical fertilizer on topsoil organic matter, bulk density and earthworm activity in a wheat–maize rotation system in Eastern China. *Soil Tillage Res.* **2016**, *156*, 140–147. [CrossRef]

50. Abbasi, M.K.; Khaliq, A.; Shafiq, M.M.; Kazmi, M.; Ali, I. Comparative effectiveness of urea n, poultry manure and their combination in changing soil properties and maize productivity under rainfed conditions in Northeast. Pakistan. *Exp. Agric.* **2010**, *46*, 211–230. [CrossRef]

51. Franke, A.; Schulz, S.; Oyewole, B.; Diels, J.; Tobe, O. The role of cattle manure in enhancing on-farm productivity, macro-and micro-nutrient uptake, and profitability of maize in the Guinea savanna. *Exp. Agric.* **2008**, *44*, 313–328. [CrossRef]

52. Sun, J.; Zou, L.; Li, W.; Yang, J.; Wang, Y.; Xia, Q.; Peng, M. Rhizosphere soil properties and banana Fusarium wilt suppression influenced by combined chemical and organic fertilizations. *Agric. Ecosyst. Environ.* **2018**, *254*, 60–68. [CrossRef]

53. Zhao, F.; Jiang, Y.; He, X.; Liu, H.; Yu, K. Increasing organic fertilizer and decreasing drip chemical Fertilizer for two consecutive years improved the fruit quality of 'Summer Black' grapes in arid areas. *HortScience* **2020**, *55*, 196–203. [CrossRef]

3

The Association between Stressful Events and Food Insecurity: Cross-Sectional Evidence from Australia

Jeromey B. Temple[ID]

Demography and Ageing Unit, Melbourne School of Population and Global Health, University of Melbourne, Melbourne 3010, Australia; Jeromey.Temple@unimelb.edu.au; Tel.: +61-3-9035-9900

Abstract: A considerable body of empirical evidence exists on the demographic and socio-economic correlates of food insecurity in Australia. An important omission from recent studies, however, is an understanding of the role of stressful life events, or stressors in explaining exposure to food insecurity. Using nationally representative data from the 2014 General Social Survey and multivariable logistic regression, this paper reports on the association between 18 discrete stressors and the likelihood of reporting food insecurity in Australia. The results, adjusted for known correlates of food insecurity and complex survey design, show that exposure to stressors significantly increased the likelihood of experiencing food insecurity. Importantly, stressors related to employment and health approximately doubled the odds of experiencing food insecurity. The results underscore the complex correlates of food insecurity and indicates that conceptually it interacts with many important social and economic problems in contemporary Australia. There is no simple fix to food insecurity and solutions require co-ordination across a range of social and economic policies.

Keywords: food insecurity; stressors; stressful life events; access to food; food equality

1. Introduction

Food insecurity is the "limited or uncertain availability of nutritionally adequate and safe foods or limited or uncertain ability to acquire acceptable foods in socially acceptable ways" [1]. In 1975, Australia ratified the United Nations International Covenant on Economic, Social and Cultural Rights, recognising the fundamental human right for its citizenry to be free from hunger [2]. More recently, in 2015, Australia further ratified the United Nations 2030 Agenda for Sustainable Development and the Sustainable Development Goals which seek to eliminate poverty and inequality, with a target of 'zero hunger' by 2030 [3].

Indeed, it is now widely understood that food insecurity is a problem facing not only low and middle-income countries, but also high-income countries such as the USA, Canada and Australia [4,5]. In Australia, approximately 4–5% of the population are estimated to be food insecure, due to a lack of financial resources, with about 40% of this group (or 2% of the population) going without food consequently [6,7]. However, the experience of food insecurity is not evenly spread throughout the Australian population, with a growing number of studies showing that constellations of socio-economic, demographic and geographic factors are associated with food insecurity. For example, young age, being divorced or separated, low income, low education, low financial resources, a high number of resident children, poor health, not owning your home, being unemployed, being an Aboriginal or Torres Strait Islander and measures of spatial disadvantage are all associated with experiencing food insecurity in Australia [7–23].

One important omission from recent studies, however, is an understanding of the role of stressful life events, or stressors, in explaining exposure to food insecurity. Stressors are events, whether anticipated or not, that can have a deleterious effect on the wellbeing of individuals and their families (e.g., onset of a serious health condition or unanticipated unemployment). Independent of known risk factors of food insecurity, an analysis of the association between stressors and food insecurity may provide evidence as to why some households beyond the bottom quintile of household income experience food insecurity in high income countries such as Australia.

International studies, mostly qualitative, have provided some evidence that stressors are associated with, or are a precursor to experiencing food insecurity. In two qualitative studies of low-income older Americans, major sickness and unexpected expenses and medical bills were key factors explaining food insecurity [24,25]. Moreover, family events such as Christmas were cited as a precursor to food insecurity, due to the financial costs associated with filial obligations such as gift giving [25]. A recent US mixed methods study provides some evidence that exposure to adverse childhood experiences (e.g., abuse, neglect, household instability) was associated with experiencing food insecurity later in adulthood [26]. A further qualitative American study found that stressful events such as those related to health and employment were related to food insecurity, but were also mediated by families 'capabilities' to offset negative consequences [27]. This finding is supported by a recent quantitative study which found that families adjusting to negative life events with low levels of income and social support were at a much greater risk of child hunger [28]. In Canada, both the onset of chronic disease and problem gambling were found to be associated with food insecurity in higher-income households [29].

Within the Australian literature, there have been few studies examining the link between stressors and food insecurity. Australian studies have, however, investigated the coping mechanisms used to avoid hunger when stressors such as homelessness, enduring social disadvantage and exogenous policy changes to welfare payments occur [20,30,31]. Generally, it is widely acknowledged that stressors may be an important determinant of food insecurity. For example, Burns (2004) has suggested "Although most persons living in poverty are at risk of food insecurity, it cannot be assumed that they are, in fact, food insecure. In addition, for many reasons, including factors such as ill health, disability, sudden job loss, and high living expenses, persons above the poverty line cannot be assumed to be food secure" [32], p. 7. Furthermore, in Temple's (2008) study of food insecurity in Australia, it is noted "It may be that in times of sudden unemployment, divorce, death or unexpected illness, greater stress is placed on family resources. The ability to negotiate these stresses is likely to contribute to the prevalence of food insecurity" [7], p. 662.

In this study, nationally representative data were used to examine the association between stressors and food insecurity. Firstly, the likelihood of food insecure persons (relative to the food secure) reporting a stressor in the previous 12 months was examined. Secondly, the prevalence of food insecurity categorised by 18 discrete stressors was calculated. Finally, multivariable logistic regression models were used to examine the association between individual stressors and the odds of food insecurity, once extensive controls were accounted for.

2. Materials and Methods

2.1. Survey Data

Data used in this study were from the 2014 General Social Survey (GSS) conducted by the Australian Bureau of Statistics (ABS) between March and June 2014. Using a face-to-face interview along with prompt cards, the ABS collected information using a Computer Assisted Interviewing (CAI) questionnaire on a range of domains to understand the "multi-dimensional nature of relative advantage and disadvantage across the population, and to facilitate reporting on and monitoring of people's opportunities to participate fully in society" [33]. The GSS was designed to provide nationally and state representative estimates across these domains. From a sample of 18,574 private dwellings, 16,145 dwellings were used due to issues of scope or uninhabited dwellings. In total, 80% fully responded, yielding a sample of 12,932 people aged 15 years and over.

The GSS included persons who were usual residents of private dwellings at the time of the survey. This sampling design meant that several populations were excluded including those living in non-private dwellings (e.g., hostels, hospitals, short-stay caravan parks). Also excluded were diplomatic or defence personnel of overseas governments stationed in Australia, those whose usual place of residence was outside of Australia, or those living in very remote areas of discrete Aboriginal and Torres Strait Islander communities. People experiencing homelessness were also excluded from the survey.

2.2. Measurement

Two questions were included in the GSS instrument to identify exposure to stressors. Firstly, the interviewer asked: "Have any of these been a problem for you or anyone close to you, during the last 12 months?". A prompt card (Card F15) was shown to respondents listing: 1. Serious illness, 2. Serious accident, 3. Death of a family member of close friend, 4. Mental illness, 5. Serious disability. Respondents were than further prompted, repeating the question with a second prompt card (Card F16) listing: 10. Divorce or separation, 11. Not able to get a job, 12. Involuntary loss of job, 13. Alcohol or drug related problems, 14. Witness to violence, 15. Abuse or violent crime, 16. Trouble with police, 17. Gambling problem, 18. Discrimination because of ethnic or cultural background 19. Discrimination for any other reason, 20. Bullying and/or harassment, 21. Removal of children, 22. Other. Using these questions, variables measuring 18 distinct stressors were generated.

Measurement of food insecurity in the GSS is included in the financial stress, resilience and exclusion module. Respondents were asked "In the last 12 months, have any of these happened because you were short of money?" A prompt card (Card K1) was shown to the respondent. Respondents who indicated that they went without meals due to a shortage of money were coded as being food insecure. The measurement of going without a meal due to a shortage of money is considered a measure of considerable financially attributable food insecurity, indicative of both inadequate food intake and food depletion [7].

2.3. Statistical Model

To examine the association between stressors and food insecurity multivariable logistic regression models were fitted. Using the raw logit coefficients, adjusted odds ratios (AOR) were calculated, which measure the change in the odds of experiencing food insecurity given an experience of each stressor, once all other factors in the model are controlled for. Regression models were estimated for each stressor independently. Given that food insecurity attributable to financial constraints is a relatively rare event, the stability of the logit coefficients were compared against those of a Scobit (Skewed Logit), Complementary Log-Log and Log Poisson regression model. The strength, significance and direction of parameter coefficients was highly comparable across all regression models, and the logit results are presented herein for simplicity.

Due to complex survey design, adjustments are necessary to generate correct variance estimates. The GSS includes 60 replicate weights on the data file to adjust for sample design and non-response. Utilizing an algorithm developed by Winter, the delete-one jackknife method was used to make the necessary replicate adjustments [34,35]. All analyses were conducted using Stata via the ABS Remote Access Data Laboratory.

Control Variables

Drawing upon previous Australian research outlined above, variables know to be associated with food insecurity were included in the regressions to control for potentially confounding effects. Specifically, the control variables included:

- Age: 15–29, 30–44, 45–59, 60+.
- Marital Status: Married, not married.

- Equivalised Household Income: The measure of household income available in the GSS is gross household income, adjusted or 'equivalised' using an equivalence scale to account for household size and placed in deciles. The ABS make this adjustment in household income to allow for welfare and financial wellbeing comparisons between households of different sizes and compositions. The categories included in the regression based upon income distribution include: 0 to 20%, 20% to 40%, 40% to 60%, 60% to 80%, 80% to 100%, not reported.
- Self-Rated Health: Poor or fair health, good or excellent health.
- Tenure: Renter, not a renter.
- University educated: Has university education, does not have university education.

Additional variables including gender and measures of geography were also included but were not found to be significant at the 95% critical level. For each stressor model, it would be inappropriate to include all control variables due to concerns regarding multicollinearity and other model misspecification issues. Specifically, for the divorce or separation model, marital status was omitted. For the illness, accident, mental illness and disability stressor models, self-rated health was omitted.

3. Results

3.1. Experiences of Stressors

Except for 'other' stressors, food insecure respondents were more likely to report experiencing each type of stressor, relative to the food secure (Table 1). Over one third of food insecure respondents reported not being able to get a job (40.5%), death of a family member or close friend (35.1%), mental illness (34.9%) and serious illness (33.3%). Large differences in the reporting of stressors between food insecure and secure respondents existed for not being able to get a job (40.5% v 16.8%) and mental illness (34.9% v 13.0%). Other considerable differences between food secure and secure respondents (with a difference in prevalence of greater than 10%) included bullying and harassment, alcohol or drug related problems, death of a family member or close friend, witness to violence, trouble with the police and serious illness. Whereas 38% of food secure persons reported no stressors in the last 12 months, only 14% of food insecure respondents did not experience stressors. In contrast, about half of the food insecure reported three or more stressors, compared with 16% of the food secure.

Table 1. Stressors reported by Food Insecurity Status, Weighted (%), 2014.

	Food Insecure (%)	Food Secure (%)		n [1]
Type of Stressor [2]				
Divorce or Separation	17.6	11.3	***	1467
Death of Family Member/Close Friend	35.1	21.4	***	2957
Serious Illness	33.3	22.3	***	3008
Serious Accident	7.7	4.5	**	612
Alcohol or Drug Related Problems	20.7	6.8	***	988
Mental Illness	34.9	13.0	***	1769
Serious Disability	13.1	6.0	***	914
Not Able to Get a Job	40.5	16.8	***	1952
Involuntary Job Loss	16.5	7.0	***	859
Witness to Violence	15.8	2.2	***	426
Abuse or Violent Crime	12.6	2.5	***	428
Trouble with the Police	14.2	2.8	***	413
Gambling Problem	6.6	2.6	***	308
Discrimination-Ethnic or Cultural Background	5.5	2.1	***	301
Discrimination-Other Reason	7.6	1.6	***	262
Bullying and/or Harassment	20.6	6.4	***	929
Removal of Children	4.8	<1%	***	141
Other	<1%	<1%		88

Table 1. *Cont.*

	Food Insecure (%)	Food Secure (%)		n [1]
Number of Stressors [3]				
None	14.0	38.1	***	4845
1	21.1	30.2	***	3807
2	15.7	15.4		1991
3	15.9	7.4	***	1011
4+	33.4	8.9	***	1278
Total	100	100		
Unweighted (n)	403	12,529		12,932

[1] Unweighted sample size per stressor; [2] Experiencing each stressor in the previous 12 months; [3] Number of stressors reported in previous 12 months. *** $p < 0.001$, ** $p < 0.01$. Significance tests denote test of proportion of exposure to each stressor by food insecurity status.

3.2. Prevalence of Food Insecurity by Stressor Type

Given that food insecure respondents were more likely to experience a range of stressors relative to their food secure peers, it is therefore not unexpected that the prevalence rates of food insecurity were much higher for those experiencing stressors (Table 2). Consistent with previous research using a similar measure, the prevalence of food insecurity with insufficient intake and food depletion was approximately 2% among the general population living in households [7]. The prevalence of food insecurity among those reporting no stressors in the previous 12 months was less than 1%. In strong contrast, the prevalence of food insecurity was very high among those reporting witness to violence (12.6%), removal of children (11.7%), abuse or violent crime (9.3%), trouble with the police (9.3%), discrimination—other reason (8.7%) and bullying or harassment (6.1%). Again, across all categories of stressors with the exception of 'other' stressors, prevalence rates of food insecurity were significantly above those who did not report any stressors or the general population level prevalence.

Table 2. Prevalence of food insecurity by stressor type, 2014.

	Weighted [1] (%)	Unweighted [2] (%)	
Type of Stressor [3]			
Divorce or Separation	3.1	5.7	***
Death of Family Member/Close Friend	3.2	4.9	***
Serious Illness	2.9	5.1	***
Serious Accident	3.4	5.9	**
Alcohol or Drug Related Problems	5.8	9.7	***
Mental Illness	5.2	8.7	***
Serious Disability	4.2	7.9	***
Not Able to Get a Job	4.6	7.7	***
Involuntary Job Loss	4.5	7.3	***
Witness to Violence	12.6	16.4	***
Abuse or Violent Crime	9.3	15.0	***
Trouble with the Police	9.3	12.6	***
Gambling Problem	5.0	9.1	***
Discrimination-Ethnic or Cultural Background	5.1	9.0	***
Discrimination-Other Reason	8.7	14.1	***
Bullying and/or Harassment	6.1	9.0	***
Removal of Children	11.7	15.6	***
Other	2.0	5.7	

Table 2. *Cont.*

	Weighted [1] (%)	Unweighted [2] (%)	
Number of Stressors [4]			
None	<1%	<1%	-
1	1.4	1.7	**
2	2.0	3.9	***
3	4.2	6.2	***
4+	7.1	11.7	***
Full Sample	2.0	3.1	***

[1] Prevalence weighted using ABS survey weights; [2] Unweighted prevalence; [3] Tests of proportions for type of stressor relative to not experiencing each stressor; [4] Tests of proportions for number of stressors relative to those reporting no stressors. 'None' is the comparison category; *** $p < 0.001$, ** $p < 0.01$, + $p < 0.1$.

Although these descriptive results indicate significant differences in the prevalence of food insecurity by exposure to stressors, it is important to control for variables that may indicate spurious statistical relationships. For example, was the prevalence of food insecurity high among those reporting bullying or harassment due to a younger age profile of those reporting this stressor? Similarly, were prevalence rates of food insecurity among those reporting a mental health stressor high because of lower average levels of economic resources available to those with mental health conditions?

3.3. Regression Results

To control for confounding effects, multivariable logistic regression models were fitted to calculate odds ratios to measure the association between each stressor and food insecurity, once extensive controls for socio-economic factors previously shown to be associated with food insecurity in Australia were accounted for. Odds ratios adjusted for control variables (AOR) and unadjusted for control variables (UOR) are presented for transparency (Table 3). Comparing the adjusted and unadjusted results, the higher magnitude of the unadjusted odds ratios indicates the importance of the control factors in explaining food insecurity. This is further discussed below.

Table 3. Odds ratios from multivariable logistic regression models of food insecurity, 2014.

	Odds Ratio (UOR) [1]	Odds Ratio (AOR) [2]	
Stressor Type Models [3]			
Divorce or Separation	1.68	1.53	*
Death of Family Member/Close Friend	1.99	2.01	***
Serious Illness	1.74	1.81	**
Serious Accident	1.78	1.55	
Alcohol or Drug Related Problems	3.58	2.35	***
Mental Illness	3.59	2.87	***
Serious Disability	2.36	2.30	**
Not Able to Get a Job	3.35	2.49	***
Involuntary Job Loss	2.62	2.59	***
Witness to Violence	8.27	4.40	***
Abuse or Violent Crime	5.67	3.26	***
Trouble with the Police	5.75	3.70	***
Gambling Problem	2.69	2.53	*
Discrimination-Ethnic or Cultural Background	2.76	2.17	*
Discrimination-Other Reason	5.04	3.75	***
Bullying and/or Harassment	3.79	2.82	***
Removal of Children	6.79	4.58	**
Other	1.00	0.66	

[1] Unadjusted Odds Ratios with no control variables included. [2] Odds Ratios adjusted for controls including age, marital status, household income, self-rated health, housing tenure and education. [3] Multivariable logistic regression models estimated for each stressor; *** $p < 0.001$, ** $p < 0.01$, * $p < 0.05$; Standard errors calculated using survey replicate weights.

Broadly repeating the descriptive prevalence rates, those reporting witness to violence (AOR = 4.40 $p < 0.001$), removal of children (AOR = 4.58 $p < 0.01$), trouble with police (AOR = 3.70 $p < 0.01$), discrimination-other reason (AOR = 3.75 $p < 0.01$), abuse or violent crime (AOR = 3.26 $p < 0.001$) and bullying/harassment (AOR = 2.82 $p < 0.001$) were approximately three or more times more likely to report food insecurity.

Among the health-related stressors, mental illness (AOR = 2.87 $p < 0.001$), serious disability (AOR = 2.30 $p < 0.01$) and serious illness (AOR = 1.81 $p < 0.01$) approximately doubled the odds of experiencing food insecurity. Similarly, difficulties in the workplace also doubled the odds of experiencing food insecurity: not able to get a job (AOR = 2.49 $p < 0.001$) and involuntary job loss (AOR = 2.59 $p < 0.001$). An experience of a serious accident in the last 12 months was not associated with food insecurity ($p > 0.05$).

Table 4 displays results from a logistic regression model measuring the association between the number of stressors reported by the respondent and food insecurity. The full parameter coefficients measuring the relative role of the control variables are also included for context. The direction, magnitude and significance of the parameter coefficients for the control variables are highly comparable across all models in Tables 3 and 4.

Table 4. Multivariable logistic regression model of number of stressors and food insecurity, 2014.

	Odds Ratio (AOR) [1]	
Number of Stressors [2]		
0	-	
1–2	1.76	*
3–4	3.75	***
5+	8.90	***
Control Variables		
Age		
15–29		
30–44	1.42	+
45–59	1.42	
60+	0.40	**
University Education		
Yes	0.39	*
Married		
Yes	0.39	***
Tenure-Renting		
Yes	3.10	***
Poor Self Rated Health		
Yes	2.28	***
Equivalent Household Income		
0–19%	-	
20–39%	0.81	
40–59%	0.52	*
60–79%	0.28	*
80–100%	0.15	**
Unknown	0.71	

[1] Adjusted Odds Ratios (AOR) with controls for all variables included in the model. [2] Count of the number of stressors reported by the respondent in the previous 12 months; *** $p < 0.001$, ** $p < 0.01$, * $p < 0.05$, + $p < 0.10$; Estimates adjusted using survey replicate weights.

Findings from this analysis showed a slightly non-linear relationship between stressors and the odds of food insecurity. Relative to those reporting no stressors, those reporting one or two stressors were about 1.8 times more likely to be food insecure (OR = 1.76 $p < 0.05$). Those reporting three or four stressors were about 3.8 times more likely (OR = 3.75 $p < 0.05$) and those reporting five or more were approximately nine times more likely to report food insecurity (OR = 8.9 $p < 0.05$). As a proxy for the severity of stressors, these findings indicate that multiple stressors play a significant role in explaining exposure to food insecurity.

Contextualizing the results in Tables 3 and 4, the control variables remain important determinants of food insecurity. Consistent with previous Australian studies, reporting food insecurity was about 60% less likely for university educated respondents (relative to those with no university education) and for those who were married (relative to the unmarried), OR = 0.39 $p < 0.05$ and OR = 0.39 $p < 0.001$, respectively. Reporting poor or fair self-rated health almost doubled the odds of experiencing food insecurity. Again, consistent with Australian studies, renters (as opposed to owners or purchasers of primary residences) were at a considerably greater risk of food insecurity in Australia (OR = 3.10 $p < 0.05$). As expected, household income (specifically equivalized household income) was strongly associated with food insecurity. Those in the top 20% of the income distribution were about 85% less likely to report food insecurity, relative to those in the bottom 20% of the distribution (OR = 0.15 $p < 0.05$).

The increased likelihood of experiencing food insecurity for those reporting multiple stressors raises the question of the composition of stressors experienced in the previous 12 months. Table 5 tabulates the types of stressors experienced by the number of stressors reported. Of those persons reporting 5 or more stressors, over half reported death of a family member or friend (59.8%), serious illness (65.9%), mental illness (60.5%), not able to get a job (67.5%) or bullying and/or harassment (51.7%). These percentages are considerably above those reported by people reporting only 1 or 2 stressors. For example, about 12% of those reporting 1–2 stressors report a mental illness shock, compared with 39% of those reporting 3–4 stressors and 61% of those reporting five or more stressors.

Table 5. Percentage of persons experiencing each stressor by number of stressors reported (%), 2014.

	Number of Stressors [1]		
	1–2	3–4	5+
Stressor Type (%) [2]			
Divorce or Separation	12.0	28.9	48.5
Death of Family Member/Close Friend	29.8	42.6	59.8
Serious Illness	29.0	50.3	65.9
Serious Accident	4.8	9.6	24.4
Alcohol or Drug Related Problems	4.1	23.8	46.3
Mental Illness	12.5	39.5	60.5
Serious Disability	6.2	16.5	26.4
Not Able to Get a Job	19.0	43.8	67.5
Involuntary Job Loss	5.7	19.4	45.3
Witness to Violence	0.7	5.8	28.9
Abuse or Violent Crime	1.0	8.3	24.3
Trouble with the Police	1.4	7.3	30.1
Gambling Problem	1.3	8.8	19.5
Discrimination-Ethnic/Cultural Background	1.0	6.1	18.9
Discrimination-Other Reason	<1%	4.9	17.9
Bullying and/or Harassment	4.2	18.0	51.7
Removal of Children	<1%	2.2	6.7
Other	<1%	<1%	1.4
Unweighted (n)	5804	1566	733

[1] Number of stressors reported in previous 12 months. [2] Percentage of respondents in each category of stressor counts (1–2, 3–4, 5+) reporting each stressor.

4. Discussion

Research in the fields of psychology and behavioural economics has emphasised the importance of stressors in explaining health and wellbeing throughout the life course [36,37]. Public health research too is increasingly recognising the important role that precariousness (through broader economic and political changes) plays in deleterious health and wellbeing outcomes [38]. Indeed, experiencing stressors and precariousness may be tied to experiences of economic and social inequality in Australia, contributing to overall food inequality [39]. Motivated by these broader frameworks, and by a limited number of American and Canadian qualitative studies, this study sought to examine the prevalence and association of 18 types of stressful events, or stressors, with food insecurity in Australia.

This analysis found that respondents reporting food insecurity were more likely to report stressors relative to food secure persons. Across 17 of the 18 stressor domains, food insecure people were significantly more likely to report experiences of a stressor. Moreover, the food insecure were significantly more likely to have encountered multiple stressors within the previous 12 months. Unsurprisingly then, the analysis herein demonstrated that the prevalence of food insecurity was considerably higher among those experiencing stressors. It was further demonstrated that once known determinants of food insecurity were controlled for, the odds of experiencing food insecurity remain highly statistically significant across 16 stressor types. Experiencing multiple stressors was also associated with significantly increased odds of food insecurity.

These findings raise the question of how stressors and precariousness can be built into policy or programs to address food insecurity? Of course, not all people who experience a stressor are at risk of food insecurity. Indeed, beyond individual levels of resilience and vulnerability, support systems from family, friends, the government and the broader community play an important role in managing the potential adverse effects of stressors [36]. However, in the absence of familial or other social-support mechanisms, how can Government support individuals at risk of food insecurity as they face potentially adverse stressors?

Solutions proposed for the broader community to protect financial wellbeing against stressors more generally include financial education, insurance and financial planning and preparedness [40]. However, for many food insecure people, lifelong disadvantage and detachment from the labour market makes such planning complex, if not unfeasible. The ability for policy to support people at risk of food insecurity also depends on the type of stressor. Of particular relevance, stressors related to both health (serious illness, mental illness, serious disability) and the labour market (not able to get a job, involuntary job loss) were strongly associated with food insecurity in this study.

Regarding labour market stressors, consideration should be given to the suitability of extant labour market programs for food insecure people. To assess this, it is necessary to firstly understand the barriers to labour force participation faced by food insecure people? Although much is known about labour market barriers more generally, there are no Australian studies that examine how policy can support unemployed food insecure people specifically. Moreover, it is well understood that higher levels of education are protective against experiences of both food insecurity and unemployment [8,9,41]. What are the barriers to education and training reported by food insecure people? These questions are being considered by the author in a subsequent analysis and underscore the complex policy solutions to food insecurity which must extend beyond food and nutrition programs alone. Relatedly, exogenous labour market shocks (e.g., unanticipated unemployment) raise the issue of the suitability of income support provided through the welfare support system. For example, the main income support payment available to unemployed people in Australia, the Newstart Allowance, has long been criticised for not providing a healthy living allowance, and the problem has compounded over time due to the method of indexation [42–44].

Onset of disability, mental health illness and other serious illness stressors were also strongly associated with food insecurity. The onset of health conditions, particularly multimorbidity and chronic conditions in Australia, has been shown to be associated with deleterious financial wellbeing [45,46]. For some Australians, analysis herein shows that health stressors may translate into a significantly higher likelihood of food insecurity. This however raises the question of the direction of the relationship between health and food insecurity. Is illness a precursor, an outcome or both with respect to food insecurity? For example, a recent scoping paper shows that a number of longitudinal studies find a bidirectional relationship between mental health and food insecurity [47]. Moreover, there is a significant literature on the detrimental mental health effects of unemployment [48]. Thus, there may be a complex relationship *between* and *within* stressors and food insecurity. Further research on the pathways between health and food security using longitudinal data is a priority. More generally, the particularly high odds ratios measuring the association between mental health stressors and food insecurity is also important given reported difficulties accessing and funding mental health care and support programs in Australia [49].

Among the strongest association between stressors and food insecurity identified in this study were for those related to violence and addiction including issues with alcohol or drug related problems and gambling. As noted previously, Canadian studies have noted gambling addiction issues as a possible precursor to food insecurity [29]. An Australian qualitative study of a charity-run soup kitchen noted issues of alcohol and illicit drug use and gambling in food insecure clients [50]. Issues of drug use (both licit and illicit) and gambling are important social problems in Australia with considerable implications for the economy as well as individual wellbeing [51,52]. The complexity of these problems and their solutions again underscore the multidimensional levers that must be employed by governments to address food insecurity.

The association between removal of children and food insecurity was very strong and highly significant. Although this result is not unexpected, interpreting this result requires some caution due to the high prevalence of Aboriginal children in out-of-home care relative to non-Indigenous children [53]. As the Aboriginal and Torres Strait Islander population are at a considerably higher risk of food insecurity in Australia, it may be that the measure of removal of children is confounding this effect [23]. Notwithstanding, just under 3% of the Australian population were Aboriginal and Torres Strait Islanders in the 2016 Census of Population and Housing and it is not clear how many Aboriginal respondents were included in the GSS. Although Aboriginal and Torres Strait Islander people are included in the GSS, variables measuring Indigenous status are not available in the datafile. The National Aboriginal and Torres Strait Islander Social Survey (NATSISS) collects similar measures of food insecurity and stressors to those collected in the GSS and the analysis presented herein could be replicated for the Aboriginal and Torres Strait Islander population.

As a proxy for the severity of stressors, reporting higher numbers of personal stressors was strongly associated with experiencing food insecurity. Descriptive statistics herein further illustrated that almost half of those reporting higher order stressors experienced death of a family member or friend, serious illness, mental illness, trouble finding employment and bullying or harassment. This raises the important point of the intercorrelation between stressors. For example, as noted above, the literature has highlighted the detrimental mental health effects of unemployment [48]. There is also a growing evidence base on experiences of violence by people living with a disability [54]. A further example of the intercorrelation between the various stressors is the relationship between onset of health conditions and difficulties finding or maintaining work and poverty [55,56]. The pathways between these stressors and food insecurity is an area that requires further research. Unfortunately, the GSS data are inappropriate to answer these questions for two reasons. First, the data are cross-sectional and retrospective questions were not asked on the timing of events. Second, the measurement of stressors in the GSS is aggregated so that it is not possible to identify whether the stressor was experienced by (i) the respondent; or (ii) somebody close to them. Detailed longitudinal data are required to disentangle these important questions for future research.

More generally, it is important to note that stressors as a risk factor for food insecurity should not lead to a disregard of other socio-economic factors and food supply characteristics placing individuals at risk. In their analysis of life events on family wellbeing, the Australian Institute of Family Studies (AIFS) notes "sole reliance on life events as indicators of the need for service provision would be unfortunate. The identification of individuals or families who are vulnerable to experiencing adverse events in the future is clearly important, but so too is the identification of families experiencing chronically destructive circumstances" [57]. In the context of food insecurity, the analyses herein should be interpreted as complementary to existing studies and further highlighting at risk population groups. This is further supported by the findings underscoring the relative importance of control variables, such as education, income and marital status, in explaining food insecurity.

Study Strengths and Limitations

The key strength of this study is that it is the first Australian and one of a few internationally that have sought to examine the experiences of a range of stressors and their association with food insecurity. This addresses an important research gap in the extant quantitative literature on food insecurity. A further important strength of this study is that it is nationally representative. Booth and Smith's (2001) key study bringing food insecurity to the fore for Australian dietitians and policy makers pointed to the key at risk populations of food insecurity in Australia [13]. Following this study, most Australian analyses of food insecurity tend to focus on population sub groups. For example, homeless or 'at risk' youth [58], students [10,59], refugees [60,61], children or families with young children [19–21], Aboriginal and Torres Strait Islanders [23,62], older Australians [14,16,22,23,63,64], those living in disadvantaged suburbs [20,65] or middle-income groups [11]. Most Australian studies also focus on cities or states: Adelaide and South Australia [9,58], Sydney and New South Wales [14,20,22,63] Brisbane Queensland [10,17,65] Melbourne and Victoria [11,15] or Tasmania and the Northern Territory [18,19]. There are very few Australian quantitative studies seeking a nationally representative view of the prevalence and correlates of food insecurity [7,16]. This study adds to that list.

Notwithstanding these strengths, there are several limitations of this study. Firstly, as the GSS data are cross-sectional, it is not possible to draw a causal link between stressors and food insecurity. Rather, the analyses show a clear association between the two, once known determinants of food insecurity have been controlled for. Second, and related to the above, due to the cross-sectional nature of the data, it is not possible to measure the complex pathways between the various stressors and food insecurity. It may be that some stressors are a precursor or outcome (or both) of food insecurity. More generally, food insecurity has been shown to be a cyclical phenomenon, varying over time. Longitudinal data are required to measure these complex pathways. A third limitation of this study relates to measurement of the experience of stressors. The GSS instrument asks whether the stressor impacted the individual respondent or someone close to them. The argument that stressors experienced by someone close to you would impact on your likelihood of food insecurity can clearly be made. For example, a spouse losing their job, or a respondent's child becoming seriously ill. Furthermore, qualitative studies provide evidence of how shocks to one person's health can impact on the food insecurity of all household members [66]. However, it may be that when the stressor is experienced by the respondent alone, the effect on the likelihood of experiencing food insecurity is stronger. Unfortunately, the GSS does not enable this disaggregation. However, this analysis would be possible for the Aboriginal and Torres Strait Islander population using NATSISS.

Furthermore, there are a range of exogenous events, such as natural disasters, that may impact exposure to food insecurity and are not measured in the GSS. This study has focussed on personal stressors only, but clearly natural disasters, even in a high-income context, will impact levels of food insecurity. For example, a recent American study found that, even after a recovery phase following Hurricane Katrina, almost one in four people reported food insecurity five years later [67]. Moreover, the personal stressors measured in the GSS exclude potentially positive life events, for example birth of a child or marriage. It may be that for some demographic groups positive life events reduce the likelihood of food insecurity, whereas for other groups it may increase exposure to food insecurity. For example, for some vulnerable populations, positive events such as birth of a child may place greater stress on family resources, leading to a higher likelihood of food insecurity. These data are currently unavailable in the GSS, and this presents an important area for future research.

A fourth limitation of this study is the measurement of food insecurity itself. Going without a meal due to financial constraints is considered a measure of considerable financially attributable food insecurity, indicative of both inadequate intake and food depletion [7]. However, food insecurity exists in circumstances beyond financial considerations alone. Indeed, a number of recent Australian studies have sought to pilot or test more comprehensive measures of food insecurity which include non-financial barriers to food [8,22,68]. These more comprehensive measures show that the prevalence of food insecurity is much higher than when measured based on financial restrictions in accessing food alone. How stressors impact non-financial forms of food insecurity is a priority for future research.

5. Conclusions

Noting these limitations and extensions, to the author's knowledge, this is one of only a few studies to examine the association of a wide range of stressors with food insecurity. Analysis herein showed specific as well as multiple occurrences of stressful events or stressors were associated with food insecurity, independent of known risk factors. These results underscore the complex determinants of food insecurity in Australia and complement existing studies which heretofore have focussed on socio-economic and demographic correlates. Further confirmation of these findings with longitudinal data is a priority, in order to establish the complex pathways in and out of food insecurity and the role of stressors as either precursors or outcomes (or indeed whether a bidirectional relationship exists). Moreover, extending this study to the Aboriginal and Torres Strait Islander population and with more comprehensive measures of food insecurity could provide further insight into stressful events and food insecurity.

Designing policy interventions to support people at risk of food insecurity is key to reducing food insecurity in Australia. Unfortunately, the results from this study suggest that addressing food insecurity is not a straightforward task for policy makers. Many of the stressors interact with important and difficult social problems in Australia, for which there are no straightforward solutions. With further longitudinal research on the pathways within and between stressors and food insecurity, appropriate interventions for those at risk of particularly deleterious stressors, could be designed in tandem with nutrition programs. By addressing food insecurity alongside the related social and economic problems identified in this study, health and economic outcomes for vulnerable populations may be improved and inequalities in health and wellbeing addressed consequently. This approach views food security as a fundamental human right, as recognised by the Australian Governments agreement with key UN accords.

Acknowledgments: Data for this study were provided to the author by the Australian Bureau of Statistics (ABS) through the ABS Universities Australia agreement.

References

1.   American Dietetic Association. Domestic food and nutrition security: Position of the American Dietetic Association. *J. Am. Diet. Assoc.* **1998**, *98*, 337–342. [CrossRef]

2.   United Nations. *International Covenant on Economic, Social and Cultural Rights*; United Nations: New York, NY, USA, 2015; Available online: https://treaties.un.org/Pages/ViewDetails.aspx?src=IND&mtdsg_no=IV-3&chapter=4&clang=_en (accessed on 30 June 2018).

3.   United Nations. *Transforming Our World: The 2030 Agenda for Sustainable Development*; United Nations: New York, NY, USA, 2015; Available online: http://www.un.org/ga/search/view_doc.asp?symbol=A/RES/70/1&Lang=E (accessed on 30 June 2018).

4.   Jones, A.D. Food insecurity and mental health status: A global analysis of 149 countries. *Am. J. Prev. Med.* **2017**, *53*, 264–273. [CrossRef] [PubMed]

5.   Smith, M.D.; Rabbitt, M.P.; Coleman-Jensen, A. Who are the world's food insecure? New evidence from the Food and Agriculture Organization's food insecurity experience scale. *World Dev.* **2017**, *31*, 402–412. [CrossRef]

6.   Australian Bureau of Statistics. *Australian Health Survey: Nutrition—State and Territory Results, 2011–2012 (Catalogue Number 4364.0.55.009)*; Australian Bureau of Statistics: Canberra, Australia, 2015.

7.   Temple, J.B. Severe and moderate forms of food insecurity in Australia: Are they distinguishable? *Aust. J. Soc. Issues* **2008**, *43*, 649–668. [CrossRef]

8.	Butcher, L.M.; O'Sullivan, T.A.; Ryan, M.M.; Lo, J.; Devine, A. Utilising a multi-item questionnaire to assess household food security in Australia. *Health Promot. J. Aust.* **2018**. [CrossRef] [PubMed]

9.	Foley, W.; Ward, P.; Carter, P.; Coveney, J.; Tsourtos, G.; Taylor, A. An ecological analysis of factors associated with food insecurity in South Australia, 2002–2007. *Public Health Nutr.* **2010**, *13*, 215–221. [CrossRef] [PubMed]

10.	Hughes, R.; Serebryanikova, I.; Donaldson, K.; Leveritt, M. Student food insecurity: The skeleton in the university closet. *Nutr. Diet.* **2011**, *68*, 27–32. [CrossRef]

11.	Kleve, S.; Davidson, Z.E.; Gearon, E.; Booth, S.; Palermo, C. Are low-to-middle-income households experiencing food insecurity in Victoria, Australia? An examination of the Victorian Population Health Survey, 2006–2009. *Aust. J. Prim. Health* **2017**, *23*, 249–256. [CrossRef] [PubMed]

12.	Pollard, C.M.; Landrigan, T.; Ellies, P.; Kerr, D.A.; Lester, M.; Goodchild, S. Geographic factors as determinants of food security: A Western Australian food pricing and quality study. *Asia Pac. J. Clin. Nutr.* **2014**, *23*, 703–713. [CrossRef] [PubMed]

13.	Booth, S.; Smith, A. Food security and poverty in Australia-challenges for dietitians. *Aust. J. Nutr. Diet.* **2001**, *58*, 150–156.

14.	Quine, S.; Morrell, S. Food insecurity in community-dwelling older Australians. *Public Health Nutr.* **2006**, *9*, 219–224. [CrossRef] [PubMed]

15.	Thornton, L.E.; Pearce, J.R.; Ball, K. Sociodemographic factors associated with healthy eating and food security in socio-economically disadvantaged groups in the UK and Victoria, Australia. *Public Health Nutr.* **2014**, *17*, 20–30. [CrossRef] [PubMed]

16.	Temple, J.B. Food insecurity among older Australians: Prevalence, correlates and well-being. *Aust. J. Ageing* **2006**, *25*, 158–163. [CrossRef]

17.	Radimer, K.L.; Allsopp, R.; Harvey, P.W.; Firman, D.W.; Watson, E.K. Food insufficiency in Queensland. *Aust. N. Z. J. Public Health* **1997**, *21*, 303–310. [CrossRef] [PubMed]

18.	Lê, Q.; Auckland, S.; Nguyen, H.B.; Murray, S.; Long, G.; Terry, D.R. Food security in a regional area of Australia: A socio-economic perspective. *Univers. J. Food Nutr. Sci.* **2014**, *2*, 50–59. [CrossRef]

19.	McCarthy, L. Household Food Security and Child Health Outcomes in Families with Children Aged 6 Months to 4 Years Residing in Darwin and Palmerston, Northern Territory Australia. Ph.D Thesis, Charles Darwin University, Casuarina, Northern Territory, Australia, 2017.

20.	Nolan, M.; Rikard-Bell, G.; Mohsin, M.; Williams, M. Food insecurity in three socially disadvantaged localities in Sydney, Australia. *Health Promot. J. Aust.* **2006**, *17*, 247–253. [CrossRef]

21.	Godrich, S.; Lo, J.; Davies, C.; Darby, J.; Devine, A. Prevalence and socio-demographic predictors of food insecurity among regional and remote Western Australian children. *Aust. N. Z. J. Public Health* **2017**, *41*, 585–590. [CrossRef] [PubMed]

22.	Russell, J.; Flood, V.; Yeatman, H.; Mitchell, P. Prevalence and risk factors of food insecurity among a cohort of older Australians. *J. Nutr. Health Aging* **2014**, *18*, 3–8. [CrossRef] [PubMed]

23.	Temple, J.B.; Russell, J. Food insecurity among older Aboriginal and Torres Strait Islanders. *Int. J. Environ. Res. Public Health* **2018**, *15*, 1766. [CrossRef] [PubMed]

24.	Wolfe, W.S.; Olson, C.M.; Kendall, A.; Frongillo, E.A. Understanding food insecurity in the elderly: A conceptual framework. *J. Nutr. Educ.* **1996**, *28*, 92–100. [CrossRef]

25.	Frongillo, E.A.; Valois, P.; Wolfe, W.S. Using a concurrent events approach to understand social support and food insecurity among elders. *Fam. Econ. Nutr. Rev.* **2003**, *15*, 25.

26.	Chilton, M.; Knowles, M.; Rabinowich, J.; Arnold, K. The relationship between childhood adversity and food insecurity: 'It's like a bird nesting in your head'. *Public Health Nutr.* **2015**, *18*, 2643–2653. [CrossRef] [PubMed]

27.	Younginer, N.A.; Blake, C.E.; Draper, C.L.; Jones, S.J. Resilience and hope: Identifying trajectories and contexts of household food insecurity. *J. Hunger Environ. Nutr.* **2015**, *10*, 230–258. [CrossRef]

28.	Jones, S.J.; Draper, C.L.; Bell, B.A.; Burke, M.P.; Martini, L.; Younginer, N.; Blake, C.E.; Probst, J.; Freedman, D.; Liese, A.D. Child hunger from a family resilience perspective. *J. Hunger Environ Nutr.* **2018**, *13*, 340–361. [CrossRef]

29.	Olabiyi, O.M.; McIntyre, L. Determinants of food insecurity in higher-income households in Canada. *J. Hunger Environ Nutr.* **2014**, *9*, 433–448. [CrossRef]

30. Booth, S. Eating rough: Food sources and acquisition practices of homeless young people in Adelaide, South Australia. *Public Health Nutr.* **2006**, *9*, 212–218. [CrossRef] [PubMed]

31. McKenzie, H.J.; McKay, F.H. Food as a discretionary item: The impact of welfare payment changes on low-income single mother's food choices and strategies. *J. Poverty Soc. Justice* **2017**, *25*, 35–48. [CrossRef]

32. Burns, C.A. *Review of the Literature Describing the Link between Poverty, Food Insecurity and Obesity with Specific Reference to Australia*; VicHealth: Melbourne, Australia, 2004. Available online: https://www.vichealth.vic.gov.au/~/media/ResourceCentre/PublicationsandResources/healthy%20eating/Literature%20Review%20Poverty_Obesity_Food%20Insecurity.ashx (accessed on 30 June 2018).

33. Australian Bureau of Statistics. *General Social Survey: Summary Results, Australia, 2014 (Catalogue Number 4159.0)*; Australian Bureau of Statistics: Canberra, Australia, 2015.

34. Winter, N. SVR: Stata Module to Compute Estimates with Survey Replication Based Standard Errors. 2008. Available online: https://ideas.repec.org/c/boc/bocode/s427502.html (accessed on 1 March 2017).

35. Wolfer, K. *Introduction to Variance Estimation*; Springer: New York, NY, USA, 1985.

36. Moloney, L.; Weston, R.; Qu, L.; Hayes, A. *Families, Life Events and Family Service Delivery*; Australian Institute of Family Studies: Canberra, Australia, 2012; pp. 1447–1469.

37. Sharam, A.; Ralston, L.; Parkinson, S. Security in retirement. The impact of housing and key critical life events. In *SISR Working Paper*; Swinburne University of Technology: Melbourne, Australia, 2016.

38. McKee, M.; Reeves, A.; Clair, A.; Stuckler, D. Living on the edge: Precariousness and why it matters for health. *Arch. Public Health* **2017**, *75*, 13. [CrossRef] [PubMed]

39. Pollard, C.; Begley, A.; Landrigan, T. The Rise of Food Inequality in Australia. In *Food Poverty and Insecurity: International Food Inequalities*; Springer: Cham, Switzerland, 2016; pp. 89–103.

40. West, T.; Worthington, A. The impact of major life events on Australian Household Financial Decision-making and portfolio rebalancing. *SSRN Electron. J.* **2016**. [CrossRef]

41. Woessmann, L. The economic case for education. *Educ. Econ.* **2016**, *24*, 3. [CrossRef]

42. Morris, A.; Wilson, S. Struggling on the Newstart unemployment benefit in Australia: The experience of a neoliberal form of employment assistance. *Econ. Labour Relat. Rev.* **2014**, *25*, 202–221. [CrossRef]

43. Saunders, P.; Bedford, M. New minimum healthy living budget standards for low-paid and unemployed Australians. *Econ. Labour Relat. Rev.* **2018**, *29*, 3. [CrossRef]

44. Saunders, P. Using a budget standards approach to assess the adequacy of Newstart allowance. *Aust. J. Soc. Issues* **2018**, *53*, 4–17. [CrossRef]

45. Kemp, A.; Preen, D.B.; Glover, J.; Semmens, J.; Roughead, E.E. Impact of cost of medicines for chronic conditions on low income households in Australia. *J. Health Serv. Res. Policy* **2013**, *18*, 21–27. [CrossRef] [PubMed]

46. McRae, I.; Yen, L.; Jeon, Y.H.; Herath, P.M.; Essue, B. Multimorbidity is associated with higher out-of-pocket spending: A study of older Australians with multiple chronic conditions. *Aust. J. Prim. Health* **2013**, *19*, 144–149. [CrossRef] [PubMed]

47. Maynard, M.; Andrade, L.; Packull-McCormick, S.; Perlman, C.M.; Leos-Toro, C.; Kirkpatrick, S.I. Food Insecurity and Mental Health among Females in High-Income Countries. *Int. J. Environ. Res. Public Health* **2018**, *15*, 1424. [CrossRef] [PubMed]

48. Modini, M.; Joyce, S.; Mykletun, A.; Christensen, H.; Bryant, R.A.; Mitchell, P.B.; Harvey, S.B. The mental health benefits of employment: Results of a systematic meta-review. *Aust. Psychiatry* **2016**, *24*, 331–336. [CrossRef] [PubMed]

49. Meadows, G.N.; Enticott, J.C.; Inder, B.; Russell, G.M.; Gurr, R. Better access to mental health care and the failure of the Medicare principle of universality. *Med. J. Aust.* **2015**, *202*, 190–194. [CrossRef] [PubMed]

50. Wicks, R.; Trevena, L.J.; Quine, S. Experiences of food insecurity among urban soup kitchen consumers: insights for improving nutrition and well-being. *J. Am. Diet. Assoc.* **2006**, *106*, 921–924. [CrossRef] [PubMed]

51. Collins, D.; Lapsley, H.M. *The Costs of Tobacco, Alcohol and Illicit Drug Abuse to Australian Society in 2004/05*; Department of Health and Ageing: Canberra, Australia, 2008.

52. Armstrong, A.R.; Thomas, A.; Abbott, M. Gambling participation, expenditure and risk of harm in Australia, 1997–1998 and 2010–2011. *J. Gambl. Stud.* **2018**, *34*, 255–274. [CrossRef] [PubMed]

53. Productivity Commission. Report on Government Services. Chapter 15: Child Protection; 2016; Productivity Commission: Melbourne, Victoria. Available online: http://www.pc.gov.au/research/ongoing/report-on-government-services/2016 (accessed on 15 June 2018).

54. Hughes, K.; Bellis, M.; Jones, L.; Wood, S.; Bates, G.; Eckley, L.; McCoy, E.; Mikton, C.; Shakespeare, T.; Officer, A. Prevalence and risk of violence against adults with disabilities: A systematic review and meta-analysis of observational studies. *Lancet* **2012**, *379*, 1621–1629. [CrossRef]

55. Callander, E.; Schofield, D.; Shrestha, R. Multi-dimensional poverty in Australia and the barriers ill health imposes on the employment of the disadvantaged. *J. Socio-Econ.* **2011**, *40*, 736–742. [CrossRef]

56. Schofield, D.; Shrestha, R.; Passe, M.; Earnest, A.; Fletcher, S. Chronic Disease and Labour Force Participation among Older Australians. *Med. J. Aust.* **2008**, *189*, 447–450. [PubMed]

57. Baxter, J.; Qu, L.; Weston, R.; Moloney, L.; Hayes, A. Experiences and effects of life events: Evidence from two Australian longitudinal studies. *Fam. Matters* **2012**, *90*, 6.

58. Crawford, B.; Yamazaki, R.; Franke, E.; Amanatidis, S.; Ravulo, J.; Steinbeck, K.; Ritchie, J.; Torvaldsen, S. Sustaining dignity? Food insecurity in homeless young people in urban Australia. *Health Promot. J. Aust.* **2014**, *25*, 71–78. [CrossRef] [PubMed]

59. Micevski, D.A.; Thornton, L.E.; Brockington, S. Food insecurity among university students in Victoria: A pilot study. *Nutr. Diet.* **2014**, *71*, 258–264. [CrossRef]

60. Gallegos, D.; Ellies, P.; Wright, J. Still there's no food! Food insecurity in a refugee population in Perth, Western Australia. *Nutr. Diet.* **2008**, *65*, 78–83. [CrossRef]

61. McKay, F.H.; Dunn, M. Food security among asylum seekers in Melbourne. *Aust. N. Z. J. Public Health* **2015**, *39*, 344–349. [CrossRef] [PubMed]

62. Pollard, C.M.; Nyaradi, A.; Lester, M.; Sauer, K. Understanding food security issues in remote Western Australian Indigenous communities. *Health Promot. J. Aust.* **2014**, *25*, 83–89. [CrossRef] [PubMed]

63. Russell, J.C.; Flood, V.M.; Yeatman, H.; Wang, J.J.; Mitchell, P. Food insecurity and poor diet quality are associated with reduced quality of life in older adults. *Nutr. Diet.* **2016**, *73*, 50–58. [CrossRef]

64. King, A.C. Food Security and Insecurity in Older Adults: A Phenomenological Ethnographic Study. Ph.D. Thesis, University of Tasmania, Tasmania, Australia, 2014.

65. Ramsey, R.; Giskes, K.; Turrell, G.; Gallegos, D. Food insecurity among Australian children: Potential determinants, health and developmental consequences. *J. Child Health Care* **2011**, *15*, 401–416. [CrossRef] [PubMed]

66. Higashi, R.T.; Lee, S.C.; Pezzia, C.; Quirk, L.; Leonard, T.; Pruitt, S.L. Family and Social Context Contributes to the Interplay of Economic Insecurity, Food Insecurity, and Health. *Ann. Anthropol. Pract.* **2017**, *41*, 67–77. [CrossRef] [PubMed]

67. Clay, L.A.; Papas, M.A.; Gill, K.; Abramson, D.M. Application of a theoretical model toward understanding continued food insecurity post hurricane Katrina. *Disaster Med. Public Health Prep.* **2018**, *12*, 47–56. [CrossRef] [PubMed]

68. Kleve, S.; Gallegos, D.; Ashby, S.; Palermo, C.; McKechnie, R. Preliminary validation and piloting of a comprehensive measure of household food security in Australia. *Public Health Nutr.* **2018**, *21*, 526–534. [CrossRef] [PubMed]

4

"A Lot of People are Struggling Privately. They don't Know where to go or They're not Sure of what to do": Frontline Service Provider Perspectives of the Nature of Household Food Insecurity in Scotland

Flora Douglas [1],*[iD], Fiona MacKenzie [2], Ourega-Zoé Ejebu [3][iD], Stephen Whybrow [4][iD], Ada L. Garcia [5][iD], Lynda McKenzie [3], Anne Ludbrook [3] and Elizabeth Dowler [6]

[1]   School of Nursing and Midwifery, Robert Gordon University, Aberdeen AB10 7QG, Scotland
[2]   Institute of Applied Health Sciences, University of Aberdeen, Aberdeen AB25 2ZD, Scotland; famackenzie68@gmail.com
[3]   Health Economics Research Unit, University of Aberdeen, Aberdeen AB25 2ZD, Scotland; oejebu@abdn.ac.uk (O.-Z.E.); l.mckenzie@abdn.ac.uk (L.M.); a.ludbrook@abdn.ac.uk (A.L.)
[4]   The Rowett Institute, University of Aberdeen, Aberdeen AB25 2ZD, Scotland; stephen.whybrow@abdn.ac.uk
[5]   Human Nutrition, School of Medicine, Dentistry and Nursing, College of Medical, Veterinary and Life Sciences, University of Glasgow, Glasgow G31 2ER, Scotland; Ada.Garcia@glasgow.ac.uk
[6]   Emeritus Professor of Food & Social Policy, Department Sociology, University of Warwick, Coventry CV4 7AL, UK; Elizabeth.Dowler@warwick.ac.uk
*   Correspondence: f.douglas3@rgu.ac.uk

Abstract: This qualitative study explored frontline service providers' perceptions of the nature of food insecurity in Scotland in 2015 to inform national policy and the provision of locally-based support for 'at risk' groups. A country-wide in-depth interview study was undertaken with informants from 25 health, social care, and third sector organisations. The study investigated informants' perspectives associated with how food insecurity was manifesting itself locally, and what was happening at the local level in response to the existence of food insecurity. Data analysis revealed three key themes. First, the *multiple faces and factors of food insecurity* involving not only increased concern for previously recognised 'at risk of food insecurity' groups, but also similar concern held about newly food insecure groups including working families, young people and women. Secondly, respondents witnessed *stoicism and struggle*, but also resistance amongst some food insecure individuals to external offers of help. The final theme identified community *participation yet pessimism* associated with addressing current and future needs of food insecure groups. These findings have important implications for the design and delivery of health and social policy in Scotland and other countries facing similar challenges.

Keywords: household food insecurity; food poverty; Scotland; low income; families; children; women; older people; qualitative

1. Introduction and Background

Household food insecurity has re-emerged as a subject of public health and social policy, civic and political concern in Scotland and the rest of the UK [1–8]. Household food insecurity is the experience associated with *"the inability to acquire or consume an adequate quality or sufficient quantity of food in socially acceptable ways, or the uncertainty that one will be able to do so"* [9]. Globally, household food insecurity is recognized as a problem in low income households in high income countries [10–13]. Household food insecurity prevalence data are not routinely captured and monitored in the UK [14] but it was estimated in 2014, in a one-off UN global survey, that 10.1% of the UK population were food insecure to some degree [15]. Despite the small sample size (1000 adults for the whole of the UK), this indicated the existence of a significant and real problem [16]. However, in the absence of food insecurity prevalence data, much of the current concern about this issue in the UK was triggered by the emergence of increased numbers, and greater visibility, of charitable emergency food assistance programmes (so-called food banks), which followed the UK economic crisis and reduced government spending in its aftermath [1–8]. The numbers of people seeking help from such sources has reached unprecedented levels since the mid-2000s [17], with the causes being politically disputed [7].

At the same time, within the Scottish context, a wide range of organisations and groups that had started to provide such support in their local communities expressed significant concern about the efficacy of food banks, both as a means of addressing household food insecurity and as a social justice issue [18].

Scotland is one of the four countries which makes up the United Kingdom, and operates with its own national government (within this context) which has responsibility over some devolved matters such as health care and education.

In North America, where it has been possible to compare routinely collected household food insecurity population survey data with national food bank use figures, food bank data are known to significantly underestimate population food insecurity prevalence. Twelve to fourteen percent of the Canadian population have reported some degree of food insecurity on an annual basis since 2005, yet only 20–30% of this food insecure group also reported using a food bank in the previous year [10,19]. Furthermore, it is well established that the capacity and capability of food banks to respond to growing demand for food assistance from low income communities is severely limited due to their dependence on corporate and public donations and volunteer labour [20,21]. These resources are quickly exhausted unless food is rationed or restricted and, because of the precarious and unpredictable nature of the food and volunteer labour supply, it is thought that many people who might benefit from food bank offerings do not get access to them, and therefore do not appear in food bank statistics [10,22,23]. This is of course in addition to those who might be missing from those figures through their active avoidance of this support due to shame and fear of stigma.

Scotland has a long running public health and social policy focus concerned with addressing health inequalities. This has been underpinned by an often explicit acknowledgement that life circumstances and socio-economic deprivation are primary drivers of those inequalities, and public services, including health and social care services, have been developed and delivered accordingly [24]. Population differences in self-reported dietary quality between the most and least deprived groups (as one specific domain of the experience of food insecurity) have also come under close scrutiny over some decades, related to the goal of addressing health inequalities [25]. The Scottish Diet Action Plan, (published in 1986) triggered a programme of recurring government funding over three decades, which is intended to enable low income families and neighbourhoods to gain access to affordable fruit and vegetables via local community food programmes. Typically, these include low cost food retailing outlets, budgeting and cooking skills training programmes, and in some cases, community food growing programmes [26]. It is important to note that these programmes were not set up to provide free food assistance.

Main Study Aim

These specific concerns about the lack of valid household food insecurity data and the possible under estimation of the magnitude of the problem through use of food bank data in its absence, combined with anxieties expressed about the efficacy and sustainability of community-based food assistance programmes in dealing with the issue, resulted in a national mixed methods study being commissioned to develop a better understanding of the nature and prevalence of household food in Scotland [27]. The study was commissioned by NHS Health Scotland, the national health promotion agency, and the Scottish Government's Rural Affairs and Environment Strategic Research programme with the aim of informing national policy and local practice.

This paper reports on the qualitative study component of the larger formative study [23], which set out to capture the perspectives and experiences of social, health and third sector practitioners, whose main role was concerned with supporting economically and socially vulnerable groups. These groups were considered to be key informants likely to have frontline, locally based experience and knowledge of that wider picture of household food insecurity within their respective communities, through their day-to-day engagement with people requiring their input because of food insecurity, but who may not necessarily be engaging with food assistance programmes. Some of the third sector practitioners were drawn from some of those long standing community food programmes described above. This work was commissioned to complement other research that was underway at the same time that was focused on capturing the perspectives of those with direct lived experience of food insecurity.

2. Materials and Methods

This was a qualitative research study informed by Grounded Theory (GT) principles and techniques [28]. The decision to use GT principles as the research framework within which to identify participants, generate, analyse and think about the data was largely pragmatic, i.e., it offered a conceptually congruent set of guidelines and principles to guide the research [29,30]. As discussed above, the study objectives had been developed on the basis of emergent concerns expressed by the policy, practitioner and civic society communities within Scotland. Consequently, an interview study was undertaken with community-based health, social care and third sector staff who were concerned with the care and support of so-called vulnerable groups. The sampling frame was discussed and agreed with the research commissioners as the study progressed. Older people and those who were, or were at risk of being, destitute (e.g., homeless groups, travelling people, asylum seekers) were of particular interest to the research commissioners. The rationale for participant selection was based on identifying professionals and practitioners who had primary responsibility for some aspect of health or social care at the individual and the community level, for groups considered to be economically and socially vulnerable and, importantly, had been operating in this role for some time, preferably prior to the aforementioned economic crisis. The research commissioners were also keen to capture the perspectives and experiences of those practitioners working within the community food programmes (as described above) who were perceived to have relevant local knowledge and experience of working alongside communities affected by varying degrees of economic deprivation and vulnerability, which was known to present a significant challenge in their ability to access to healthy foods.

Two interview topic guides were developed to guide the discussions and to enable the researchers to combine inductive and deductive reasoning to generate and analyse the data. The guides themselves were generated based upon the main study objectives and a series of iterative discussions between the research commissioners and the research team. Topics in the interview guides included participants' views about:

- what it means to live in household food insecurity in Scotland;
- which population groups were considered most affected by food insecurity;
- the main drivers of household food insecurity
- community responses to those trends and;
- notions of effective intervention/policy changes required to reduce the numbers of people seeking help with feeding.

Informants from community food programmes were also asked about how their organisation was alleviating food poverty at the current time, what they thought they might be doing to alleviate food insecurity in their community in the future, and their ideas or views about alternative models, or means required to address food insecurity.

The study was based on the conceptual definition of household food insecurity, which recognises the experience of food insecurity as one that negatively impacts nutritional and psycho-social domains of human existence, i.e., *"the inability to acquire or consume an adequate quality or sufficient quantity of food in socially acceptable ways, or the uncertainty that one will be able to do so"* [9].

The study protocol and associated materials were reviewed and endorsed by the University of Aberdeen's Rowett Research Institute's Human Studies Ethical Review PanelProject Review No. 2015-Douglas-01. The manuscript was written in accordance with the RATS qualitative research review guidelines [31].

A combination of purposive and maximum variation sampling was used to recruit informants to the study. As a national study, it was important to try to capture views from the different types of professional groups of interest across the whole country. Therefore we sought to engage with individuals from the different professional groups in urban, remote and rural contexts, the length and breadth of the country.

The majority of interviews took place by phone and lasted between 30 min to an hour. Two researchers (F.D. and F.McK.) undertook the interviews, and data collection stopped at the point that it became clear no new data was emerging from the interviews. All interviews were audio recorded and transcribed verbatim with informants' consent.

Data were analysed using a thematic content analysis approach. This method is commonly used for health-related research and is particularly useful for exploring questions about meaningful issues amongst a particular study group of interest [30,32]. The basis of this approach is to reduce the multiple individual responses and identify common patterns or themes in the data, as well as so-called 'deviant case' issues. At the initial stage of the analysis, a sample of interview transcripts was read and re-read independently by two researchers to identify the key concepts and themes, and a draft coding index was drawn up. The researchers met to discuss their initial analysis: areas of difference were identified and where different ideas about what particular instances of the interview discourse represented, these were discussed and agreed. The final version of the thematic index was also agreed through discussion, and all transcripts were coded manually. Memos and notes of emerging themes, issues and patterns were also recorded during this process and were referred to during the analysis. Constant comparison method was used throughout to confirm coding consistency and assignation of coded data to the emergent themes and categories, and to check that possible new themes were not being overlooked. Every attempt was made to search for disconfirming data within the data set. Data were also scrutinised for the possibility of dominant and/or marginalised viewpoints.

3. Results

Ten informants representing community food programmes and 15 informants from organisations concerned with the care and support of vulnerable groups were recruited to the study. The combined sample of informants was drawn from across Scotland and represented some of the key organisations and services that were being delivered in diverse urban, rural and remote locations. (see Appendix A for a detailed breakdown of the study participants' characteristics). The community food programme informants were people who worked in programmes that were offering multiple services, including low cost food retailing, and/or training and development programmes and/or community growing and gardening schemes. This group also contained three NHS-employed community food development staff. Although not originally set up for this purpose, six community food programmes also begun offering a take-home free food parcels (i.e., similar to a food bank service). One informant representing a recently opened food bank also took part. The 15 health, social care, and third sector participants, were drawn from a range of community-based care and support services agencies. It is important to note that those interviewed were also targeted on the basis of having been in their current post over a number of years so that they could provide insights from practice about the current position compared to their pre-recession experience.

Three major themes that emerged from this analysis are discussed in this paper, i.e., the *faces and factors of food insecurity* in Scotland associated with emergent food insecure groups, and those groups previously recognised to be at risk; *stoicism and struggle* witnessed at the individual level amongst people affected by food insecurity, and the community *participation yet pessimism* that surfaced in relation to the challenge of responding to expressed local feeding needs now and into the future.

3.1. Faces and Factors of Food Insecurity

Two fundamental issues explored at the beginning of each interview were informants' perspectives about who they believed to be, and encountered to be, most obviously affected by household food insecurity and what they believed was causing their food insecurity. The most common responses that surfaced here were not only more concern and anxiety for groups previously well known to them but also great concern for groups they had never previously considered to be affected by food insecurity.

Families with young children, young people and women were identified as emergent groups and sections of particular concern. This anxiety is illustrated by the following quotes from two different development workers based in urban locations in the north and central parts of Scotland:

> *I've got families that the parents do without, so that the child has got what they need to have, and it means that society is becoming even more uneven than it used to be before.* (Development Worker, urban),

and:

> *You've got people making choices about the kids clothing and shoes or a meal, you've got adults, women in particular I suspect, not eating properly so the kids are fed.* (Development Worker, urban).

While both quotes typify concerns for parents and children in general, the second quote illustrates the particular concern for women with children, some of whom were believed to be sacrificing their own food resources to ensure their children could eat. Some reported specific concerns about pregnant women.

The notion that families with young children were more obviously affected by food insecurity now compared to the past was linked to their having insufficient household incomes. Much of the public discourse about the rise of food banks in the UK has been linked to changes in UK government policy and related social security entitlements that were associated with unemployment (job seekers) or sickness or disability benefits. Yet many of our informants described supporting or encountering people who were working but not earning enough to cover their necessary household bills, illustrated here:

> *We have families, I have a lot of experience with people who work very hard and work long hours, to support their families, and still at the end of the week don't have enough money for basic food* (Rural, voluntary org, family worker).

Not only were people described as living on low incomes from their employment, but the issue of unpredictable levels of income was also flagged as an underlying determinant of the food insecurity. In this next illustrative quote, this welfare support worker who was based in a rural community in mid-east Scotland talks about her frustration that her clients were very keen to find work but were unable to survive on the hourly rates and number of hours on offer from local employers:

> *. . . one of the bigger employers in this area is a market gardener, who employs people through agencies, very often on short term contracts. They'll be zero hour contracts and certainly, because it's off season at the moment, a lot of people get signed off or maybe only get one shift a week, so they may be in employment, however, their income is so low that they actually can't pay their bills.* (Welfare support, rural).

Indeed, it was notable that local food production and food processing work featured in other rural participants' accounts as examples of industries which offered very low and unpredictable levels of pay for their workers.

However, picking up on the experiences of some other community-based development workers, we also found degrees of frustration expressed about recent policy changes to UK social security entitlement, which was perceived to be driving people into destitution as their benefits were reduced or removed for periods of time. These changes were viewed by many as a primary cause of household food insecurity: an argument typified in this quote:

> *He said that his benefits had changed, and he'd had to make a new claim or something, and there was a delay in getting his benefits. And this is often what we're told; that people have a delay, they've got to make a new claim, they get less money than they think they would get, they've got to wait an extra week or a fortnight to get the money. And in the meantime they often don't have anything, and they don't have any fall back.* (Social worker, island).

A few participants also talked about policy changes that were counterproductive to the aim of getting people off government support and into paid employment. These quotes from a community-based nurse located in a remote island community, and an urban-based development worker illustrate this notion of people cycling back into debt and poverty as they tried to move into paid work and off social security:

> *Younger people, who are of working age, have a much more variable source of income. If they're in employment that's fine; they might be in low employment and things are difficult. If they're moving in and out of employment, and in and out of the benefits system, it seems to me that it's very precarious* (Nurse, rural/remote).

and

> *The problem is that when they start work their first pay day may not be for four weeks. They then have got to work out how they're going to survive for that period. For many of them, the only solution is actually getting into debt of some kind. There's meant to be all kind of safety nets around that but that's just not happening in practical terms* (Development worker, urban).

These quotes also highlight the common concern expressed by our informants about younger people being amongst those new groups perceived to be most badly affected by and at risk of household food insecurity. In the next quote, the same community-based nurse, cited above, raises the issue of their existing vulnerability as an economically disadvantaged group being exacerbated by poor social support, in this case, emanating from people having to move away from the island to find work:

> *There could be any, they're working age people, and I would say that it's more typical for the younger end of working age, but it could be older people, in the working age group, who've had some other life crisis, like their family has broken up. They've had to move away from their family and from the way that they used to do things.* (Nurse, remote island).

During the time period in which the interviews took place there had also been an economic downturn in some industries in Scotland, including the oil and gas energy sector. This was linked to the experience reported by a few urban-based informants of having dealt with or being aware that previously high income earners were struggling as a consequence of losing their jobs and not being able to feed themselves, despite having a lot of expensive possessions, highlighted by this quote:

> *I've actually had people coming in with the best cars, the best fancy phones and whatever - not a lot, but I have had, coming in with all the flashiest of stuff saying that they've got a problem. The problem is they can't pay their bills. It doesn't matter that their bills are ten times higher than maybe somebody else's bills, they still come to the end of the month and they can't pay, you know? . . . So it's kind of like hidden, I suppose. It's not what you expect.* (Community Food Programme Development, urban).

This quote (above) also touches on an issue that was remarked upon by many of the informants (regardless of income status) in terms of the 'hidden' nature of food insecurity; a theme that is picked up again later in the paper.

The situation for older people which was of initial, primary concern from the research commissioner's perspective, was more nuanced. Generally speaking, this study found most informants expressed less concern about older than younger people. This was often described in terms of an acknowledgement that while many older people lived on a low income, it was a predictable and relatively stable income that people had learned to live within and budget accordingly. In addition, older people were viewed as possessing all the necessary additional resources need to provide a constant, if limited, food and meal supply in the home, i.e., had the necessary food preparation, storage and cooking equipment that had been accumulated over their lifetimes. Older people were considered better able to cope with household food insecurity as illustrated here:

> … *we very seldom have to help them [older people] out with money or with food.* (Nurse, rural/remote).

Mention was also made of older people not appearing at food banks in great numbers, which was interpreted by some to mean they were not in need of help. Interestingly, this was something that the research commissioners had noted, but had viewed as an indication of there being a problem, not a reassurance that all was well.

However, there were a minority of informants who were working directly with older people in their homes who were concerned about what they were seeing in practice (e.g., noticing that their clients' cupboards and fridges had little or no food during home visits) that led them to believe that some of their older clients were food insecure. These older people were also commonly described as denying they were having a problem with this and commonly refused offers of a referral to a food bank. Older carers were also highlighted as a group of concern.

However, even groups normally in regular contact with health and social care services were reported as being more badly affected by food poverty compared to the past, illustrated thus:

> *Definitely an increase in people who are long term sick who'd sort of settled down to a lifestyle where they understood their income so you may have had somebody who for 15 years had been in receipt of a benefit that was related to their ill-health who found themselves unchallenged around that, their rent was being paid, their council tax was being paid and they understood how much they had to live on every week.* (Development worker, urban).

This quote also illustrates a commonly cited participant observation that financial instability and unpredictability appeared to have become the norm for many people who were in receipt of social security payments due to long term ill health, and which was perceived to have occurred as a consequence of changes to government policy. Those changes to the previous pattern of timing and level of payment had made household income difficult to manage as a result.

These perceptions about the prevalence of insufficient and unpredictable income in Scottish households fit with informants' views about what it means to be food insecure in Scotland; i.e., lacking choice and being compelled to seek out cheap, nutrient poor food to survive, illustrated in this quote from an urban-based community food initiative informant:

> *I suppose the general idea is that you don't have enough food to eat but my thinking is, it's not the right food, not nutritious food that people can't afford. Or they're making choices out of necessity as to what's available rather than what they would probably like to eat. As you know, a lot of people—you see it in the supermarkets when they're reducing the food there are people queuing up just waiting for the food to be reduced.* (Community food programme informant, mixed/urban rural).

3.2. Stoicism and Struggle

It is important to stress that this study was concerned with community caregivers or support workers views' of their clients' food security status and that we were not able to explore their clients' perspectives directly during this particular study. However, this research was concerned to understand how those care givers were drawing conclusions about their clients, and what evidence they used to conclude that individuals were dealing with food insecurity. We found informants were using a wide range of different information sources, including perceptions of their clients' behaviours and attitudes, and assessments about their physical appearance, as well as their dialogue with them. It was from these data that the theme of widespread individual (and private) *struggle and stoicism* emerged.

The behaviours and attitudes participants cited ranged from actions intended to keep up appearances of being able to manage, to denial of there being a problem in the household, through to overt refusal of food bank referrals. This notion of private and long-term struggle is illustrated by this quote from a community nurse who was working in a part of the country where large numbers of long term unemployed people live:

.., a lot of people are struggling privately. They don't know where to go or they're not sure of what to do, you know, or they've been sanctioned. Can you appeal this, can you, you know, do different things about that, and they're struggling day to day. "Oh today I've got some money, tomorrow I don't have anything." They'll not worry about tomorrow, because they're managing with today; that kind of idea (Outreach community nurse, mixed urban/rural).

A few informants talked about seeing people they had been dealing with over time looking progressively unwell and noticing or being concerned about their clients' appearance, the lack of food they observed in some of their clients' homes, and noticing that basic household furniture and fittings were missing from their houses (presumably sold to raise money for food), as things that led them to believe that some people were struggling with food poverty, illustrated thus:

You know on a couple of occasions we have seen people come in who are clearly you know, look unwell and you know are struggling, (Housing Regeneration Manager, urban).

These discussions of private struggles were also underpinned by notions of underlying pride that, from the perspective of the interview participants, prevented people seeking help, highlighted here:

I think for people that are too proud to come forward ... you know, older people who worked all their lives, who don't expect to find themselves in the kind of poverty that they find themselves in (Manager Counselling Charity, urban).

Many also talked about people they considered to be food insecure being consumed with embarrassment during conversations the informant had initiated that were intended to help, illustrated thus:

The number of people that have been referred to myself that have been working and they have described financial hardship for a number of reasons and I've offered to make these referrals to the food banks, whichever one is more accessible for them, and they really just become very embarrassed. And then when I probe just that wee bit further about how they're going to provide for their families and themselves they kind of say that they're going to rely on their families and friends to do that. (Community link worker, urban).

Perhaps another reflection of the widespread private stoicism described above was the finding that participants who were involved with the delivery or management of community food programmes had noticed increased recent uptake of, and interest in, any food and budgeting training and cooking skills development courses. It seems that this had happened 'organically' as there had been no significant increase in their promotion and marketing of those courses. Yet people were signing up to them. They also noticed increased demand for their low cost food retailing services (fruit and vegetables). Moreover, a few had noticed more people growing their own food in community gardens and allotments, and that demand for community growing spaces was increasing. This was interpreted by some to mean that people were taking active, self–initiated steps to mitigate their situation.

Conversely, a few participants reported finding some people were more willing and able to ask for help, and/or accepting of their referrals to food banks to help them acquire food, compared to their previous experience. This effect was theorised to have occurred because they believed emergency food aid centres, such as food banks, were more commonly known and talked about compared to the past. In effect, using a food bank had become more socially acceptable making it easier for some people to accept this type of help when offered.

3.3. Participation Yet Pessimism

To reiterate, we deliberately set out to engage with professionals and third sector workers who had long term experience of supporting groups who were considered to be vulnerable due to their economic or social circumstances, or had health care needs, or who had long standing and established experience of designing and running community-based food programmes intended to enable low income households to purchase, prepare and consume healthy foods. Yet we found that both groups had in-depth knowledge and experience of the role and operation of food banks within their local communities. In exploring responses to food insecurity at the community level, the overriding theme to emerge was that the community had actively *participated* in attempting to support local people in food crisis, but was *pessimistic* and sceptical about its effectiveness as a solution now or in the future.

All the community food programmes that we engaged with for this study had been operating for over a decade prior to this study, without a food bank, and all reported a very similar experience in relation to dealing with local requests for help with feeding. All had added a food bank operation to their range of programmes or services in recent months in response to those appeals. Those appeals appear to have come from two groups: health and social care professionals who had lobbied them for emergency food parcels on behalf of patients or clients they believed were in food crisis; and direct requests from local people in food crisis, who knew of their previous existence as a local, low-cost food programme.

Yet there were mixed views amongst community food programme informants about the role of food banks and the impact that they had in addressing household food insecurity in Scotland. Overriding participants' narratives about the community responses were notions of pessimism, scepticism and concern about the role and efficacy of food banks as a solution to household food insecurity. This next illustrative quote highlights the dilemma expressed by many of the deep concern they had for members of the local community who were perceived to be suffering, feeling the need to help them, but at the same time being aware that a food bank response did not address the problem:

> *I feel outrage that people have to go through this kind of terrible suffering, food poverty, in this age! And, you know, I'm sure there are many people kind of saying the same thing. You know, I'm very satisfied that I've got this kind of work, where I feel I can make a difference now and again, but I'm also overwhelmed by the fact that I know that's just almost a drop in the ocean. There are many, many people that need help and support* (Welfare support assistant, mixed urban rural).

The sense of anger expressed in this quote was also apparent in other community food informants' accounts. This anger and frustration was centred not only on the individual suffering witnessed day-to-day but was also focussed on their organisations feeling obliged to help and becoming a de facto social safety net as a consequence. This next quote highlights some resentment directed towards mainstream (government-funded) organisations and agencies about expectations that were perceived to have been placed on poorly-resourced charities to help alleviate local suffering:

Well, I think it's one of the few areas that I'm aware of that the only response is, "Go to the voluntary sector." I can't think of very many other services that are related to similar sorts of outcomes, where the response is, "Go to a food bank, go to the voluntary sector," especially food banks, who get very little money from anywhere. I think part of the problem is that it's a free service that's been offered that we may have to challenge, in the future. I can't think of anything else, in a similar situation, where people say, "Go to your local church, they'll help you out," which is what people are, in effect, saying about food banks, you know, main stream services, main stream agencies, Local Authority's and whoever else. I find that very, very worrying (Community food programme informant, mixed urban).

In addition, there was an overriding sense of pessimism amongst informants that this picture and these trends in household food insecurity were about to change in the short-term. Most believed it was likely to become worse rather than better, particularly when the additional proposed changes to the social security system were enacted in the near future. This proposed change referred to here is the introduction of new UK Government policy associated with the so-called Universal Credit system of social security payment that would see the scrapping of fortnightly payment of separate types of security payments such e.g. family tax credits, housing benefit unemployment benefit etc. in favour of a single, monthly payment system. This fear and pessimism is illustrated here:

And I don't know what would happen to the other half; I'm really frightened, and because, as I say, we have designed and promoted ourselves as a place of last resort for funders, you know, it's the only option available; the last option available. I don't know what would happen [to them]. (Community Food Program, urban).

Some informants predicted future expansion of the food bank service on the basis that there would be an ongoing need to support hungry people, highlighted in this quote:

I think food poverty in Scotland isn't something that's going to be resolved overnight. I think it's going to be a long ... there's going to need to be looking at like longer term more sustainable solutions but I feel that until these things are achieved, food banks are now kind of part of the dialogue and will be for, maybe longer term, until adaptions are made to the welfare system and especially with regard to sanctions. But as a result of that, food banks will be ... will have a kind of longer-term role to play (Community food programme, urban).

Almost all the community food programme informants indicated they did not believe that food banks were a positive development or an effective or sustainable solution, but could not envisage them becoming redundant soon. Some talked about wishing to develop a different 'model' of local assistance, in the future, that would enable people to buy low-cost, healthy food according to their individual dietary needs and preferences, as opposed to being handed a free food parcel. All community food programme informants talked about trying to ensure that their clients had access to as nutritious a food parcel as they were able to supply. Most also commented at some point in their interview about the limited nature (in terms of nutritional quality and dietary preference) and lack of choice their clients had in the food were given. In the context of these discussions, it was also interesting to note that a few informants also talked about the unpredictable and limited nature of the food supply available to them (sourced from public and corporate donations, and allocations from franchised food surplus distributors) and the challenge they had in meeting the needs of their local community. This next quote illustrates the limited and unhealthy nature of the food informants received from a national food surplus redistribution operation:

The council gave us money to join (food surplus distributor), but as to date since we started with (food surplus distributor), the amount of produce we've been able to use is less than 20 kg a week. Because we can't take chilled produce, we can't take frozen produce, so the ambient temperature ... they've given us a lot more than that but the biggest item by weight we've had has been diet Irn-Bru (soft drink). I would actually use that as an example of something with no nutritional value whatsoever. The second biggest item we've had, not by weight but by quantity, has been salt and vinegar crisps (CFI mixed urban/rural).

One social care informant, working with young people at risk of homelessness, described his frustration associated with observing that the components of food bank parcels did not necessarily match the healthy eating on a budget training that his young clients were being directed towards:

Well, we've tried to work with food banks. We haven't always found that entirely easy to be honest. We've produced a range of recipes and that sort of thing aimed at healthy eating on a budget and not all of the food banks are providing a great balance of food within the food boxes and that's not in any way to throw any blame at them, they can only allocate what they get, but access to fresh food and things can be quite difficult. We've done a range of training workshops with young people primarily aimed at teaching people how to create meals that don't require cooking but it's hard to get that matched up well with the contents of the food boxes. (Homeless organisation, urban).

Moreover, it also became apparent when talking to the community food programme informants that food banks were not well placed to meet the needs of people with a long term health condition or conditions seeking help from them.

Whilst food banks were predicted to remain a response to the existence of hungry people in local communities, overall, informants believed it was action to increase the levels and predictably of people's income that would make the biggest impact on food insecurity in Scotland. Support for young people to get into employment and get access to decent housing were also high on the list of things informants mentioned here. While a few described their aspirations that locally grown food would be part of the answer, they expressed disbelief that it ever would be for those on very low incomes, as it was considered well out of reach, cost wise, for those people.

4. Discussion

While this study revealed observations and concerns about groups of people historically well known to services due to their economic and social vulnerability, or frank destitution, this study also revealed widespread perceptions and concern about groups (particularly) families with young children and young people never previously considered to have been so obviously affected by food insecurity in affluent contexts. Income insufficiency was thought to be the primary cause of this by the majority of our study participants. This was related to the nature of work i.e., low wages, and insufficient and unpredictable hours of work, as well as changes to social security entitlement changes that previously boosted the take-home pay of those in low wage employment. While concepts of food insecurity and those affected by it, described in this study, did include descriptions of destitute life circumstances and/or crisis situations involving obvious hunger, those accounts also included concern for a growing number of people living within communities who were perceived to be dealing with food insecurity but were not necessarily totally insolvent or going hungry per se. This was characterized by our study participants as something they associated with having to eat (or survive) on cheap, poor quality foods due to having insufficient household income. Concerns about groups and households not obviously experiencing destitution but who are still considered to be at risk of food insecurity, due to inadequate income, has also been highlighted elsewhere [33,34].

The UK's Joseph Rowntree Foundation, for example, has found that those living in the lowest income decile households in the UK are routinely spending 20–23% of their household income on food and non-alcoholic beverages compared to 11% allocated to this expenditure by those living in average to above average income households [35]. Our quantitative study found those living in households with below 60% average income were routinely spending between 18–23% on food and non-alcoholic beverages in Scotland between 2005 and 2012 [27]. Caraher and Furey also estimated that the lowest income decile group in the UK would have to spend 40% of their household income if they were to buy what they describe as a consensually healthy diet in the year ending 2016/2017 [16]. Furthermore, the cost of purchasing healthy food and beverages (compared to unhealthy foods) has been steadily been rising in the UK since 2002, and predictions that healthy diets will become less affordable over time suggests, as Jones et al. also argue, that there are significant implications for individual food security and population health going forward [36]. It should perhaps be no surprise therefore, that low income households in Scotland are consistently failing to achieve population healthy eating targets in Scotland [37].

In addition, while hunger due to destitution is no less a public health and social concern in its own right in the UK and elsewhere, food insecurity without hunger in high income countries (like Scotland) is increasingly understood to be the more common experience, but also as damaging to health [33,38,39]. Recent UK research indicates that the numbers of people who report skipping meals in the previous year due to economic constraints had risen from 13% in 1983 to 28% in 2012 [40]. Our participants' observations and experiences of encountering an increasing number of people and groups of people affected by food insecurity, characterized by many of them to be synonymous in the Scottish context with having to eat cheap, nutrient poor food to deal with household income insufficiency, and is also consistent with this finding.

These findings therefore have important implications for public health and social policy makers, researchers and practitioners concerned with population health improvement and promotion, who are facing growing health care costs associated with non-communicable diseases. There is growing, evidence-based recognition that chronic compromises in dietary quality (due to the experience of food insecurity), rather than periodic episodes of hunger, are not only the more common experience of food insecurity in high income countries like Scotland, but also the more likely cause of a wide range of negative physical and mental health outcomes [41]. Food insecurity is known to increase the risk of a range of chronic, non-communicable health conditions and mental health related problems such as depression [42–44]. It is also notable that Scotland ranks second behind the US (in the top 20 OECD countries) in terms of the population prevalence of overweight and obesity. The Scottish Public Health Observatory has estimated that a fifth of all cases of obesity here can be attributed to living in deprivation [45]. Living in poverty in high income countries increases the risk for overweight and obesity [46], and while the mechanisms behind this are not fully understood, it is suggested that those living in poverty consume large quantities of highly energy dense foods (and therefore excessive calories) due to their appealing combination of affordability and palatability [45,47]. Therefore it maybe that policy interventions aimed at maximizing household income, such as those currently being tested in the Scottish context associated with addressing child poverty [48] and a universal basic income [49], hold more promise in addressing the root causes and health consequences of food insecurity, compared with an emergency food-based policy response.

It is also important to remember that those living in destitution (and their food security status) remain a significant public health concern in the UK [17,50], and those interviewed for this study were acutely aware of this, regularly highlighting their observations of increased hardship and concern about the significant challenges faced by those groups they were more commonly used to dealing with in their work. This increase in adversity was frequently linked to changes to social security entitlements associated with unemployment and sickness benefits due to changes in UK government policy [48,51]. In relation to older people, the target group of concern at the outset of this research, the mixed picture that emerged here reinforces the need for vigilance and continued close monitoring of this group in relation to food insecurity. Whilst pensioner poverty has declined in Scotland in recent times [51] and some older people were perceived and observed to be living without obvious barriers to food resources, from our study participants' perspectives there was still cause for concern. That older people are not turning up at food banks in the same numbers of younger people is not an indication that all is well with this group.

Stoic struggle, and resistance to the notion of being thought of as being unable to feed oneself, was featured amongst accounts of encounters with older people, and other groups too. This study found that professional offers of referrals to food banks were being turned down by some who had given such cause for concern. This resistance to being considered or revealed as being incapable of feeding oneself should be no surprise when considering Poppendieck's and Chilton's arguments that, relying on charity (to feed oneself) not only undermines basic human dignity, but also risks drawing public attention to one's reduced capability as family providers, protectors and consumers [22,52]. In consumer societies like the UK, this defective status represents a significant challenge to an individual's self-worth and wellbeing [53]. Indeed, the experience of living in poverty is known to be accompanied by feelings of great shame and fear of stigma [54]. Moreover, the drive to 'keep up appearances' and pretence to appear 'normal' and 'respectable' is universally experienced in cultures of widely varying economic circumstances throughout the world [55]. There is certainly a growing body of experiential studies, investigating food bank users' perspectives, that has revealed that their use is the action of last resort, and is commonly accompanied by feelings of great shame and powerlessness [56–61]. This apparently human instinct, to hide individual household food insecurity from public and professional scrutiny, has significant implications for the design and delivery of policies intended to address it. For example, vigilance needs to be maintained through research and service evaluations to reduce the risk that people and households struggling to cope with food insecurity are missing out on support they are entitled or eligible to receive, by those front line service providers who interact with them.

Whilst families with young children were considered to be amongst those groups giving cause for concern amongst our participants, a few expressed specific anxiety about the food security status of mothers and pregnant women. Women with children, living in very low income households, are believed to be at particular risk in relation to coping with food insecurity and its potential impacts on their own food intake and health [62–64]. Moreover, it is not uncommon for mothers to try to optimise their children's dietary intake at the expense of their own diets [65]. Women have been found to be less likely to present at a food bank for help in the UK [7,61], but are notably more likely to report moderate or severe food insecurity in population surveys compared to men [66]. While Loopstra and Lalor (2017) reported in their recent study of UK food bank users that men were the largest group of users (39%), lone mothers with children were the next most prominent group (13%), with households with three or more children particularly prominent amongst this group and the most vulnerable to severe food insecurity [67]. Therefore, the fears expressed by our participants appear plausible.

Almost all the community food programmes we engaged with had been operating without a food bank for over a decade but reported very similar experiences in relation being compelled to add this facility to their service offerings in response to locally expressed need in recent times. Nevertheless, there were mixed views amongst study participants about the extent to which they thought their food banks were effectively addressing their clients' needs, a finding which concurs with the lived experiences of food bank users reported elsewhere [56–60]. There was also some concern expressed in this study in relation to food banks not being able to meet the needs of people with a long term health condition or conditions. This is an important issue to take note of, as people with long term conditions are disproportionately represented in UK food bank use statistics. For example, the 2017 Loopstra and Lalor survey of food banks in the UK found that 63% of food bank user respondents had a health condition, and a further 5% had someone living with a health condition in the household [67]. The experience of living with food insecurity is known to adversely affect individuals' ability to manage their health condition and achieve optimal health outcomes [68–70]. Furthermore, there is also an emerging trend in the UK to suggest that more people are relying on food bank parcels on a regular basis, as opposed to this being a one off, rarely-used food crisis support [56,71]. Therefore, there is a need to undertake research with people in Scotland and the rest of the UK, who are living with a long term condition or conditions and who are affected by chronic or periodic food insecurity, to develop a better understanding of these experiences and their impacts.

These findings raise important considerations for public health and health care policy addressing household food insecurity in Scotland. Whilst Scottish Government investment in feeding assistance programmes like food bank operations and children's holiday feeding programmes, through their Fairer Food Fund [72], might make a short term difference to those subsets of the food insecure population using them, this investment will not reach the remainder who either do not access or have no access to such support.

Almost all the study food programme informants were pessimistic about any prospect of a future reduction in demand for food banks. There is certainly evidence to indicate that those predictions have been well founded [73]. Concerns were also expressed about the sustainability of some food banks in relation to local demand outstripping supply and in relation to being unable to provide healthy nutritious food in sufficient quantity and quality to supply the needs of people seeking help from them; concerns that have been highlighted elsewhere [21,22,72,74].

This study has some important limitations that need to be borne in mind. For example, the relatively small number of participants we were able to reach within the study timeframe means that it is problematic to generalize to all possible participants throughout Scotland. However, we attempted to gain the perspectives of as varied and relevant a sample of participants as possible (as described in Section 2) and argue that the findings are theoretically generalizable for two reasons. Firstly, there is a dearth of existing studies that has explored social, health care and third sector practitioner's perspectives and experiences of these issues. Secondly, after the study was finished we found from a series of knowledge exchange events that took place throughout Scotland, that our respondents and their narratives were not atypical [75].

A further limitation is that the study was not designed to engage with people directly affected by the lived experience of food insecurity. As discussed above, some additional work was being undertaken to explore that lived experience perspective in a separate but simultaneous piece of work in Scotland. Nevertheless, there is still a significant gap in the published literature particularly with respect to those individuals and households perceived to be experiencing food insecurity and believed to be at risk of food insecurity by practitioners and professionals working in health and social care arenas, but who are choosing not to use, or are having difficulty accessing, feeding assistance programmes. This study does not purport to represent the views of people with lived experience food insecurity, but to provide important insights into the perspectives and experiences of those frontline health and social care service providers, including those third sector and community-based programmes. These individuals are more commonly and historically used to dealing with groups and individuals who are financially or socially vulnerable; for example, who are not necessarily destitute but affected by in-work poverty, and, or who have routine health care needs. To the best of our knowledge, this is the first study of its kind to represent these views, for much of the emerging, published studies focusing on household food insecurity in the UK have been directed towards the experiences and perspectives of food assistance programme providers.

Finally, it was beyond the scope of this study to measure the extent of food insecurity but the findings stress the need to monitor food insecurity. A routine population survey tool could be added to an existing survey, such as the Scottish Health Survey, as the means by which policy can be informed by a more accurate picture of the population food insecurity prevalence, particularly given the evidence presented here of there being groups and individuals thought to be in need of help with feeding, due to income insufficiency, but who are not engaging with feeding programmes that might benefit them. However, routine surveys may still fail to capture fully the experiences of hard-to-reach groups.

5. Conclusions

This study set out to understand the nature of food insecurity beyond food bank provider's experiences and it revealed widespread concern for highly vulnerable groups more commonly known to be affected or at risk of destitution; and this remains a pressing public health issue. However, it also identified concern about groups, particularly families with young children, young people, women, and some older people, who were never previously considered to have been so obviously affected by food insecurity. The notion of food insecurity underpinning this view point was frontline observations of households having to survive on cheap, poor quality foods due to insufficient income; a conclusion that may explain why low income households have been consistently failing to achieve dietary targets in Scotland over some decades. The study also revealed a sense of commonplace stoic and private struggle within some food insecure households that seemed designed to avoid revealing their condition to public view. This apparently basic human instinct to try to conceal lived experiences of food insecurity from public and professional scrutiny has significant implications for the design and delivery of policies intended to address it. Furthermore, community-created and delivered food-based responses, that have been accessed by those willing and able to use them, were understood by those setting up and operating them to be insufficient and ineffective in addressing the root causes, and for those with health conditions, not well suited to meet their needs. Therefore, these findings point to some important public health, health care, and social policy implications.

Focusing on optimizing food bank operations seems unlikely to impact on the experience of food insecurity for those people who are unable or unwilling to access a food bank. Even for those who do access food banks, their operation can be viewed as alleviating the symptoms of food insecurity rather than addressing its causes. However, in Scotland, this has recently been a primary response to addressing food insecurity at the local level, through the provision of competitive grant funding to food bank operators. Policies that focus on income maximization, on the other hand, would seem to hold more promise in enabling more people to feed themselves, according to the perspective of frontline service providers interviewed in this study. In addition, we believe it is important to capture and monitor the experience of food insecurity both quantitatively through routine population surveys, as is the case already in Canada and the US, but also qualitatively through regular engagement with people with direct, lived experience of food insecurity, both those who use and don't use food banks, through research and dialogue. Both types of data are required to develop and monitor policy interventions intended to address food insecurity and to understand the impact of any policy changes arising.

Author Contributions: Conceptualization, F.D., O.-Z.E., A.L.G., S.W., L.M., A.L. and E.D.; methodology F.D., A.L.G., E.D. and F.M.; validation F.D. and F.M.; formal analysis F.D. and F.M.; data curation F.M.; writing—original draft preparation F.D.; writing—review and editing F.D., F.M., A.L.G., A.L. and E.D.; supervision F.D.; project administration F.D.; funding acquisition F.D., O.-Z.E., L.M., S.W., A.L. and E.D.

Acknowledgments: We would like to acknowledge Bill Gray and Dionne MacKinnon (BG NHS Health Scotland and DMcK, formerly of NHS Health Scotland) for their professional review and support during the project and our study participants for their time and expertise. We are also grateful to the anonymous reviewers of our paper for their time and extremely helpful contributions to this work.

Appendix A

Table A1. Service Provider Informant Details.

Type of Organisation	Role of Interviewee	Project or Service Description	Location	Population Group Served
Service Provider	Staff nurse, Vulnerable Populations Team	Health Service representative supporting vulnerable adults	Greater Glasgow & Clyde	Vulnerable adults of all ages (16 and over)
Service Provider	Pre School Educational Home Visitor. Provides support & education to parents regarding their children's development needs	Education & children's services	Fife	Vulnerable parents regarding their children's development needs
Service Provider	Deputy manager of advice and information service for vulnerable groups	Supports homeless or those at risk of homelessness	Grampian	Homeless & other groups at risk of homelessness
Service Provider	Family worker supporting vulnerable families via parent and toddler groups	Supports vulnerable families	Highlands	Vulnerable families with young children
Service Provider	Principal adult social worker for vulnerable groups	Supports disabled and other vulnerable adults	Orkney	Disabled and other vulnerable adults
Service Provider	Welfare Support Assistant for unemployed people	Supports unemployed people back into work	Fife	Unemployed people
Service Provider	Community Health Improvement Advisor	Promotes healthy eating and the prevention of chronic illnesses	Grampian	Vulnerable adults of all ages (16 and over)
Service Provider	Community Links Practitioner working in Primary Care—supports all patients in GP practice	Supports vulnerable patients	Greater Glasgow & Clyde	All patients in GP practice in community
Service Provider	Manager. Supports vulnerable groups in city	Supports people back into work. Counselling services	Grampian	Vulnerable adults of all ages (16 and over)
Service provider	Adult befriending Service co-Ordinator. Supports adults who are socially isolated in community	Supports vulnerable adults in community	Orkney	All adults who are socially isolated in community

Table A1. *Cont.*

Type of Organisation	Role of Interviewee	Project or Service Description	Location	Population Group Served
Service Provider	Assistant Chief Executive. Supports vulnerable young people	Supports young people at risk of homelessness back into employment	Highlands	Young people at risk of homelessness
Service Provider	Development officer. Supports vulnerable adults	Supports vulnerable adults in community	Grampian	Vulnerable adults of all ages (16 and over)
Service Provider	Re-generation manager. Supports vulnerable adults	Supports vulnerable adults in community	Greater Glasgow & Clyde	Vulnerable adults of all ages (16 and over)
Service Provider	Administrator. Supports vulnerable adults	Supports vulnerable adults in community	Grampian	Vulnerable adults of all ages (16 and over)
Service Provider	Integration Development worker. Supports asylum-seekers and refugees	Supports asylum-seekers and refugees	Greater Glasgow and Clyde	Asylum-seekers and refugees

Table A2. Community Food Programme Informant Details.

Type of Organisation	Role of Interviewee	Project or Service Description	Health Board Area	Population Group Served
Community Food Initiative: Community food programme with food bank	Manager of community food and health initiative	To improve people's health by providing them with nutritious food and cooking and nutrition classes	Greater Glasgow & Clyde	Vulnerable adults on a low income
Community Food Initiative: Food bank only	Manager of food bank	Food bank	Greater Glasgow & Clyde	Vulnerable children and adults on a low income
Community Food Initiative: Community food programme without food bank	Project Assistant at voluntary community health project	Voluntary community project which promotes healthy eating/living	Forth Valley	Vulnerable adults on a low income
Community Food Initiative: Community food programme with food bank	Chief Executive. Supports vulnerable adults	To improve health and wellbeing and to increase employability	Grampian	Vulnerable adults on a low income
Community Food Initiative: Community food programme without food bank	Community Food Development Worker for community food and health project	Supports people at risk of homelessness, offenders or those at risk of offending	Fife	Vulnerable adults on a low income

Table A2. *Cont.*

Type of Organisation	Role of Interviewee	Project or Service Description	Health Board Area	Population Group Served
Community Food Initiative: Community food programme without food bank	Manager of a healthy living centre	Tries to alleviate food poverty through their education and promotion work	Greater Glasgow & Clyde	Vulnerable adults on a low income
Community Food Initiative: Food bank only	Development worker at the foodbank	Promotes healthy eating in local schools and nurseries and runs cookery classes	Greater Glasgow & Clyde	Vulnerable children and adults living in community
Community Food Initiative: Community food programme with food bank	Foodbank coordinator at national voluntary organisation	Food bank and drop-in advice service	Dumfries and Galloway	Vulnerable children and adults on a low income
Community Food Initiative: Community garden	Volunteer coordinator at community food and health project	Promotes healthy eating via cookery classes and workshops. Sells cheap fruit and veg	Fife	All residents living in the local village
Community Food Initiative: Community food programme with food bank	Food and Health Development Worker for this Community food and health project	Supports vulnerable people living in food poverty. Promotes healthy eating via cookery classes	Lothian	Disadvantaged groups in deprived areas of city—mainly serves families with young children

References

1. Cooper, N.; Purcell, S.; Jackson, R. Below the Breadline: The Relentless Rise of Food Poverty in Britain. Available online: https://oxfamilibrary.openrepository.com/bitstream/handle/10546/317730/rr-below-breadline-food-poverty-uk-090614-en.pdf;jsessionid=2DBEBAA5229576B20714001FDF50F88C?sequence=1 (accessed on 2 December 2018).

2. UK Parliament. Hansard Report of House of Commons Food Banks Debate 18th December. Available online: http://www.publications.parliament.uk/pa/cm201314/cmhansrd/cm131218/debtext/131218-0003.htm (accessed on 20 August 2018).

3. Ashton, J.R.; Middleton, J.; Lang, T. Open letter to prime minister david cameron on food poverty in the UK. *Lancet* **2014**, *383*, 1631. [CrossRef]

4. Duggan, E. The Food Poverty Scandal that Shames Britain: Nearly 1m People Rely on Handouts to Eat–and Benefit Reforms May Be to Blame. Available online: https://www.independent.co.uk/news/uk/politics/churches-unite-to-act-on-food-poverty-600-leaders-from-all-denominations-demand-government-u-turn-on-9263035.html (accessed on 2 December 2018).

5. Sosenko, F.; Livingstone, N.; Fitzpatrick, S. *Overview of Food Aid Provision in Scotland*; Scottish Government Edinburgh: Edinburgh, UK, 2013.

6. Lambie-Mumford, H. *The Right to Food and the Rise of Charitable Emergency Food Provision in the United Kingdom*; University of Sheffield: Sheffield, UK, 2014.

7. MacLeod, M.A.; Curl, A.; Kearns, A. Understanding the prevalence and drivers of food bank use: Evidence from deprived communities in Glasgow. *Soc. Policy Soc.* **2018**, 1–20. [CrossRef]

8. All-Party Parliamentary Inquiry into Hunger. *Feeding Britain: A Strategy for Zero Hunger in England, Wales, Scotland and Northern Ireland*; Children's Society: London, UK, 2014.

9. Radimer, K.L.; Olson, C.M.; Campbell, C.C. Development of indicators to assess hunger. *J. Nutr.* **1990**, *120* (Suppl. 11), 1544–1548. [CrossRef] [PubMed]

10. Tarasuk, V.; Dachner, N.; Hamelin, A.M.; Ostry, A.; Williams, P.; Bosckei, E.; Poland, B.; Raine, K. A survey of food bank operations in five canadian cities. *BMC Public Health* **2014**, *14*, 1234. [CrossRef] [PubMed]

11. Martin-Fernandez, J.; Grillo, F.; Parizot, I.; Caillavet, F.; Chauvin, P. Prevalence and socioeconomic and geographical inequalities of household food insecurity in the paris region, France, 2010. *BMC Public Health* **2013**, *13*, 486. [CrossRef] [PubMed]

12. Pfeiffer, S.; Ritter, T.; Hirseland, A. Hunger and nutritional poverty in Germany: Quantitative and qualitative empirical insights. *Crit. Public Health* **2011**, *21*, 417–428. [CrossRef]

13. Reeves, A.; Loopstra, R.; Stuckler, D. The growing disconnect between food prices and wages in Europe: Cross-national analysis of food deprivation and welfare regimes in twenty-one EU countries, 2004–2012. *Public Health Nutr.* **2017**, *20*, 1414–1422. [CrossRef]

14. Food Foundation. Household Food Insecurity: The Missing Data. 2016. Available online: https://foodfoundation.org.uk/wp-content/uploads/2016/11/FF-Food-insecurity-4pp-V3.pdf (accessed on 1st September 2018).

15. Taylor, A.; Loopstra, R. *Too Poor to Eat: Food Insecurity in the UK*; Food Foundation: London, UK, 2016; Available online: http://foodfoundation.org.uk/wp-content/uploads/2016/07/FoodInsecurityBriefing-May-2016-FINAL.pdf (accessed on 2 December 2018).

16. Caraher, M.; Furey, S. The cultural and economic dimensions of food poverty. In *The Economics of Emergency Food Aid Provision*; Palgrave Pivot: Cham, Switzerland, 2018; pp. 1–24.

17. Loopstra, R. Rising food bank use in the UK: Sign of a new public health emergency? *Nutr. Bull.* **2018**, *43*, 53–60. [CrossRef]

18. Faith in Community Scotland. Beyond Foodbanks? Growing a Food Justice Movement. Available online: https://www.faithincommunityscotland.org/beyond-foodbanks-2015-conference-outputs/ (accessed on 1 September 2018).

19. Loopstra, R.; Tarasuk, V. The relationship between food banks and household food insecurity among low-income Toronto families. *Can. Public Policy* **2012**, *38*, 497–514. [CrossRef]

20. Bazerghi, C.; McKay, F.H.; Dunn, M. The role of food banks in addressing food insecurity: A systematic review. *J. Community Health* **2016**, *41*, 732–740. [CrossRef]

21.   Iafrati, S. We're not a bottomless pit: Food banks' capacity to sustainably meet increasing demand. *Volunt. Sect. Rev.* **2018**, *9*, 39–53. [CrossRef]

22.   Poppendieck, J. *Sweet Charity?: Emergency Food and the End of Entitlement*; Penguin: New York, NY, USA, 1999.

23.   Thompson, C.; Smith, D.; Cummins, S. Understanding the health and wellbeing challenges of the food banking system: A qualitative study of food bank users, providers and referrers in London. *Soc. Sci. Med.* **2018**. [CrossRef] [PubMed]

24.   The Scottish Government. Equally Well—The Report of the Ministerial Task Force on Health Inequalities. Available online: https://www2.gov.scot/Resource/Doc/229649/0062206.pdf (accessed on 5 November 2018).

25.   Fraser, P.L.F.B.; Douglas-Hamilton, J. Eating for Health: A Diet Action Plan for Scotland; Scottish Executive 1996. Available online: https://www2.gov.scot/Resource/0040/00400745.pdf (accessed on 5 November 2018).

26.   Lang, T.; Dowler, E.; Hunter, D.J. *Review of the Scottish Diet Action Plan: Progress and Impacts 1996–2005*; NHS Scotland Edinburgh: Edinburgh, UK, 2006.

27.   Douglas, F.; Ejebu, O.Z.; Garcia, A.; MacKenzie, F.; Whybrow, S.; McKenzie, L.; Ludbrook, A.; Dowler, E. *The Nature and Extent of Food Poverty in Scotland*; NHS Health Scotland: Glasgow, UK, 2015.

28.   Strauss, A. *Basics of Qualitative Research: Techniques and Proceduare for Developing Grounded Theory*; Sage: Thousand Oaks, CA, USA, 1998.

29.   Hussein, M.E.; Hirst, S.; Salyers, V.; Osuji, J. Using grounded theory as a method of inquiry: Advantages and disadvantages. *Qual. Rep.* **2014**, *19*, 1–15.

30.   Green, J.; Thorogood, N. *Qualitative Methods for Health Research*; Sage: London, UK, 2010.

31.   Clark, J. How to peer review a qualitative manuscript. *Peer Rev. Health Sci.* **2003**, *2*, 219–235.

32.   Ritchie, R.; Lewis, J.; Nicholls, C.M.; Ormston, R. *Qualiative Research Practice: A Guide for Social Science Students and Researchers*; Sage: London, UK, 2013.

33.   Tarasuk, V. Discussion Paper on Household and Individual Food Insecurity. Available online: https://www.researchgate.net/profile/Valerie_Tarasuk/publication/245946029_Discussion_Paper_ on_Household_and_Individual_Food_Insecurity/links/566eefd508ae4bef40611e55.pdf (accessed on 1 September 2018).

34.   Patil, S.P.; Craven, K.; Kolasa, K.M. Food insecurity: It is more common than you think, recognizing it can improve the care you give. *Nutr. Today* **2017**, *52*, 248–257. [CrossRef]

35.   Joseph Rowntree Foundation. *UK Poverty 2017: A Comprehensive Analysis of Poverty Trends and Figures*; Joseph Rowntree Foundation: York, UK, 2017.

36.   Jones, N.R.; Conklin, A.I.; Suhrcke, M.; Monsivais, P. The growing price gap between more and less healthy foods: Analysis of a novel longitudinal uk dataset. *PLoS ONE* **2014**, *9*, e109343. [CrossRef] [PubMed]

37.   Food Standards Scotland. *The Scottish Diet Needs to Change: Situation Report Update*; Food Standards Scotland: Aberdeen, UK, 2018.

38.   Butcher, L.; Ryan, M.; O'Sullivan, T.; Lo, J.; Devine, A. What drives food insecurity in Western Australia? How the perceptions of people at risk differ to those of stakeholders. *Nutrients* **2018**, *10*, 1059. [CrossRef] [PubMed]

39.   Ward, P.R.; Verity, F.; Carter, P.; Tsourtos, G.; Coveney, J.; Wong, K.C. Food stress in Adelaide: The relationship between low income and the affordability of healthy food. *J. Environ. Public Health* **2013**, *2013*, 968078. [CrossRef]

40.   Lansley, S.; Mack, J. *Breadline Britain: The Rise of Mass Poverty*; Oneworld Publications: London, UK, 2015.

41.   Gundersen, C.; Ziliak, J.P. Food insecurity and health outcomes. *Health Aff. (Millwood)* **2015**, *34*, 1830–1839. [CrossRef]

42.   Tarasuk, V.; Mitchell, A.; McLaren, L.; McIntyre, L. Chronic physical and mental health conditions among adults may increase vulnerability to household food insecurity-3. *J. Nutr.* **2013**, *143*, 1785–1793. [CrossRef]

43.   Maynard, M.; Andrade, L.; Packull-McCormick, S.; Perlman, C.; Leos-Toro, C.; Kirkpatrick, S. Food insecurity and mental health among females in high-income countries. *Int. J. Environ. Res. Public Health* **2018**, *15*, 1424. [CrossRef] [PubMed]

44.	Martin, M.S.; Maddocks, E.; Chen, Y.; Gilman, S.E.; Colman, I. Food insecurity and mental illness: Disproportionate impacts in the context of perceived stress and social isolation. *Public Health* **2016**, *132*, 86–91. [CrossRef] [PubMed]

45.	Grant, I.; Fischbacher, C.; Whyte, B. *Obesity in Scotland: An Epidemiology Briefing*; Scottish Public Health Observatory: Edinburgh, UK, 2007.

46.	Butland, B.; Jebb, S.; Kopelman, P.; McPherson, K.; Thomas, S.; Mardell, J.; Parry, V. Foresight. Tackling Obesities: Future Choices. Available online: https://assets.publishing.service.gov.uk/government/uploads/system/uploads/attachment_data/file/287937/07-1184x-tackling-obesities-future-choices-report.pdf (accessed on I1 September 2018).

47.	Drewnowski, A. Obesity, diets, and social inequalities. *Nutr. Rev.* **2009**, *67*, S36–S39. [CrossRef] [PubMed]

48.	Scottish Government. *Child Poverty (Scotland) Act 2017*; Scottish Government: Scotland, UK, 2017.

49.	Scottish Government, Citizen's Income. Available online: http://www.parliament.scot/parliamentarybusiness/CurrentCommittees/103211.aspx (accessed on 5 November 2018).

50.	Fitzpatrick, S.; Bramley, G.; Sosenko, F.; Blenkinsopp, J. *Destitution in the UK 2018*; The Joseph Rowntree Foundation: York, UK, 2018; Available online: https://www.jrf.org.uk/report/destitution-uk-2018?gclid=EAIaIQobChMI96jcnoaE3wIVGeR3Ch2wBA3iEAAYASAAEgJuhPD_BwE (accessed on 5 November 2018).

51.	Joseph Rowntree Foundation. Poverty in Scotland: Briefing Paper. Available online: https://www.jrf.org.uk/report/poverty-scotland-2018 (accessed on 30 July 2018).

52.	Chilton, M.; Rose, D. A rights-based approach to food insecurity in the United States. *Am. J. Public Health* **2009**, *99*, 1203–1211. [CrossRef] [PubMed]

53.	Bauman, Z. *Consuming Life*; John Wiley & Sons: Hoboken, NJ, USA, 2013.

54.	Shildrick, T. *Poverty Propaganda: Exploring the Myths*; Policy Press: Bristol, UK, 2018.

55.	Walker, R.; Kyomuhendo, G.B.; Chase, E.; Choudhry, S.; Gubrium, E.K.; Nicola, J.Y.; Lødemel, I.; Mathew, L.; Mwiine, A.; Pellissery, S. Poverty in global perspective: Is shame a common denominator? *J. Soc. Policy* **2013**, *42*, 215–233. [CrossRef]

56.	Holmes, E.; Black, J.L.; Heckelman, A.; Lear, S.A.; Seto, D.; Fowokan, A.; Wittman, H. "Nothing is going to change three months from now": A mixed methods characterization of food bank use in greater vancouver. *Soc. Sci. Med.* **2018**, *200*, 129–136. [CrossRef]

57.	Middleton, G.; Mehta, K.; McNaughton, D.; Booth, S. The experiences and perceptions of food banks amongst users in high-income countries: An international scoping review. *Appetite* **2018**, *120*, 698–708. [CrossRef]

58.	Garthwaite, K.A.; Collins, P.J.; Bambra, C. Food for thought: An ethnographic study of negotiating ill health and food insecurity in a uk foodbank. *Soc. Sci. Med.* **2015**, *132*, 38–44. [CrossRef]

59.	Purdam, K.; Garratt, E.A.; Esmail, A. Hungry? Food insecurity, social stigma and embarrassment in the UK. *Sociology* **2016**, *50*, 1072–1088. [CrossRef]

60.	Van der Horst, H.; Pascucci, S.; Bol, W. The "dark side" of food banks? Exploring emotional responses of food bank receivers in the netherlands. *Br. Food J.* **2014**, *116*, 1506–1520. [CrossRef]

61.	Douglas, F.; Sapko, J.; Kiezebrink, K.; Kyle, J. Resourcefulness, desperation, shame, gratitude and powerlessness: Common themes emerging from a study of food bank use in Northeast Scotland. *AIMS Public Health* **2015**, *2*, 297. [CrossRef] [PubMed]

62.	Tarasuk, V.S. Household food insecurity with hunger is associated with women's food intakes, health and household circumstances. *J. Nutr.* **2001**, *131*, 2670–2676. [CrossRef] [PubMed]

63.	Ivers, L.C.; Cullen, K.A. Food insecurity: Special considerations for women. *Am. J. Clin. Nutr.* **2011**, *94*, 1740S–1744S. [CrossRef] [PubMed]

64.	Pederson, A.; Haworth-Brockman, M.; Clow, B.; Isfeld, H.; Liwander, A. *Rethinking Women and Healthy Living in Canada*; Centre of Excellence for Women's Health: Vancouver, BC, Canada, 2013.

65.	Hall, S.; Knibbs, S.; Medien, K.; Davies, G. *Child Hunger in London: Understanding Food Poverty in the Capital*; Greater London Authority: London, UK, 2013.

66.	Jung, N.M.; de Bairros, F.S.; Pattussi, M.P.; Pauli, S.; Neutzling, M.B. Gender differences in the prevalence of household food insecurity: A systematic review and meta-analysis. *Public Health Nutr.* **2017**, *20*, 902–916. [CrossRef] [PubMed]

67.	Loopstra, R.; Lalor, D. *Financial Insecurity, Food Insecurity, and Disability: The Profile of People Receiving Emergency Food Assistance from the Trussell Trust Foodbank Network in Britain*; Trussell Trust: Oxford, UK, 2017.

68.   Galesloot, S.; McIntyre, L.; Fenton, T.; Tyminski, S. Food insecurity in Canadian adults: Receiving diabetes care. *Can. J. Diet. Pract. Res.* **2012**, *73*, e261–e266. [CrossRef] [PubMed]

69.   Seligman, H.K.; Davis, T.C.; Schillinger, D.; Wolf, M.S. Food insecurity is associated with hypoglycemia and poor diabetes self-management in a low-income sample with diabetes. *J. Health Care Poor Underserved* **2010**, *21*, 1227. [PubMed]

70.   Gucciardi, E.; Vahabi, M.; Norris, N.; Del Monte, J.P.; Farnum, C. The intersection between food insecurity and diabetes: A review. *Curr. Nutr. Rep.* **2014**, *3*, 324–332. [CrossRef] [PubMed]

71.   Garratt, E. Please sir, I want some more: An exploration of repeat foodbank use. *BMC Public Health* **2017**, *17*, 828. [CrossRef] [PubMed]

72.   The Scottish Government. Tackling Food Poverty. Available online: https://news.gov.scot/news/tackling-food-poverty-1 (accessed on 5 November 2018).

73.   Trussell Trust. UK Food Bank Use Continues to Rise. Available online: https://www.trusselltrust.org/2017/04/25/uk-foodbank-use-continues-rise/ (accessed on 6 August 2018).

74.   Loopstra, R.; Tarasuk, V. Food bank usage is a poor indicator of food insecurity: Insights from Canada. *Soc. Policy Soc.* **2015**, *14*, 443–455. [CrossRef]

75.   Mason, J. Making convincing arguements with qualitative data. In *Qualitative Resaerching*; Sage: London, UK, 2002.

5

Undeserving, Disadvantaged, Disregarded: Three Viewpoints of Charity Food Aid Recipients in Finland

Anna Sofia Salonen [1,*] , Maria Ohisalo [2] and Tuomo Laihiala [1]

1   Faculty of Social Sciences, University of Tampere, 33014 Tampere, Finland; tuomo.laihiala@uta.fi
2   Y-Foundation, 00531 Helsinki, Finland; maria.ohisalo@ysaatio.fi
*   Correspondence: anna.salonen@uta.fi

Abstract: Since the economic recession of the 1990s, Finland has experienced the proliferation of charity food aid as a means of helping people who are afflicted by poverty. However, so far little research has been conducted regarding the food aid recipients. This article gives discursive, demographic, and experiential insights into charity food provision and reception in Finland. Drawing on quantitative survey data, online discussion data related to news published on Finnish newspapers' web pages, and observation and interviews with food aid recipients, this article sheds new light on Finnish food aid recipients from three perspectives. First, public perceptions about food aid often portray food recipients as dishonourable and responsible for their own poverty. Secondly, the survey data shows that the main reason for people resorting to charity food aid is deep economic disadvantage, and further, that there is an unequal accumulation of disadvantage among the food aid recipients, illustrating internal diversity. Third, observational and interview data show that from the food recipients' perspective, the food aid system has only a limited ability to answer even their immediate food needs, and for the recipients, food aid venues can become not only socially significant, but also socially demanding and emotionally burdening places.

Keywords: food aid; charity; Finland; welfare state; food aid recipient; deservingness; disadvantages; inequality

---

1. Introduction

Despite the almost thirty years of charitable food aid in Finland, so far little research has been conducted about the aid recipients. There have been a few studies examining the clientele of church diocese work and the food aid users at individual food banks [1–5]. This trend has changed only recently, as three studies have taken the initiative to explore Finnish charity food aid particularly from the users' perspectives [6–8]. In this article, we use the existing data from these three studies to give a comprehensive picture of what is known so far about people receiving food aid in Finland.

Recent decades have witnessed the growth of food aid across the affluent world [9,10]. The global expansion of this phenomenon raises serious questions concerning food insecurity, public policy, and the future of welfare states. Food aid has prompted a lot of research in different parts of the world. However, there is still a need for more research on the various societal contexts in which food aid proliferates and on the viewpoints of the aid users [11] in terms of both who they are and how they perceive the aid they receive. With the concept of charity food aid, we refer to the phenomenon where non-governmental organizations (NGOs) provide free food to people who are living in poor social and economic situations; in contrast to statutory welfare provision, the food aid is voluntarily organized by the NGOs.

The Nordic welfare state context makes the Finnish case peculiar in relation to the many other countries where food aid has proliferated. In principle in Finland, the state is assumed to provide universal social security against social risks, such as poverty, for all its citizens. However, since the recession of the 1990s, Finland has experienced the proliferation of charity-based food aid provision as a means of helping people who are afflicted by poverty, indicating that the welfare state does not feed everybody. In Finland, food aid was initially considered a short-term response to the consequences of the recession of the 1990s, but it has gradually grown into an unorganized field, with hundreds of actors sharing food throughout the country. Over a quarter of a century, breadlines have become one of the most visible and well-known portrayals of poverty in Finland [12,13].

In the first cross-national study of charity food aid in the 1990s, it was stated that food aid is characteristic of residual welfare states, whereas the universalist Nordic welfare states have been able to safeguard social rights, such as the human right to food [14]. However, the Finnish case has challenged this perception. In her recent study comparing food aid and its implications for the welfare state in Finland and Scotland, Mary Anne MacLeod found that the rise of food assistance in Finland is coupled with the dilemmas of welfare state identity. Food poverty and food aid are considered marginal to the welfare state; food aid questions the effectiveness of the welfare system, and it is associated with societal failure. According to MacLeod's study, in Finland, food is positioned as a public good, and thus charitable models of food aid provision are perceived as a threat to the social democratic welfare regime [15].

On the state level, it has been argued that the necessity for charity food aid contravenes the Finnish Constitution, which declares that everyone should have the right to a life of dignity guaranteed by the state. Section 19 in the Finnish constitution, 'the right to social security', explicitly lays the foundation for public social policy and social security, and points out the responsibility of the public authorities to safeguard social welfare and health. Finland has also signed the UN covenant on the Right to Food (RTF), which should guarantee freedom from hunger together with access to safe and nutritious food [9]. In other words, charity food aid raises particular disputes in the context of a Nordic welfare state that is presumed to guarantee basic social security for all its citizens.

Tellingly, food aid has even been called the 'open wound' of the welfare state [16] (p. 255). In public debates, it has been considered a deviant practice, since there should be no need for food aid in an affluent Finnish society with a comprehensive social security system. At the same time, the efforts of churches and NGOs to provide food aid have been applauded. The perception of food aid thus holds an ambivalent position in Finnish public discourse: charitable food assistance is not fitting for the Nordic welfare state, but it is an appropriate way for churches to help the needy [17]. Thus, Finland marks an interesting case where the strong constitutional responsibilities of the state meet widespread unofficial aid provided by a lively and diverse non-governmental sector.

Due to this particular discrepancy between the strong welfare state ideal and strong grassroots charity aid, the connection between professional social work and food aid is in principle absent in Finland. There is no referral system between charity food providers and social services, and it has even been considered unconstitutional for social workers to inform or guide their clients to charity food aid services [18,19]. In other words, there are no explicit connections between food aid and public social policy. Illustrative of this gap on the state level is the fact that the administration of the EU's food aid programme in Finland was first set up under the Ministry of Agriculture and Forestry—and later the Ministry of Employment and the Economy—instead of the Ministry of Social Affairs and Health ([13], p. 476). Interestingly, however, many of the non-governmental organizations providing food aid receive some public funding—from local municipalities, for example—to support their non-profit work. Nevertheless, this funding is not targeted at food aid per se, but to the infrastructures and general activities of the organizations. In practice, then, food aid is often publicly supported, though only partly and indirectly.

On the grassroots level, the characteristic features of Finnish charity food aid are a low-level of organization and a lack of eligibility control. Unlike in many other countries, there are hardly any intermediaries in Finland that could collect and store food and redeliver it to local charities. Instead, local actors most often collect, store, and redistribute the food independently and according to their own individual practices [20]. The methods of providing assistance vary across the individual food aid organizations, but very often food aid provision is based on the principles of low threshold and the absence of means tests. Some food aid providers might ask to see proof of the recipient's status as unemployed or a pensioner, for example, but a detailed income assessment is rarely conducted. The basic principle is that asking for food aid is in itself a sign that the recipient deserves the aid. Thus, in many assistance venues, technically anyone can ask for and receive charity food aid.

Due to a lack of coordination, shared practices, or comparable statistics, only rough approximations can be drawn about the volume of food aid in Finland. A 2013 survey estimated that food assistance was available in over 220 of the more than 300 municipalities throughout the country [20]. The food aid is distributed via various faith-based and other NGOs. The food comes from two main sources: the EU food aid programme and food companies and grocery stores donating their surplus food. In addition, public institutions such as schools have recently started to give out surplus meals to charities. Based on the assessment of food aid distributors, approximately 20,000 people received food aid rather regularly in 2013 [20]. However, a national-level survey asking whether respondents had used food aid at least once a year found that more than four times that number had received food aid [21]. The Evangelical-Lutheran Church in Finland gave food in the form of free or cheap meals or food packages to roughly 56,000 people in 2015 [22]. These are significant figures in a country with a population of approximately 5.5 million people. For comparison, in 2015, 634,000 people, or 11.7% of the Finnish population, were considered low-income—that is, they belonged to the population living on less than 60% of the equivalent median money income of all households [23].

Overall, the Finnish food aid system can be described as an unorganized yet widespread practice of unofficial, last-resort aid targeted at people living in difficult social and economic situations. Moreover, the system has no strict criteria for eligibility. This peculiar situation raises many questions. First of all, the lack of objective criteria for food eligibility provokes a normative debate concerning deservingness—that is, who should get what, and why [24,25]. Who should be granted the moral entitlement to use assistance that is in principle available to everyone, but which is at the same time contrary to the Finnish welfare ethos? Second, the situation raises a policy question concerning the populations involved in this widespread yet abnormal form of aid. In the absence of guidelines and practices shared between different food aid providers, it is very hard to estimate who the food assistance recipients are or to determine their reasons for using food aid. Third, such an unregulated and unofficial setting calls for an exploration of the experiences of the recipients. What are the repercussions of food aid use for these individuals? Without research addressing these questions, preconceptions flourish and colour the public and policy discussions on the issue.

In this article, we examine the Finnish charity food aid recipients from three distinct perspectives. First, we present findings from a study that analyses the online perceptions of food aid recipients to illustrate the discursive landscape in which Finnish charity food aid is rooted. Second, drawing on quantitative survey data collected among food aid recipients, we bring new light to the often-held assumptions about who the food aid recipients actually are. Third, we use observation and interview material from Finnish food banks to illustrate how the aid is experienced by the recipients. By bringing these findings together, we aim to provide a holistic picture of the food aid recipients in Finland. Together, the findings presented in this article provide discursive, demographic, and experiential insights into charity food provision and reception in the Finnish context, thus giving a novel account of charity food aid in an affluent, Nordic welfare state from the viewpoint of the people whom this aid concerns the most.

2. Materials and Methods

In this article, we present findings from recently conducted studies that utilize data from three sources. First, we present findings from online discussion data related to news published on Finnish newspapers' web pages to understand how the food aid recipients are perceived in public discourses. The data consist of 1294 comments collected from online discussions that were connected to news articles about food aid in nine prominent Finnish newspapers (*Aamulehti, Helsingin Sanomat, Iltalehti, Ilta-Sanomat, Länsiväylä, Metro, Satakunnan Kansa, Taloussanomat, Turun Sanomat*) in 2014 and 2015. The data were analysed with close reading, and a topic model was created with GUI Topic Modelling -programme to cover all the relevant themes. The themes that occurred in the data were interpreted in the light of Wim van Oorschot's criteria for deservingness, including need (the greater the level of need, the more deserving), control (poor people's control over their neediness, or their responsibility for it), identity (the identity of the poor, i.e., their proximity to the rich or their "pleasantness"), attitude (poor people's attitude towards support, or their docility or gratefulness), and reciprocity (the degree of reciprocation by the poor, or having earned support) [25]. The data collection and analysis is described in detail in [6].

Second, we present data from a quantitative survey that researched both the socio-economic status of food aid recipients and the accumulation of the recipients' disadvantages (see the Supplementary Materials for the English version of the survey form). This is the first and so far only study where the socio-economic position and disadvantages of the Finnish aid recipients has been studied with larger-scale survey data. The data were collected in a national food aid study ($N = 3474$) in 2012–2013 from 37 different charity food aid distributions in 11 Finnish municipalities. The food aid venues chosen for this study were known to be the largest in Finland in terms of the number of food aid recipients. As the number of people receiving food aid in Finland is unknown, the demographic sample does not necessarily represent all the food aid recipients in the country. However, the results from different municipalities are relatively uniform, indicating that the data sample captures a good overall picture of the food recipients. Surveys were distributed in three different languages—Finnish, Russian, and English—and the researchers who collected the surveys helped the respondents in translating them according to the situation. The study targeted the subjective well-being of the food aid recipients. The data were analysed with SPSS (IBM Corporation, Armonk, NY, USA) using multivariate methods, namely factor analysis, cluster analysis, and cross tabulations. The data collection and analysis is described in detail in [7].

Third, we present findings from a qualitative study that consist of observational notes from over seven months of participant observation in four food assistance organizations, written documents related to the operation of the organizations, and open-ended interviews with 25 food aid recipients. The data were collected from four food charity organizations in the city of Tampere, Finland, in 2012 and 2013. The selection of one of the large cities in Finland enabled the researchers to uncover possible variations in the different kinds of food aid venues and to reach a wider group of food recipients. The data were analysed with qualitative methods, such as qualitative inductive content analysis and grounded theory, where conceptions of different incidents, venues, people, and occasions were constructed and compared in order to develop a comprehensive understanding of the phenomenon. The data collection and analysis is described in detail in [8]. In this article, we discuss the findings that relate to the ability of food aid to meet the needs of the recipients.

In the subsequent sections, we first present the findings from these different data sets and then draw a synthesis of this recent body of knowledge on Finnish food aid recipients: we discuss how they are perceived by the public, who they actually are, and how they themselves see their own social position and the phenomenon they are engaged in (Figure 1). In the discussion section, we discuss these combined findings to show how they raise some significant issues regarding food aid recipients.

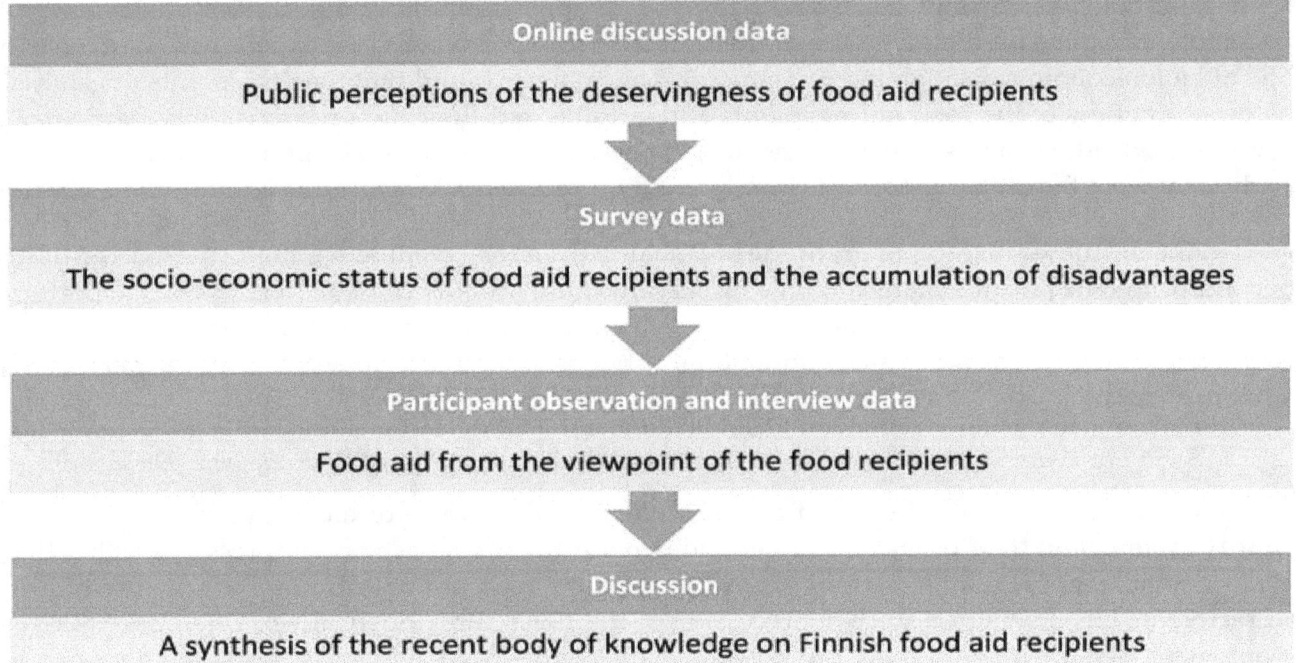

Figure 1. The outline of the study.

3. Results

3.1. Public Perceptions of Food Aid Recipients' Deservingness in Online Discussions

The online discussion data shows that Finnish food aid recipients are exposed to strong public criticism and blame. Of the themes covered in the discussions, the most prominent was the issue of need: the discussants questioned whether the food recipients were in need of food aid, for example, by suggesting that the recipients squander their money and then request assistance. The emphasis on need is surprising given that the needs-based arguments of deservingness do not fit well with the Finnish welfare state context.

The analysis of the online discussion data shows that the discussants differed based on how they related to the need of the food aid recipients and how they perceived the causes and reasons for the food aid use. The discussants who considered the food aid recipients to be in genuine need expressed their desire to help and give support and encouragement to the disadvantaged. Those who acknowledged the need but also blamed the recipients for their situation considered obtaining charity food aid acceptable only if the recipients were genuinely in need of help. However, the needs and motives of most of the recipients were questioned, and they were presumed to be caused by lifestyle choices. Furthermore, some of the online discussants maintained that food aid represents a systemic problem: in a good society, charity food aid should not be needed. The poor life situation of an individual is a matter for society and the welfare state rather than the fault of the individual. Finally, some of the discussants questioned the food recipients' need and pigeonholed them as undeserving scroungers.

Another central topic that surfaced in the discussions was the question of who is responsible for poverty. Unlike in previous quantitative research that found Finnish people tend to see poverty as a structural problem [26,27], a significant number of the online discussants considered the situation of the food aid recipients to be self-inflicted. The recipients' need was often questioned, and the recipients were considered a dishonourable group responsible for their own poverty. In its considerable resemblance to traditional aid for the poor, Finnish charity food aid enables this kind of discussion about deservingness, which fits poorly with an institutional welfare state.

Not all online discussants condemned the charity food aid recipients. Some defended the recipients' deservingness and considered them unfortunate, disadvantaged people who have to rely on charity food as a result of society's failures. Empathy, solidarity, and positive attitudes towards the recipients can be predicted by the discussant's personal or other close experiences with charity food aid and economic disadvantage in general. The analysis found that the discussants questioned the deservingness of the food aid recipients and emphasized their own responsibility particularly when the food aid recipients were not considered to belong to the same social group as them. The most conditional were the attitudes towards immigrant food recipients.

Unlike in studies that found gratitude and shame to be the prominent emotions expected of the food aid recipients [28], the Finnish online discussants rarely required the food recipients to perform emotional or attitude-related responses towards the aid or the aid providers. Instead, the food aid itself was seen by the discussants as humiliating, either for the food recipient or from the perspective of wider society.

3.2. The Socio-Economic Status of Food Aid Recipients and the Accumulation of the Recipients' Disadvantages

Perceptions of the extent of food aid in Finland, the position of aid recipients in the social security system, and their usage of services and benefits are often based on impressions rather than on systematic, empirical information. According to many food aid distributors, the picture of food aid recipients has diversified since the recession of the 1990s. Previously, it was often unemployed or homeless men queuing for food, but nowadays the charity food aid venues bring together people from a variety of backgrounds. The findings of the national food aid study presented here provide empirical evidence of the recipients' socio-economic position and disadvantages.

The socio-economic status of people receiving food aid was outlined with 11 questions. To begin with age, the biggest age group of food aid recipients was 46–65-year-olds. Young people tend not to be highly represented in Finnish food aid venues. There are several reasons for this; for example, students receive subsidized meals at the university level, and many of them complement their income by working part-time during their studies. Thus, the people receiving food aid seem to be older compared to the demographic structure of Finland in general (see Appendix A for the results compared to the general population of Finland).

Unlike in many other disadvantaged groups, the gender division among food aid recipients was nearly non-existent. There was only a small majority of women (51.7%, N = 1704) receiving food aid, even though men tend to be overrepresented in many disadvantaged groups. The majority of the people receiving food aid were native Finns (87.3%, N = 2817).

One stereotype about people receiving food aid in Finland is their assumed low educational background. However, the data partly challenge this supposition. In the food aid venues, there were more people with only a basic level of education (39.6%, N = 1270) and fewer people with a higher education background (20.4%, N = 656) compared to the general population in Finland. Nevertheless, the relative amount of the people with an upper secondary level education (40%, N = 1282) was nearly the same as it is among the wider Finnish population.

In terms of employment status, food aid recipients were characterized by a weak labour market position. Roughly four fifths of them were either pensioners (38.4%, N = 1260) or unemployed or laid off (38.4%, N = 1260). One in seven respondents were at home (7.3%, N = 240) or students (6.6%, N = 215). Many of the student respondents were working while studying, but their main occupation was recorded as 'student'. The phenomenon of the working poor is seen in food aid, as one in ten food aid recipients were people working part-time or on a fixed-term contract (5.6%, N = 185), or full-time (3.7%, N = 120).

In terms of housing, the majority of the respondents (78%, $N = 2570$) lived in a rented property, and only 16% ($N = 527$) owned their own home. On the national level in 2011, the percentages were nearly the reverse: 59% lived in owner-occupied dwellings, whereas only 29% of the people lived in rented dwellings. Homeless respondents (3.3%, $N = 109$) and people living in supported housing (2.8%, $N = 92$) were a small minority. However, these figures exceed the national levels, as roughly 8000 (0.15%) people in Finland were homeless at that time. The size of the household was measured by asking the number of adults and children living in the household. Of the respondents, over three fifths (60.5%, $N = 2024$) lived alone, whereas on the national level two fifths live in one-adult households [29].

In terms of the frequency of food aid use, nearly one third ($N = 952$) of the food aid recipients obtained charity food weekly. One quarter (25.9%, $N = 816$) received food aid approximately every two weeks, and one fifth (20.1%, $N = 633$) received food aid roughly once a month. Under a quarter (23.9%, $N = 752$) of the respondents received food aid only couple of times a year. A majority of the recipients of the food aid got the food for themselves (47.6%, $N = 1544$), but over two fifths (42.6 %, $N = 1380$) picked up food for themselves and their families. One in ten (9.8%, $N = 317$) got the food for themselves and other non-family members.

In terms of the money left over after each month's compulsory outgoings, the results show that nearly half of the respondents (44.5%, $N = 1316$) were left with 0–100 euros. One third (30.9%, $N = 913$) had 101–300 euros, and a quarter (24.7%, $N = 730$) had more than 301 euros per month.

It is known from Finnish national-level surveys that disadvantages tend to accumulate in three main dimensions: economic, social, and health [30]. When researching the disadvantages of the respondents, the findings show that the same dimensions found in studies representing the Finnish population were also found among the food aid recipients (Table 1). The results are statistically significant. One quarter of the respondents had not experienced severe economic disadvantage or accumulated disadvantages, although they were less well off when compared with the wider population. Typically, people belonging to this group were pensioners and the working poor living on social assistance or a guarantee pension and experiencing high levels of scarcity. Most of the people (three quarters) receiving food aid had deep economic problems, such as difficulties in making ends meet and paying debts. These were mainly young people, students, and people with families.

Notably, over two fifths of the people receiving charity food aid suffered from several simultaneous disadvantages. They not only had problems with their economic situation but also health disadvantages, such as poor mental and/or physical health and lower levels of life satisfaction. In addition, they experienced social disadvantages such as hunger, loneliness, and depression. In this group, the homeless, unemployed, substance abusers, and people with the least disposable income were overrepresented.

Overall, based on the data, people receiving food aid in Finland are a heterogeneous group. However, the group has a poorer employment status compared to the wider Finnish population, and is older, less educated, and on a lower income. People receiving food aid mostly suffer from economic deprivation. They are also more likely to live alone. Moreover, two fifths of the food aid recipients live with accumulated economic, social, and health disadvantages.

Table 1. Accumulation of disadvantages and people affected by economic, social, and health disadvantages.

How Do Disadvantages Accumulate?	Less well-off compared to the wider population, no accumulated disadvantage, 24.7% (N = 693)	Severe economic disadvantage (without other disadvantages), 33.7% (N = 945)	Strongly accumulated economic, social, and health disadvantage, 41.5% (N = 1163)
What does it mean?	Does not suffer from severe economic or accumulated disadvantage	Suffers from severe economic disadvantage, but not from social or health disadvantages; has difficulties in making ends meet and paying debts; is dissatisfied with the current standard of living and has experiences of insufficient support	Severe economic disadvantages; disadvantages in mental and physical health and lower levels of life satisfaction; social disadvantages such as hunger, loneliness, and depression
Who is affected?	Pensioners and the working poor living on social assistance or a guarantee pension and experiencing high levels of scarcity	Young people, students, and people with families	The homeless and people living in supported housing, the unemployed and laid-off, substance abusers, people considering themselves disadvantaged, people with the least money to spend freely, and people using last-resort social support

3.3. The Food Recipients' Viewpoint of Food Aid

The sections above illustrate that while the public perception of food aid recipients mostly presents these people as a homogeneous group, in reality food aid recipients come from various walks of life, and they experience disadvantages of various degrees and intensities. What, then, do these people themselves think about the assistance they receive? The qualitative data on the food aid recipients' perspectives of the assistance further complement the above findings. As in the survey data, the informants of the qualitative study were a heterogeneous group that came from various backgrounds. The common denominator for the informants was a low income and the concomitant need for material assistance. For these recipients, using food aid was a practical coping mechanism for dealing with a weak social and economic situation; it was relief that helped in managing everyday scarcity.

However, even though food aid alleviates the immediate food needs of the recipients, the study found out that there are limitations in the food aid system's ability to satisfy these needs. The finding is in line with previous research that suggests food aid does not address the root causes or structural problems behind food insecurity [31–33]. Furthermore, the study found that the food aid system has only a limited ability to meet the immediate food needs of the recipients. This was particularly the case due to the detachment of the food resources in the food assistance venues under study from the needs of the food recipients. Much of the food delivered to these venues was market surplus, and thus its quality and quantity was dependent on what happened to be left over from the primary food markets. Moreover, some of the venues also redistributed food from the EU's food programme, which did not completely align with the needs of the food recipients.

There were problems regarding both the amounts of food available and the quality of food: even though there was occasionally plenty of food available, the food recipients had difficulties in utilizing it. Thus, the occasional abundance of food highlights the inconsistency between the food needs and the food supply in the food aid venues. In terms of the material needs of the food recipients, food aid seems to be able to alleviate only the direct, immediate food needs of these people, and even those only insofar as the needs correspond with what happens to be available.

In addition to their food needs, many informants mentioned social reasons for coming to food aid venues, such as meeting other people, spending time, and enjoying the additional social and religious programmes that some of the food aid providers integrated in the food delivery events. This finding is in line with the quantitative survey study, which found that 53% of the respondents agreed with the statement that it is important for them to meet other people in the food aid venues [34].

Recently, the communal and social aspect of food assistance has gained prominence in Finnish public discussions about food assistance. There are efforts to remodel food aid to provide the participants with communal experiences. However, the findings of this study reveal that from the perspective of the food aid recipients, the communal and social aspect of food aid is not only a positive feature. Occasionally, the low threshold and lack of eligibility control that aimed at inclusiveness resulted in adverse outcomes, such as mutual surveillance among participants and both subtle and hash negotiations over who should receive food first. Thus, the study highlights that food banks are communities with various communal qualities, and not all of them are positive. For the recipients, food aid venues can be socially significant yet socially demanding and emotionally burdening places. From the perspective of the recipients, it is thus important to acknowledge that these venues are about 'more than bread'—both in the good, and in the bad.

In addition to the material and social challenges faced by the food aid recipients, the study found that the informants encountered restrictions on their ability to express their needs, expectations, and experiences related to the assistance. For example, the recipients could only subtly express criticism towards the quality or practical usability of the food items, even in matters regarding food safety. To give an example, one informant delicately noted when he realized that the expiry date of a food item had passed a while ago: 'I really don't dare to eat those meat products. I am not picky, but ... ' In the context of food aid, the exercise of consumer choice was restricted and even resented. In everyday discussions, criticism was aimed at individuals who were considered choosy. One interviewee remarked aptly how, in the food aid context, '[y]ou have to be something like a piggy. You eat what comes. Yes. [. . .] If you choose, you starve!' The interviewee thus hints that in a food bank, exercising choice regarding food might lead to receiving nothing. As a further example, one recipient lamented how 'there are those finicky ones, who [do not eat particular food stuffs even though they] are not allergic, or anything. But if they can afford to...' Implicit in this statement is the idea that food aid recipients do not have the right to choose the content of the aid. As the latter part of the comment suggests, refusing certain food items indicates that one is not really in need of aid, which hints at the discussions of deservingness presented above.

The recipients' limited choices were also present in their limited ability to withdraw from food aid use. This became apparent in situations where the informants spoke about the social and emotional stress that food aid use caused for them. For example, one recipient stated, 'I feel that it would be easier not to come. But how do I cope then? Where do I get [food] then? I don't know where I would then get [food], and I don't know what I should do. But it is like, it is already quite depressing.' The restricted agency of the food recipients means that due to their harsh economic situations, they rarely have a chance to decide whether or not make use of the assistance food without tremendous disadvantages. However, they rarely have the ability to express their needs, outlooks, and feelings related to the assistance, either. In many ways, their needs and aspirations remain overlooked.

4. Discussion

The above findings shed new light on the recipients of Finnish food aid from various perspectives. First, public perceptions of food aid in the online discussions often portray the recipients as dishonourable and responsible for their own poverty. At the same time, the quantitative data reveal that the main reason for people resorting to charity food aid is deep economic disadvantage. Furthermore, the quantitative data show that there is an unequal accumulation of disadvantage, illustrating the internal diversity within food aid recipients. Finally, observational and interview data show that from the food recipients' perspective, food aid provision disregards the material and social needs of the food recipients. The assistance system has only a limited capacity to meet even the recipients' immediate food needs, and for the food assistance recipients, food aid venues can become not only socially significant, but also socially demanding and emotionally burdening places.

Together, these findings point out some significant issues regarding food aid recipients. First, the findings from the online discussions indicate that from perspective of outsiders, the food aid recipients are often seen as a homogeneous group, alien to the majority population. Paradoxically, the life situations of the food aid recipients are often evaluated by arguing that there should not be severe poverty in a Finnish welfare state. As a result, if and when one is afflicted by poverty, the need for help is questioned and the individual is blamed [35]. Hence, it is important to gather empirical data to understand who the food recipients really are and what their socio-economic status is. The survey data of the food aid recipients bring facts to the public discussion, where the stereotypical picture of a food aid recipient is an uneducated, poor, typically male substance abuser standing in a breadline. The data can reveal the inner diversity of this group and the fact that many of the recipients are living in weak social and economic positions when compared to the wider Finnish population.

Second, the quantitative data reveal that food aid recipients suffer from economic, social, and health disadvantages. In addition, qualitative data show that they suffer from disadvantages in the form of social exclusion from the consumer practices of the wider population. Further, the findings indicate the inner polarization among food aid recipients: the survey data show that there is an accumulation of disadvantages in certain groups, while the qualitative analysis of the experiences of the food recipients highlight experiences of social exclusion and being left without.

Finally, on the level of public perceptions, food aid recipients are judged based on their perceived deservingness. However, at the same time, from the perspective of the food recipients the question arises of whether the available food aid meets their needs in the first place. The study of the food aid from the perspective of the Finnish food assistance recipients highlights the ambivalent social position that the recipients hold. First of all, they are excluded from ways of acquiring food that are customary in contemporary society. At the same time, they are dependent on the consumer practices of the affluent population that secure the continuous flow of excess. Second, socialization into the food aid community might promote the institutionalization of food aid on the individual level and entrench the food aid recipients' social exclusion from wider society. Food aid serves as an instrument for polarization that distances the life worlds of the disadvantaged people and the well-off majority. As seen in the findings from the online discussions, the public perceptions of food aid recipients feed back into these experiences and aggravate the social divide.

5. Conclusions

There are certain limitations to this study that should be taken into account when interpreting the findings. First of all, the data used in this article were collected some years ago already, and thus they do not present the most recent situation. From a research perspective, it is unfortunate that there are no up-to-date data readily available. On the other hand, this situation well illustrates the ad hoc and unorganized field of food aid in Finland. There are no registers or any other reliable data available about food aid recipients in Finland. Charity food aid recipients comprise one of the so-called hard-to-survey populations [36]: people receiving food aid tend to be hard to find or contact, as they are not found via post or phone surveys; they are occasionally difficult to persuade to participate, as going to food aid is stigmatizing for many; and being anonymous is important for some [37]. Furthermore, they can be difficult to interview, as there is not always a common language, some might be illiterate, some might be intoxicated, and some might be generally reluctant to take part in research. These are only some of the difficulties faced in interviewing food aid recipients. We have relied on data from 2012–2013, because they represent the first and so far only consistent quantitative information about the Finnish food aid users.

Second, it is worth noting that the data from the online discussions about food aid is not representative when it comes to the general populations' perceptions and attitudes. About 80% of Finns follow online media sources. Still, relatively few readers use the opportunity to comment on and discuss the news online. Strong opinions and active debaters gain the most visibility online [38]. However, keeping this limitation in mind, the online discussions provide an interesting viewpoint to approach public perceptions about food aid, because they offer—albeit in aggravated form—an indication of the traits that represent the general public's attitudes. Furthermore, the mindsets expressed online have the potential to spread outside the online debates, and thus it is helpful to be aware of them.

Third, since this article uses existing sources of data that have been each collected for the particular purposes of the original studies, one should be cautious when discussing the combined findings. In this article, we have settled on discussing the connections between different data sets descriptively instead of conducting cross-data analyses about each domain of the results. The discussion of the findings shows that different data sources complement each other, and together they help to paint a more nuanced picture of the reality in which food aid takes place in Finland and where the food aid recipients make do. Further research is needed that more thoroughly integrates discursive, demographic, and experiential insights into charity food provision and reception.

Despite these limitations, the study offers valuable insights into Finnish food aid, as it brings together the current body of knowledge about Finnish food aid recipients. In doing so, it shows that unlike in other Nordic countries such as Norway and Sweden, where the food aid clientele often represents the very margins of society [39,40], the recipients in Finland make up a relatively wide and diverse group. The food aid recipients are more typically of an older age, lower education, and lower income compared to the wider Finnish population. They are also more likely to have a weaker employment status and live in a one-person household. At the same time as the public debates about their deservingness, the food recipients themselves suffer from (often accumulated) economic, social, and health disadvantages. For them, the aid is important—if not necessary—to cope in their everyday life, even though they simultaneously struggle to make use of the aid, which does not always fall in line with their wants and needs.

Despite the general image of Finland as an affluent welfare state, there are tens of thousands of people who need to resort to charitable food aid in order to cope in their everyday lives. In February 2018, the annual fundraising campaign of the Finnish Lutheran Church, called the 'Common Responsibility Campaign' (*Yhteisvastuukeräys*), launched its annual campaign with the theme of hunger and poverty. With the domestic part of the proceeds, the campaign aims to provide one-off subsidies and food aid for low-income households in Finland. With its poignant hashtag #foodtrends, the campaign underlies the ambiguity of today's Finnish society where some people feast while others fast or starve [41]. This example illustrates that the issue of food aid is far from diminishing in Finnish society. Rather, it is becoming institutionalized, and it is gaining public recognition. One distinguishing feature of Finnish food aid has been the relative absence of a charitable culture attached to the aid; this is in contrast to the United States and Canada, for example, where private individuals and corporations are invited and encouraged to donate food for charitable purposes through prominent popular campaigns [42,43]. In the future, the proliferation of visible 'hunger campaigns' in Finland might influence who receives food aid, how the aid is experienced, and how its recipients are perceived by the public. More research is needed about food aid recipients in this changing landscape.

With charity food aid, the issues of poverty and food insecurity have been shifted to the margins and the purview of NGOs and third-sector voluntary aid. However, it is ideally a public responsibility to take care of people who experience poverty. Leaving the responsibility for the care of this vulnerable group to voluntary and religious actors indicates a neglect of the constitutional and basic rights of these people, especially the right to food [10,13].

Poor relief is always stigmatizing. People who receive last-resort charitable aid are exposed to public judgement, which is likely to weaken their well-being. Charity food aid also provokes discourses of deservingness that are alien to the universalist welfare model [24]. In the light of the findings, there is a legitimate need for assistance. However, this need cannot be met solely by giving people food as charity. Rather than deservingness, the focus of public concern ought to be on how the official social security system could be developed so that it can respond to the life situations of those who are afflicted by poverty. Mapping the actual needs and reasons for food aid use requires more research knowledge on the life worlds of the people who live in vulnerable social and economic positions.

Finally, charitable food aid venues are often one of the only places where the most deprived members of society can be found. This fact could be used as an asset when planning more effective ways to tackle poverty and food insecurity. Information and research knowledge about food aid in general, and food aid recipients' wellbeing and experiences in particular, should be systematically gathered and made available in order to alleviate poverty and food insecurity more effectively.

Author Contributions: Conceptualization, A.S.S.; Methodology, A.S.S., M.O. and T.L.; Formal Analysis, M.O. and T.L.; Investigation, A.S.S., M.O. and T.L.; Writing-Original Draft Preparation, A.S.S. and M.O; Writing-Review & Editing, A.S.S., M.O. and T.L.; Project Administration, A.S.S.

Appendix A

Table A1. Socio-economic background of food aid recipients compared to the general population in Finland (2012–2013).

	Food Aid Recipients		General Population of Finland
	N	**%**	**%**
Age (in full years)			
16–25	199	6	12.2
26–35	356	10.7	12.6
36–45	512	15.4	12.1
46–55	789	23.7	13.7
56–65	893	26.9	14.2
Over 65	574	17.3	18.8
Gender			
Male	1592	48.3	49.1
Female	1704	51.7	50.9
Nationality			
Finnish	2817	87.3	96.4
Other	410	12.7	3.6
Education			
Comprehensive school	1270	39.6	32
Upper secondary school/Vocational school	1282	40	40
University	656	20.4	28
Employment status			
At home	240	7.3	
Pensioner	1260	38.4	
Unemployed or laid off	1260	38.4	
Student	215	6.6	
Working fixed term or part-time	185	5.6	
Working under permanent contract	120	3.7	
Housing			
Home owner	527	16	59
Rental accommodation	2162	65.6	29.1
Council accommodation	408	12.4	
Supported living	408	2.8	
Homeless	109	3.3	0.15
Recipient of food aid during the last year			
A few times a year	752	23.9	-
Approximately once a month	633	20.1	-
Approximately every other week	816	25.9	-
Every week	952	30.2	-
Getting food			
Only for myself	1544	47.6	-
For myself and my family	1380	42.6	-
For myself and others	317	9.8	-
Number of adults in a household			
1	2024	60.5	41
2 or more	1324	39.5	59
Number of children in a household			
0	2403	71.6	
1	412	12.3	
2 or more	543	16.2	
Money (€) left after each month's compulsory outgoings			
0	607	20.5	
1–100	709	24	
101–300	913	30.9	
301–500	429	14.5	
Over 500	301	10.2	

References

1. Iivari, J.; Karjalainen, J. *Diakonian Köyhät. Epävirallinen Apu Perusturvan Paikkaajana*; Stakes: Helsinki, Finland, 1999.
2. Jokela, U. *Diakonian Paikka Ihmisten Arjessa*; Diak: Helsinki, Finland, 2011.

3. Juntunen, E.; Grönlund, H.; Hiilamo, H. *Viimeisellä Luukulla. Tutkimus Viimesijaisen Sosiaaliturvan Aukoista ja Diakoniatyön Kohdentumisesta*; Kirkkohallitus: Helsinki, Finland, 2006.

4. Kettunen, P. *Leipää vai Läsnäoloa? Asiakkaan Tarve ja Diakoniatyöntekijän Työnäky Laman Puristuksessa*; Kirkon Tutkimuskeskus: Tampere, Finland, 2001.

5. Siiki, A. Myllypuron ruokajono—Esimerkki hyvinvointiköyhyydestä. In *Toisten Pankki. Ruoka-Apu Hyvinvointivaltiossa*; Hänninen, S., Karjalainen, J., Lehtelä, K., Silvasti, T., Eds.; Stakes: Helsinki, Finland, 2008; pp. 127–161.

6. Laihiala, T. Kokemuksia ja Käsityksiä Leipäjonoista: Huono-Osaisuus, Häpeä ja Ansaitsevuus. Ph.D. Thesis, University of Eastern Finland, Kuopio, Finland, February 2018.

7. Ohisalo, M. Murusia Hyvinvointivaltion Pohjalla: Leipäjonot, Koettu Hyvinvointi ja Huono-Osaisuus. Ph.D. Thesis, University of Eastern Finland, Kuopio, Finland, June 2017.

8. Salonen, A.S. Food for the Soul or the Soul for Food: Users' Perspectives on Religiously Affiliated Food Charity in a Finnish City. Ph.D. Thesis, University of Helsinki, Helsinki, Finland, October 2016.

9. Riches, G.; Silvasti, T. (Eds.) *First World Hunger Revisited. Food Charity or The Right to Food*, 2nd ed.; Palgrave Macmillan: Basingstoke, UK, 2014.

10. Riches, G. *Food Bank Nations. Poverty, Corporate Charity and the Right to Food*; Routledge: London, UK; New York, NY, USA, 2018.

11. Caraher, M.; Cavicchi, A. Old crises on new plates or old plates for new crises? Food banks and food insecurity. *Br. Food J.* **2014**, *116*. [CrossRef]

12. Hiilamo, H. Rethinking the role of church in a socio-democratic welfare state. *Int. J. Sociol. Soc. Policy* **2012**, *32*, 401–414. [CrossRef]

13. Silvasti, T. Food aid—Normalising the abnormal in Finland. *Soc. Policy Soc.* **2015**, *14*, 471–482. [CrossRef]

14. Riches, G. Hunger, food security and welfare policies: Issues and debates in first world societies. *Proc. Nutr. Soc.* **1997**, *56*, 63–74. [CrossRef] [PubMed]

15. MacLeod, M. Understanding the Rise of Food Aid and Its Implications for the Welfare State: A study of Scotland and Finland. Ph.D. Thesis, University of Glasgow, Glasgow, UK, June 2018.

16. Silvasti, T. Elintarvikejärjestelmä globalisoituu—Ruokaturvasta yksityinen liikesuhde? In *Toisten Pankki. Ruoka-apu Hyvinvointivaltiossa*; Hänninen, S., Karjalainen, J., Lehtelä, K., Silvasti, T., Eds.; Stakes: Helsinki, Finland, 2008; pp. 241–262.

17. Silvasti, T.; Karjalainen, J. Hunger in a Nordic welfare state: Finland. In *First World Hunger Revisited. Food Charity or the Right to Food?* 2nd ed.; Riches, G., Silvasti, T., Eds.; Palgrave Macmillan: Basingstoke, UK, 2014; pp. 72–86.

18. Demokraatti.fi. Available online: https://demokraatti.fi/polemiikki-vantaan-sosiaalitoimi-ohjaa-leipajonoihin-arajarvi-loukkaavaa/ (accessed on 10 October 2018).

19. Kaks.fi. Available online: https://kaks.fi/uutiset/polemiikki-uutiset-professori-pentti-arajarvi-vantaan-leipajonotapauksesta-kyse-vakavasta-oireesta/ (accessed on 10 October 2018).

20. Ohisalo, M.; Eskelinen, N.; Laine, J.; Kainulainen, S.; Saari, J. *Avun Tilkkutäkki. Suomalaisen Ruoka-Apukentän Monimuotoisuus*; RAY: Helsinki, Finland, 2014.

21. Lehtelä, K.-M.; Kestilä, L. Kaksi vuosikymmentä ruoka-apua. In *Suomalaisten Hyvinvointi 2014*; Vaarama, M., Karvonen, S., Kestilä, L., Moisio, P., Muuri, A., Eds.; Terveyden ja Hyvinvoinnin Laitos: Helsinki, Finland, 2014; pp. 270–281.

22. Kirkkohallitus. *Kirkon Diakoniarahaston Avustustoiminta v. 2015. Kirkon Diakoniarahasto*; Kirkkohallitus: Helsinki, Finland, 2016; Available online: Http://sakasti.evl.fi/sakasti.nsf/0/E3537B3D390324C5C22578E10047CB71/$FILE/KDR%202015.pdf (accessed on 14 January 2017).

23. Tilastokeskus. Available online: https://www.stat.fi/til/tjt/2015/01/tjt_2015_01_2017-03-03_kat_001_fi.html (accessed on 26 November 2018).

24. Larsen, C.A. The Institutional Logic of Welfare Attitudes: How Welfare Regimes Influence Public Support. *Comp. Political Stud.* **2008**, *41*, 145–168. [CrossRef]

25. Van Oorschot, W. Who should get what and why? On deservingness criteria and the conditionality of solidarity among the public. *Policy Politics* **2000**, *28*, 33–48. [CrossRef]

26. Niemelä, M. Perceptions of the causes of poverty in Finland. *Acta Sociol.* **2008**, *51*, 23–40. [CrossRef]

27. Kallio, J.; Niemelä, M. Kuka ansaitsee tulla autetuksi? Kansalaisten asennoituminen toimeentulotuen saajiin Suomessa vuonna 2015. *Janus* **2017**, *25*, 144–159.

28.   Van der Horst, H.; Pascucci, S.; Bol, W. The 'dark side' of food banks? Exploring emotional responses of food bank receivers in the Netherlands. *Br. Food J.* **2014**, *116*, 1506–1520. [CrossRef]

29.   Findikaattori: Asuntokuntien Koko. Available online: https://findikaattori.fi/fi/93 (accessed on 10 October 2018).

30.   Vaarama, M.; Karvonen, S.; Kestilä, L.; Moisio, P.; Muuri, A. *Suomalaisten Hyvinvointi 2014*; Terveyden ja Hyvinvoinnin Laitos: Helsinki, Finland, 2014.

31.   Poppendieck, J. *Sweet Charity? Emergency Food and the End of Entitlement*; Penguin Books: New York, NY, USA, 1999.

32.   Tarasuk, V.; Eakin, J.M. Charitable food assistance as symbolic gesture: An ethnographic study of food banks in Ontario. *Soc. Sci. Med.* **2003**, *56*, 1505–1515. [CrossRef]

33.   Tarasuk, V.; Eakin, J.M. Food assistance through 'surplus' food: Insights from an ethnographic study of food bank work. *Agric. Hum. Values* **2005**, *22*, 177–186. [CrossRef]

34.   Kainulainen, S. Ruoka-avun hakijoiden hyvinvointi. In *Kuka Seisoo Leipäjonossa?* Ohisalo, M., Saari, J., Eds.; KAKS—Kunnallisalan Kehittämissäätiö: Helsinki, Finland, 2014; pp. 59–69.

35.   Goffman, E. *Stigma. Notes on the Management of Spoiled Identity*; Penguin Books: London, UK, 1963.

36.   Tourangeau, R.; Edwards, B.; Johnson, T.; Wolter, K.; Bates, N. *Hard-to-Survey Populations*; Cambridge University Press: Cambridge, UK, 2014.

37.   Laihiala, T.; Kallio, J.; Ohisalo, M. Personal and social shame among the recipients of charity food aid in Finland. *Res. Finn. Soc.* **2017**, *10*, 73–85.

38.   Pöyhtäri, R.; Haara, P.; Raittila, P. *Vihapuhe Sananvapautta Kaventamassa*; Tampere University Press: Tampere, Finland, 2013.

39.   Farnes, S.B.H. Fattigdom og Frivillig Velferd i Norge En Kvalitativ Studie av Brukere ved Robin Hood Huset i Bergen. Master's Thesis, Sosiologisk Institutt, Universitetet i Bergen, Bergen, Norway, 2014.

40.   Engebrigtsen, A.I.; Haug, A.V. *Evaluering av Tilskuddsordningen for Humanitære Tiltak til Tilreisende EØS-Borgere som Tigger*; NOVA Notat 2/2018; Norsk Institutt for Forskning om Oppvekst, Velferd og Aldring: Oslo, Norway, 2018.

41.   DeLind, L.B. Celebrating hunger in Michigan: A critique of an emergency food program and an alternative for the future. *Agric. Hum. Values* **1994**, *11*, 58–68. [CrossRef]

42.   Salonen, A.S. Religion, poverty and abundance. *Palgrave Commun.* **2018**, *4*, 1–5. [CrossRef]

43.   Caplan, P. *Feasts, Fasts, Famine: Food for Thought*; Berg Occasional Papers in Anthropology, No. 2; Berg Publishers: Oxford, UK, 1994.

6

Health-Promoting Food Pricing Policies and Decision-Making in Very Remote Aboriginal and Torres Strait Islander Community Stores in Australia

Megan Ferguson [1,2,*] [ID], Kerin O'Dea [3], Jon Altman [4], Marjory Moodie [5] and Julie Brimblecombe [2,6] [ID]

[1] School of Public Health, The University of Queensland, Brisbane 4072, Australia
[2] Wellbeing and Preventable Chronic Diseases, Menzies School of Health Research, Darwin 0811, Australia; julie.brimblecombe@monash.edu
[3] Division of Health Sciences, University of South Australia, Adelaide 5001, Australia; Kerin.O'Dea@unisa.edu.au
[4] Alfred Deakin Institute for Citizenship and Globalisation, Deakin University, Burwood 3125, Australia; jon.altman@anu.edu.au
[5] Deakin Health Economics, Centre for Population Health Research, Deakin University, Geelong 3220, Australia; marj.moodie@deakin.edu.au
[6] Faculty of Medicine, Nursing and Health Sciences, Monash University, Melbourne 3168, Australia
* Correspondence: megan.ferguson@uq.edu.au

Abstract: Aboriginal and Torres Strait Islander people living in remote communities in Australia experience a disproportionate burden of diet-related chronic disease. This occurs in an environment where the cost of store-purchased food is high and cash incomes are low, factors that affect both food insecurity and health outcomes. Aboriginal and Torres Strait Islander storeowners and the retailers who work with them implement local policies with the aim of improving food affordability and health outcomes. This paper describes health-promoting food pricing policies, their alignment with evidence, and the decision-making processes entailed in their development in community stores across very remote Australia. Semi-structured interviews were conducted with a purposive sample of retailers and health professionals identified through the snowball method, September 2015 to October 2016. Data were complemented through review of documents describing food pricing policies. A content analysis of the types and design of policies was undertaken, while the decision-making process was considered through a deductive, thematic analysis. Fifteen retailers and 32 health professionals providing services to stores participated. Subsidies and subsidy/price increase combinations dominated. Magnitude of price changes ranged from 5% to 25% on fruit, vegetables, bottled water, artificially sweetened and sugar sweetened carbonated beverages, and broadly used 'healthy/essential' and 'unhealthy' food classifications. Feasibility and sustainability were considered during policy development. Greater consideration of acceptability, importance, effectiveness and unintended consequences of policies guided by evidence were deemed important, as were increased involvement of Aboriginal and Torres Strait Islander storeowners and nutritionists in policy development. A range of locally developed health-promoting food pricing policies exist and partially align with research-evidence. The decision-making processes identified offer an opportunity to incorporate evidence, based on consideration of the local context.

Keywords: food security; diet-related chronic disease; policy; food pricing

1. Introduction

Aboriginal and Torres Strait Islander people living in remote areas generally experience the poorest health outcomes and hold the worst economic position in Australia [1,2]. Aboriginal and Torres Strait Islander people experience unemployment at 4.2 times, and have an average disposable income 70% of, non-Indigenous Australians [3]. Poverty is greatest for Aboriginal and Torres Strait Islander people living in very remote areas and is growing [2]. The life expectancy of Aboriginal and Torres Strait Islander people is approximately 10 years less than non-Indigenous Australians. The majority of this gap is due to chronic disease, especially cardiovascular disease and cancer, and injury for the 35–74 years age group [4]. The gap is largest in remote areas where Aboriginal and Torres Strait Islander people experience a burden 2.4 times that of non-Indigenous people [5]. Dietary intake is a key risk factor contributing to this gap [4,5].

Nutrient-rich traditional, non-market food continues to contribute to dietary intake [6], though the rapid nutrition transition resulting from colonization has led to a population diet high in sugar, salt and fat and low intakes of vegetables, fruit and other nutrient-rich foods [7]. In remote Aboriginal and Torres Strait Islander communities, Western foods are predominantly purchased from the single retail food outlet, referred to as the store, operating in a challenging, remote environment, which contributes to the high cost of food. Many stores are community-owned, providing a unique opportunity for local policy development [8].

The remote store landscape has undergone considerable change in the last decade, particularly in policy and services. In 2008, a Close the Gap statement of intent was agreed to by a number of Aboriginal and Torres Strait Islander people and organizations and the Australian Government [9]. In the same year, the Council of Australian Governments released the Closing the Gap Strategy that aimed to achieve health equity within 25 years [10] and in 2009 developed the National Strategy for Food Security in Remote Indigenous Communities which linked food security (i.e., the ability to acquire appropriate and nutritious food in a regular and socially acceptable manner) and nutrition with the national Closing the Gap targets [11]. Two years prior to this in the Northern Territory (NT) of Australia, the Northern Territory Emergency Response was implemented and included a number of measures indirectly related to food 'security'. One of these was for the compulsory income management of welfare recipients [12] (i.e., restriction of available cash and purchase of specific products), which has since been extended beyond the NT [13]. A second measure was the introduction of a regulatory framework for the operation of remote stores, including minimum standards relating to food security; this remains effective today [14]. The Australian National Audit Office reports however, that government policies have made minimal contribution to addressing food insecurity in remote communities [15]. Reports on the Closing the Gap targets show mixed outcomes, though importantly that the target to close the life expectancy gap is not on track [10] and that outcomes are worse in remote than non-remote areas [2]. The Productivity Commission highlights the importance of developing an evaluation culture in Aboriginal and Torres Strait Islander policy where policy evaluation informs future policy [16].

During this time of policy change there has also been a growth in organizations that provide retail management services to remote community storeowners, alongside an increasing recognition of the role that the stores play in the health of the communities [17–21]. The historical tension between economic and health outcomes may be giving way as organizations publicly demonstrate valuing health outcomes as an objective of sustainable business [19,21–25]. In remote Aboriginal and Torres Strait Islander community stores, there are examples of local policies (i.e., the rules of operation determined by the governing body [26]), which aim to promote health outcomes within a sustainable business model [24,25,27]. There is significant opportunity in this dynamic remote retail context to work with storeowners and the systems they operate within to influence local store food policy to create health-promoting environments.

Food pricing is considered one of the more effective practices to influence consumer purchasing patterns [28]. Health-promoting food pricing policies exist in remote stores, but there is little understanding of the decision-making process informing their design development including the magnitude of the price increase or decrease and promotion of the policy [29]. Policy analysis can help understand the process of design development and thereby identify opportunities to strengthen design and improve health outcomes through the store [30,31]. Policy development models have evolved to consider trade-offs between multiple and often conflicting objectives [32]; they may have utility in understanding efforts in the remote retail context where governing bodies deal with the dual and potentially conflicting objectives of consumer health outcomes alongside commercial viability of stores. Decision-making which incorporates evidence will hopefully lead to consideration of a greater range of policy options and result in more effective outcomes [33].

This paper describes health-promoting food pricing policies including their alignment with evidence, and the decision-making processes in their development in very remote Aboriginal and Torres Strait Islander community stores in Australia. We specifically refer to 'food policy' as the local-level food policy implemented in stores aimed at modifying the price of food/beverages in order to promote health.

2. Methods

2.1. Context

Approximately 175 stores supply food in some of the 1187 discrete Indigenous communities in remote locations across Australia [8,34]. A total of 92,960 Aboriginal and Torres Strait Islander people and a small number of non-Indigenous people reside in these communities. Seventeen communities have a population greater than 1000 and almost 75% are located in very remote locations [34]. Our study included very remote communities only [35]. These are located largely in the NT, Queensland (Qld), South Australia (SA) and Western Australia (WA). Some stores are owned by the government or are privately owned, though the most common model is of incorporated community ownership where Aboriginal and Torres Strait Islander residents comprise the membership. These stores function as either not-for-profit or business enterprises and are often responsive to community priorities. The owners of community-owned stores employ a store manager/s or engage the services of a retail organization to manage the store's operation, with the latter model accounting for approximately 55% of stores in remote Aboriginal and Torres Strait Islander communities in Australia [17–21]. In addition to operating an effective retail operation, a number of stores and retail organizations aim to employ local Aboriginal and Torres Strait Islander people and promote positive nutrition outcomes and healthy lifestyles [8].

2.2. Design

A qualitative study was conducted that applied a methodology informed by Thow's framework used in the Pacific Region. This framework was informed by policy theories related to lesson drawing to understand the form of food policies and how to engage with policy-makers [30]. It was successfully used to describe the common elements of policy processes across the diversity of policy processes identified in different countries in the Pacific Region. Our methodology was informed by this framework as we similarly anticipated a diversity of policy processes across different remote communities, states and territories and governance models. We first focused on determining the range of pricing policies in place in remote stores and secondly on an understanding the stages of the process [32], the people involved [30,33], identification of objectives [32], consideration of assessment criteria applied [32] including a list of pre-determined criteria previously used in food policy assessment (i.e., feasibility, sustainability, acceptability, importance, effectiveness, unintended consequences [36–39]), and the evidence considered.

2.3. Data

Purposive sampling was employed, informed by the snowball method, to maximize coverage of the types of policies implemented. Participants were: (i) retailers, who were the store managers employed by the owners of a community store or store managers and retail management staff employed by a retail organization, and (ii) health professionals, including public health nutritionists (hereafter, nutritionists) and others working in roles with stores employed by a retail organization, government or non-government organization. Participants were required to identify that they had knowledge of health-promoting food pricing policy in remote Aboriginal and Torres Strait Islander community stores. At least one retailer and where applicable, the nutritionist from each of five retail organizations representing the majority of these entities, and all nutritionists in service provision and food supply policy known to Megan Ferguson and Julie Brimblecombe operating in remote NT, Qld, SA and WA, were invited to participate. Participants were invited by email from the lead researcher or by a potential participant in the study. This study did not seek to quantify policy implementation by store, store governance model or state/territory.

A semi-structured interview guide was used in all interviews. It focused on two sets of data. The first was the health-promoting food pricing policies in stores. We included price increases and subsidies in the form of price discounts, rewards, vouchers and free product give-away. We excluded takeaway food outlets as a setting and government policy instruments that might impact on food purchases such as income management. The second set of data focused on the decision-making process for one of the policies reported. Interviews lasted on average 50 min, and were conducted by Megan Ferguson, a nutritionist who has worked in both the remote health and retail sectors. This background was important in terms of understanding the context and relating to participants' experiences. Interviews were conducted in English, in person or by phone. In one case, responses to the interview questions were e-mailed by a participant. Participants provided consent and all interviews were audio-recorded, transcribed verbatim and returned to participants for checking. Documents describing food pricing policies were sourced or provided by participants and used to complement interview data. Data were uploaded and managed in NVivo (QSR International Pty Ltd. Version 11, Melbourne, Victoria, Australia, 2012). Ethical approval for this study was provided by Human Research Ethics Committees in the NT (HREC NTDHMSHR 2012–1711; CAHREC HREC-12-13; CDU HREC H12096), Qld (FNQ HREC HREC/16/QCH/35-1041) and WA (WACHS HREC 2016/13; WAAHEC 715; KAHPF 2016-006). Informed consent was obtained from all participants.

2.4. Analysis

The dataset was reviewed independently by two researchers, Megan Ferguson and Julie Brimblecombe, who have extensive research, policy and practice experience in the remote retail and health sectors. This strengthened the analysis by ensuring research quality and relevance. The authors discussed and agreed on the coding framework. The data were coded by Megan Ferguson and the findings reviewed with Julie Brimblecombe.

Firstly, a data content analysis relating to the types and design of food pricing policies was conducted, with allowance for additional codes. The coding framework included the following: Under the three pre-determined codes, *subsidy, price increase, subsidy/price increase combination*; the sub-codes relating to each code of *targeted food or beverage, magnitude of price change, duration, administration, complementary strategies, other design elements*; and, a fourth emergent code, *business fundamentals*. Secondly, a deductive, thematic analysis of the decision-making process was conducted to identify why, how and who was involved.

3. Results

3.1. Participants

Between September 2015 and October 2016, 47 interviews were conducted with 15 retailers, 28 nutritionists and four health professionals servicing communities in NT, Qld, WA and SA. Forty-two more people were invited to participate by Megan Ferguson; two delegated the interview invitation to staff under their supervision, 21 did not respond to the email invitation and 19 declined, with the most common response being that they did not have sufficient knowledge relevant to the study objectives.

3.2. Health-Promoting Food Pricing Policies

The most commonly implemented food pricing policies across very remote Australia were subsidies and subsidy/price increase combinations as shown in Table 1. These policies mostly targeted fruit, vegetables, bottled water, artificially sweetened and sugar sweetened carbonated beverages, in addition to groups of foods broadly referred to as 'healthy/essential' foods and 'unhealthy' foods. Magnitude of price changes ranged from 5% to 25%. The policies were largely ongoing. A number of these, predominantly those targeting fruit, vegetables and 'healthy/essential' and 'unhealthy' foods, had been in place for many years including in some locations for over 35 years, where the beverage policies were first introduced in 2010. Short-term discounts were applied more recently and were usually up to two weeks duration. Stores generally funded the long-term policies, such as fruit and vegetables discounts, while more recently implemented policies were partly funded by the suppliers and manufacturers. Pricing policies were at times supported by one or more merchandising strategies involving product availability (e.g., specific brand, quality), placement (e.g., shelf space allocation, planograms) and promotion (e.g., in-store announcements, use of local celebrities), though implementation of these strategies seemed more ad hoc than planned. Promotion of the ongoing pricing policies did not occur and was identified as a missed opportunity in communicating the policy to customers.

> *"I reckon that it is not visible to the average person in terms of what pricing policies stores have . . . and therefore not as effective. . . . I don't think that translates to the customer that they're getting a good deal on whatever they're getting a good deal on."* (Interviewee 47, Health professional)

Finally, retailers and health professionals stressed the requirement of efficient and effective retail operations as the key condition for the development of health-promoting pricing policies.

3.3. Decision-Making

3.3.1. Process of Decision-Making

The process of decision-making reported included some level of deliberation and procedure, though this was generally described as flexible. The processes described by those in retail organizations were more structured with specific stages of development, than those described for stores operating independently. However, there were often more people involved in the decision-making processes of retail organizations than in individual community stores.

Table 1. Health-promoting food pricing policies in very remote Aboriginal and Torres Strait Islander community stores in Australia.

Food/Beverage Targeted	Impact on Selling Price	Duration	Administration
Subsidy—Price discount			
Fruit and vegetables—all fresh	**Approximately 20% to 25% discount or equal to, to ≤30% of urban retail prices**	**Ongoing**	**Store**
Fruit and vegetables—all fresh, frozen, canned and dried	**Approximately 20% discount**	**Ongoing**	**Store**
Water—bottled	**Various, example $0.53, $1.00 and $2.00 for 600 mL**	**Ongoing**	**Store and manufacturer**
Fruit and vegetables—a small range of fresh items	5% to 10% discount or comparable to urban retail prices	Short-term, rotating	Store and supplier
Dairy products—fresh milk, yoghurt and cheese	Approximately 20% discount	Ongoing	Store
Dairy products—low-fat fresh milks	Low-fat milk retailed for the price of full cream milk	Ongoing	Store; Store and manufacturer
Bread—multigrain and wholemeal bread	$1.00 less than white bread	Ongoing	Store
Healthy foods [1]	n/a	Ongoing and short-term	Store; Store and supplier
Beverages—bottled water and artificially sweetened soft-drink	Various, example bulk packs of bottled water retailing for less than the equivalent volume achieved in single units	Short-term, rotating	Store and manufacturer
Subsidy—Reward			
Fruit and vegetables—fresh; fresh, frozen, canned and dried	Various, example a $10 fruit and vegetable gift following a $20 fruit and vegetable purchase	Short-term, including feasibility assessment	Store; Health organization [2]
Fruit, vegetables, meat [3] and bottled water	$25 voucher for health assessment participation	Ongoing	Health organization
Subsidy—Free			
Water—chilled via a bubbler outside the store	Free	Ongoing	Store
Price increase			
Sugar sweetened carbonated beverages	19% increase	Ongoing	Store
Sugar sweetened carbonated beverages	$0.30 increase per 375 mL can and $1.00 per 1.25 L bottle	Ongoing	Store
Subsidy/price increase combination			
Reduction on healthy foods and increase on unhealthy foods [1]	**n/a**	**Ongoing**	**Store**
Reduction on artificially sweetened carbonated beverages and increase on sugar sweetened carbonated beverages	**Various ranging from 6% to 22%, and in places a widening gap** [4]	**Ongoing**	**Store; Stores and manufacturer**

Note: The policies most commonly reported are in bold (i.e., subsidy on fruit and vegetables—all fresh; fruit and vegetables—all fresh, frozen, canned and dried; water—bottled and subsidy/price increase combination on healthy and unhealthy foods and artificially sweetened carbonated and sugar sweetened carbonated beverages). All values are in AUD (AUD1.00 = USD0.77 in 2016). [1] Healthy and unhealthy foods were not specified though healthy foods often reported to include commodity groups which were largely though not solely considered to be healthy/core foods such as fruit, vegetables, bread, milk, meat, eggs and infant foods, or items deemed to be essential food items such as tea, sugar and margarine and unhealthy foods often reported to include foods commonly considered to be discretionary foods such as crisps, confectionery, chocolate, biscuits, bakery lines and sugar sweetened beverages. [2] Health organization is a local or regional Aboriginal health organization. [3] Meat included lean and non-lean cuts of meat. [4] It was unclear if this price gap always included a price increase to sugar sweetened carbonated beverages.

3.3.2. Decision-Makers

Three groups of people were identified as being involved in policy development, namely retailers, nutritionists employed by retail organizations, and Aboriginal and Torres Strait Islander and non-Indigenous store committee/board members. There were a few cases where nutritionists or health professionals employed by the health sector contributed directly to the process. Retailers and/or nutritionists employed by retail organizations reported that they primarily identified the need for, and designed policies, though the need for a policy was said to be identified sometimes by Aboriginal and Torres Strait Islander storeowners.

"...we are working with (X) communities at the moment to reduce the sale of full sugar soft drink. And I must note the communities or the storeowners approached us about it. So we talk about the health stats every quarter. But now that there's more education around you know, the impacts of diet and poor health and those things. Now storeowners are saying, 'What can we do to improve these outcomes?'" (Interviewee 40, Retailer)

Policies were reported to be approved by the store committee/board, and at times, by retailers. Examples were provided where store committees/boards were reported to actively direct and monitor policy, whereas others provided support or opposition to policy proposals initiated by retailers.

3.3.3. Policy Objectives

Price manipulation was seen by most participants as a means to increase purchases of healthy foods and to reduce purchases of unhealthy foods and hence improve the quality of dietary intake, with participants acknowledging the high rates of overweight and obesity, diet-related chronic diseases and lower life expectancy of Aboriginal and Torres Strait Islander people. A second policy objective described, although to a lesser extent, was one of addressing equity and providing access to healthy food at prices comparable to that of all Australians.

These two objectives were not considered in isolation, with operating costs and commercial viability raised largely, though not solely, by retailers as significant pertinent factors. The cost of food to the store was seen as a significant barrier in implementing health-promoting pricing policies. Participants described the balance required between pricing and profit. Examples were described where storeowners chose to invest their profits in reduced food prices. It was proposed that there is an opportunity to reframe the discourse around profit, by engaging new terms such as 'retailing for health.'

3.3.4. Decision-Making Criteria

Participants were first asked about the use of six predetermined criteria in policy-making in their context. They were then asked which criteria they considered most important to the process and to identify any gaps in the criteria used. These predetermined criteria were feasibility, sustainability, effectiveness, importance, acceptability and unintended consequences. In describing which criteria were applied, participants described the meaning these criteria had in their context.

Feasibility and sustainability were reported by both retailers and health professionals to be considered in the policy-making processes. A feasible policy was described as one which is achievable in both economic and practical terms, including being a good fit with the existing system, aligning with the available human resource skill set and capacity and the supply of product and infrastructure required to deliver the policy. A sustainable policy was considered to be one which could be continued or scaled-up. A small number of health professionals viewed sustainability as the need for a policy to have appeal to, or be aligned with government policy.

The potential effectiveness of a policy was considered by both retailers and health professionals in policy-making though often with a caveat, such as they 'assumed', 'hoped', or 'thought' a policy might be effective, rather than describing having confidence in a policy's potential effectiveness. Participants referred to policy as being influenced by the poor population-level health status of Aboriginal and

Torres Strait Islander people and current and recommended dietary intake. Rarely however, was research-informed evidence of effectiveness reported to inform policy development.

Participants reported less consideration of the criteria of importance and acceptability. Importance included an assessment of how worthwhile a policy was considered, which was almost solely related to health outcomes. Acceptability related to a policy's appropriateness to the recipients (i.e., customers) and implementers (i.e., store managers). Both retailers and health professionals reported that it was important to have community buy-in, or that policies be community-driven or at least community-partnered and support capacity enhancement of Aboriginal and Torres Strait Islander storeowners.

Unintended consequences were rarely reported as being considered, though where they were, this was by both retailers and health professionals.

"Unintended consequences—I don't think we really considered at all. It's definitely not, if we do, if we drop the price of milk, what will happen next? I don't think we considered that at all. We, our presumption is always that they (i.e., customers) will continue to spend more money in the store." (Interviewee 9, Retailer)

Unintended consequences were perceived as factors that may positively or negatively impact on a health or business outcome. Organization or store brand image and positive or negative publicity were highlighted as emerging unintended consequences that were perceived to impact on business outcomes and recently informed policy development. In relation to health outcomes, one retailer referred to the group of Aboriginal and Torres Strait Islander storeowners he worked with, considering equity across the population in policy development.

Participants were asked to nominate criteria that they considered most important to decision-making and any gaps. All six pre-determined criteria were considered important to decision-making, with the exception that approximately half of the retailers considered assessment of unintended consequences as unnecessary. The order of importance placed on these criteria was generally considered to be context- and policy-specific. No new criteria were identified.

3.3.5. Evidence Informing Decision-Making

There was limited use of research-informed evidence in the processes reported. The three key forms of information used largely originated from the retail sector. Firstly, health professionals, more so than retailers, noted the 'diffusion of ideas' or benchmarking as a method which commonly informed local policy. Policy was also informed by food price survey reports and urban store pricing. Secondly, retailers and health professionals referred to the use of store sales in a variety of ways: to conduct retail modelling to inform policy design, to measure retail performance and sales of a targeted product when a pricing policy is implemented, and to provide ongoing monitoring to staff and storeowners in relation to top sellers or targeted products. A reliable point-of-sale system was seen as a requirement for implementing pricing policies, as was the importance of understanding data and disseminating user-friendly reports.

"So a Board that's not getting nutritional reports back to them, from the store is really not being told enough of the key information. ... So that it's always in their mind and they can see what the store's doing and then they start to think about their own, well, what if we did this, why can't we do that, you know. 'Cause management (i.e., retailers) doesn't have all the answers." (Interviewee 23, Retailer)

The third key information source described was retail, and especially remote retail, industry knowledge. Retailers often described their thinking as influenced by employing the strategies known to work in the retail industry to promote or disincentivize targeted products to shape a health-promoting environment.

3.4. Strengthening the Decision-Making Process

3.4.1. Supporting Roles of Decision-Makers

The Aboriginal and Torres Strait Islander and non-Indigenous store committee/board members, retailers and nutritionists, and the relationships between these decision-makers were considered crucial to the process. Opportunities to enhance the current process were proposed: (i) to further support/engage Aboriginal and Torres Strait Islander storeowners, staff and customers in the identification and design of policies, and (ii) to support greater participation of nutritionists, by addressing barriers which included nutritionists either not having the opportunity or not recognizing a role for themselves or their capacity to contribute to policy-making.

Suppliers, whilst not considered to be central to the decision-making process, appeared to have an increasing support role as shown in Table 1. Some suppliers were reported to be supportive having shared values; others, however, were seen as having a poor understanding of the context and promoted unhealthy products even as retailers tried to secure deals on healthy products.

3.4.2. Accessing and Strengthening the Evidence Base

Retailers and health professionals identified three forms of evidence as being potentially useful to the process. The first was accessing research-informed evidence through user-friendly dissemination methods.

> "...all the journal articles and big reports and what not are nice, but even people within our (health) organization wanted like almost sound bites, like stories and we needed options in the community and say, 'This is what's been done before, here's the stories and you can choose from these options.'" (Interviewee 11, Health professional)

The second was further development of locally-informed evidence through improved evaluation and timely feedback to communities. Time and resources were identified as the limiting factor in conducting quality evaluation, not the lack of data. Notably, retailers and health professionals referred to reduced capacity to support activities such as evaluation owing to government funding cuts, resulting in the loss of nutritionist positions in retail and non-government organizations dedicated to working with stores. The third was a better understanding of the factors that drive purchasing decisions, including income and cost of living data and the impact of price on the purchasing of targeted products. Participants sensed that price elasticity of demand varied for different products, that price impacted differently across population groups and that customer response to price is changing. There was also a sense that customers generally may not have all the necessary information available to them in a useable form to make an informed purchasing decision in relation to price.

4. Discussion

Health-promoting food pricing policies implemented in very remote Aboriginal and Torres Strait Islander community stores in Australia were dominated by subsidies and subsidy/price increase combinations. These had a small to moderate impact on food prices of fruit, vegetables, bottled water, artificially sweetened and sugar sweetened carbonated beverages, and broadly used 'healthy/essential' and 'unhealthy' food classifications. Decision-making was a deliberative process, which evaluated policy feasibility and sustainability, though generally lacked incorporation of research-informed evidence.

4.1. Designing Health-Promoting Food Pricing Policy

The dominance of subsidies and subsidy/price increases reported in this study is in line with recommendations to support healthier choices in low socioeconomic populations with the subsidy/price increase combination possibly mitigating concerns about the potential regressive nature of taxes [40,41]. The range of products targeted only partially align with the current evidence. The lack of criteria applied to the 'healthy' category for example, results in a misalignment with guidelines for good health and a lost opportunity to promote a healthy diet. Targeting artificially sweetened carbonated beverages may not support positive health outcomes as reducing the price of these is unlikely to decrease the consumption of sugar sweetened carbonated beverages [42–45]. Additionally, there are calls for a greater focus on policy targeting discretionary foods [43,46]. Magnitude of price changes were at best in line with recommendations for modifying purchasing [47]. Equity was the objective of decision-making in some cases, and the magnitude of the price changes went some way to achieving this [48]. The ongoing nature of most policies which are not routinely advertised to customers prevented the use of price as a signal to customers; this was described by participants and supported by others as a significant missed opportunity [49].

Food pricing policies in this context which aim to improve health would be more aligned with research evidence if there was: (i) further targeting of products (e.g., specify healthy foods, foods likely to have a greater response to price changes [43]); (ii) increased magnitude of price change [47,50]; (iii) use of price and price promotion to send a signal to customers, such as through a price increase alone or dynamic, rotating subsidies and promoting the change in price to customers [29,47,49,51]. Policies need to be assessed within the local context and may require new avenues for funding, such as by manufacturers, suppliers and wholesalers, by government or through evaluation of current food pricing policy or funds dispersal.

4.2. Enhancing Policy Development Processes

This analysis indicates that the process of decision-making was deliberative [32]. Improved health, and to a lesser extent equity, were key objectives in the decision-making process. These objectives of health and equity inform policy development differently, including the sources of evidence required. Whilst assessment of effectiveness was considered a priority, participant response and the design of current policies, indicates limited use of research-informed evidence. Although consideration of unintended consequences was not universally viewed as important to the process, research-informed evidence would go some way to inform the assessment of this criterion whether it was explicitly included or not. Acceptability and importance were not well-considered criteria, although they were regarded a priority and likely to be best addressed through further engagement with Aboriginal and Torres Strait Islander storeowners and others they elect to involve. Given articulating and communicating problems is a crucial stage in decision-making [32], the processes reported in this context are likely to be improved with further assessment of the criteria, acceptability, importance, effectiveness and unintended consequences of potential policies. The processes were generally focused on a single policy rather than evaluation of a suite of options. They were based on analysis of retail data, informed by an assessment of cost in terms of retail impact though not cost-effectiveness, nor health impact, and limited in terms of robust monitoring and evaluation. Greater incorporation of research-informed evidence into the design of food pricing policies which have an objective of dietary or health improvement, is likely to result in more effective policy, and was called for by study participants [33].

Complex policy with multiple and potentially conflicting objectives, is likely to create tension [32]. There appears to be a shift in the well-documented tension between commercial profit and health outcomes in remote stores [22,23]. Opportunities exist for well-designed health-promoting food pricing policies to be considered within the suite of business practices by storeowners, and precedent has been set for this as described in our study. Currently, retailers are front and center of the decision-making process in remote stores, hence the reliance on retail-focused evidence and criteria in the decision-making process. Current processes offer opportunities to further progress health-promoting policy, such as using the role of benchmarking against other stores and organizations as a potential mechanism for dissemination of good practice. Mechanisms to support decision-makers to access research-informed evidence and to assess acceptability, importance and unintended consequences of policies for the local context could lead to more effective health-promoting policies.

This might involve a greater role for Aboriginal and Torres Strait Islander storeowners and nutritionists in decision-making.

4.3. Strengths and Limitations

This study has captured the views and experiences of retailers and health professionals across remote Aboriginal and Torres Strait Islander communities in Australia. Effort was made to ensure retailers operating in independent stores were included, though without a census of all stores, this is a more challenging cohort to identify and locate. The resources for this study did not allow for the conduct of interviews in remote communities with Aboriginal and Torres Strait Islander store committee/board members. Interviewing those persons known to work closely with storeowners provided insight into the roles and processes which could be further explored. Participants were invited to contribute where health-promoting food pricing policies were implemented and as such, this is likely to represent the best-case scenario rather than the situation in all remote Aboriginal and Torres Strait Islander community stores. The case considered was food pricing policies, and the process of policy development may be different to that of other health-promoting food policies in stores.

5. Conclusions

Remote Aboriginal and Torres Strait Islander community stores provide a crucial setting if health outcomes of their customers are to improve. While owners and operators face major challenges, community ownership provides an opportunity to make a difference to the foods purchased from community stores. The urgency of the situation for Aboriginal and Torres Strait Islander storeowners and those who work to support them is not unlike that of low- and middle-income countries currently leading the way in implementing food-related policies [31,52]. This study identifies opportunities that exist to further shape the store food environment through incorporation of research-informed evidence. In doing so, it offers lessons on how locally-developed and -implemented policies can be formulated to shape other food retail environments for health outcomes. However, addressing equity and positively shaping healthy retail environments should not be a task for storeowners and retailers alone. There is a role for government, manufacturers and wholesalers to work with Aboriginal and Torres Strait Islander storeowners and those who support their efforts, to implement evidence-informed policy to support healthy environments.

Author Contributions: Conceptualization, M.F.; data curation, M.F.; formal analysis, M.F., J.B.; validation, J.B., K.O., J.A. and M.M.; investigation, M.F.; resources, M.F.; writing—original draft preparation, M.F.; writing—review and editing, K.O., J.A., M.M, J.B.; supervision, J.B., K.O., J.A. and M.M.; project administration, M.F.; funding acquisition, M.F.

Acknowledgments: The authors are grateful to the study participants for providing such valuable insights into food policy decision-making in stores across very remote Australia. We are grateful to Anthony Gunther for his review of the manuscript.

References

1. Vos, T.; Barker, B.; Begg, S.; Stanley, L.; Lopez, A.D. Burden of disease and injury in Aboriginal and Torres Strait Islander Peoples: The Indigenous health gap. *Int. J. Epidemiol.* **2009**, *38*, 470–477. [CrossRef]
2. Markham, F.; Biddle, N. *Income, Poverty and Inequality, CAEPR 2016 Census Paper No. 2*; Centre for Aboriginal Economic Policy Research; The Australian National University: Canberra, Australia, 2018.
3. Australian Institute of Health and Welfare. *The Health and Welfare of Australia's Aboriginal and Torres Strait Islander Peoples 2015*; Cat. No. IHW 147; AIHW: Canberra, Australia, 2015.

4.   Australian Institute of Health and Welfare. *Australia's Health 2016*; Australia's Health Series No. 15. Cat. No. AUS 199; AIHW: Canberra, Australia, 2016.

5.   Australian Institute of Health and Welfare. *Australian Burden of Disease Study: Impact and Causes of Illness and Death in Aboriginal and Torres Strait Islander People 2011*; AIHW: Canberra, Australia, 2016.

6.   Ferguson, M.; Brown, C.; Georga, C.; Miles, E.; Wilson, A.; Brimblecombe, J. Traditional food availability and consumption in remote Aboriginal communities in the Northern Territory, Australia. *Aust. N. Z. J. Public Health* **2017**, *41*, 294–298. [CrossRef]

7.   Brimblecombe, J.; Ferguson, M.; Liberato, S.; O'Dea, K. Characteristics of the community-level diet of Aboriginal people in remote northern Australia. *Med. J. Aust.* **2013**, *198*, 380–384. [CrossRef]

8.   House of Representatives Aboriginal and Torres Strait Islander Affairs Committee. *Everybody's Business Remote Aboriginal and Torres Strait Community Stores*; Commonwealth of Australia: Canberra, Australia, 2009.

9.   Australian Human Rights Commission. Close the Gap: Indigenous Health Equality Summit—Statement of Intent. Available online: https://www.humanrights.gov.au/publications/close-gap-indigenous-health-equality-summit-statement-intent (accessed on 18 September 2017).

10. Commonwealth of Australia, Department of the Prime Minister and Cabinet. *Closing the Gap Prime Minister's Report 2017*; Commonwealth of Australia: Canberra, Australia, 2017.

11. Council of Australian Governments. National Strategy for Food Security in Remote Indigenous Communities. Available online: http://webarchive.nla.gov.au/gov/20130329094202/http://www.coag.gov.au/node/92 (accessed on 18 September 2017).

12. Altman, J.; Klein, E. Lessons from a basic income programme for Indigenous Australians. *Oxf. Dev. Stud.* **2017**, *46*, 132–146. [CrossRef]

13. Parliament of Australia. Social Services Legislation Amendment (Cashless Debit Card) Bill 2017. Available online: http://www.aph.gov.au/Parliamentary_Business/Committees/Senate/Community_Affairs/CashlessDebitCard (accessed on 18 September 2017).

14. Australian Government. *Stronger Futures in the Northern Territory: A Ten Year Commitment to Aboriginal People in the Northern Territory July 2012*; Commonwealth of Australia: Canberra, Australia, 2012.

15. Australian National Audit Office. *Food Security in Remote Indigenous Communities*; Commonwealth of Australia; Commonwealth of Australia: Canberra, Australia, 2014.

16. Productivity Commission. *National Indigenous Reform Agreement, Performance Assessment 2013-4*; Commonwealth of Australia: Canberra, Australia, 2015.

17. Regional Merchandising Solutions. Homepage. Available online: http://regionalmerchandising.com.au/ (accessed on 19 December 2016).

18. Outback Stores. Map of Stores. Available online: http://outbackstores.com.au/map-of-stores/ (accessed on 19 December 2016).

19. Community Enterprise Queensland. Store Locations. Available online: http://www.ceqld.org.au/store-locations/ (accessed on 17 July 2017).

20. The Arnhem Land Progress Aboriginal Corporation. Where We Operate. Available online: http://www.alpa.asn.au/pages/Where-we-operate.html (accessed on 19 December 2016).

21. Mai Wiru. Mai Wiru Stores. Available online: http://www.maiwiru.org.au/stores (accessed on 19 December 2016).

22. Department of Health. *FoodNorth: Food for Health in North Australia*; Government of Western Australia: Perth, Australia, 2003.

23. Brimblecombe, J. *Enough for Rations and a Little Bit Extra: Challenges of Nutrition Improvement in an Aboriginal Community in North-East Arnhem Land*; Charles Darwin University: Darwin, Australia, 2007.

24. The Arnhem Land Progress Aboriginal Corporation. Nutrition Policy. Available online: http://www.alpa.asn.au/pages/Nutrition-Policy.html (accessed on 9 February 2014).

25. Outback Stores. Nutrition Strategy. Available online: http://outbackstores.com.au/wp-content/uploads/2013/09/Nutrition-Strategy.pdf (accessed on 11 February 2014).

26. Guba, E.G. The effect of definitions of policy on the nature and outcomes of policy anlaysis. *Educ. Leadersh.* **1984**, *42*, 63–70.

27. Nganampa Health Council and Ngaanyatjarra Pitjantjatjara Yankunytjatjara Women's Council. *Mai Wiru—Process. and Policy Regional Stores Policy and Associated Regulations for the Anangu Pitjantjatjara Lands*; Nganampa Health Council and Ngaanyatjarra Pitjantjatjara Yankunytjatjara Women's Council: Alice Springs, Australia, 2002.

28. Chandon, P.; Wansink, B. Does food marketing need to make us fat? A review and solutions. *Nutr. Rev.* **2012**, *70*, 571–593. [CrossRef]

29. Ferguson, M.; O'Dea, K.; Holden, S.; Miles, E.; Brimblecombe, J. Food and beverage price discounts to improve health in remote Aboriginal communities: Mixed method evaluation of a natural experiment. *Aust. N. Z. J. Public Health* **2016**, *41*, 32–37. [CrossRef]

30. Thow, A.M.; Swinburn, B.; Colagiuri, S.; Diligolevu, M.; Quested, C.; Vivili, P.; Leeder, S. Trade and food policy: Case studies from three Pacific Island countries. *Food Policy* **2010**, *35*, 556–564. [CrossRef]

31. Thow, A.; Quested, C.; Juventin, L.; Kun, R.; Khan, A.; Swinburn, B. Taxing soft drinks in the Pacific: Implementation lessons for improving health. *Health Promot. Int.* **2011**, *26*, 55–64. [CrossRef]

32. Walker, W.E. Policy analysis: A systematic approach to supporting policymaking in the public sector. *J. Multi-Crit. Decis. Anal.* **2000**, *9*, 11–27. [CrossRef]

33. Hanney, S.; Gonzalez-Block, M.; Buxton, M.; Kogan, M. The utilisation of health research in policy-making: Concepts, examples and methods of assessment. *Health Res. Policy Syst.* **2003**, *1*, 2. [CrossRef] [PubMed]

34. Australian Bureau of Statistics. *Housing and Infrastructure in Aboriginal and Torres Strait Islander Communities*; Cat. No. 4710.0; ABS: Canberra, Australia, 2007.

35. Australian Bureau of Statistics. 1270.0.55.005—Australian Statistical Geography Standard (ASGS): Volume 5—Remoteness Structure, July 2016. Available online: http://www.abs.gov.au/AUSSTATS/abs@.nsf/Lookup/1270.0.55.005Main+Features1July%202016?OpenDocument (accessed on 7 December 2018).

36. Braun, K.L.; Nigg, C.R.; Fialkowski, M.K.; Butel, J.; Hollyer, J.R.; Barber, L.R.; Bersamin, A.; Coleman, P.; Teo-Martin, U.; Vargo, A.M.; et al. Using the ANGELO Model to Develop the Children's Healthy Living Program Multilevel Intervention to Promote Obesity Preventing Behaviors for Young Children in the US-Affiliated Pacific Region. *Child. Obes.* **2014**, *10*, 474–481. [CrossRef] [PubMed]

37. Snowdon, W.; Lawrence, M.; Schultz, J.; Vivili, P.; Swinburn, B. Evidence-informed process to identify policies that will promote a healthy food environment in the Pacific Islands. *Public Health Nutr.* **2010**, *13*, 886–892. [CrossRef] [PubMed]

38. Snowdon, W.; Potter, J.; Swinburn, B.; Schultz, J.; Lawrence, M. Prioritizing policy interventions to improve diets? Will it work, can it happen, will it do harm? *Health Promot. Int.* **2010**, *25*, 123–133. [CrossRef] [PubMed]

39. Swinburn, B.; Gill, T.; Kumanyika, S. Obesity prevention: A proposed framework for translating evidence into action. *Obes. Rev.* **2005**, *6*, 23–33. [CrossRef]

40. Thow, A.; Jan, S.; Leeder, S.; Swinburn, B. The effect of fiscal policy on diet, obesity and chronic disease: A systematic review. *Bull. World Health Organ.* **2010**, *88*, 609–614. [CrossRef] [PubMed]

41. Purnell, J.Q.; Gernes, R.; Stein, R.; Sherraden, M.S.; Knoblock-Hahn, A. A systematic review of financial incentives for dietary behavior change. *J. Acad. Nutr. Diet.* **2014**, *114*, 1023–1035. [CrossRef]

42. Ball, K.; McNaughton, S.A.; Le, H.N.; Gold, L.; Mhurchu, C.N.; Abbott, G. Influence of price discounts and skill-building strategies on purchase and consumption of healthy food and beverages: Outcomes of the Supermarket Healthy Eating for Life randomized controlled trial. *Am. J. Clin. Nutr.* **2015**, *101*, 1055–1064. [CrossRef]

43. Brimblecombe, J.; Ferguson, M.; Chatfield, M.D.; Gunther, A.; Liberato, S.; Ball, K.; Moodie, M.; Miles, E.; Magnus, A.; Ni Mhurchu, C.; et al. Effect of a price discount and consumer education strategy on food and beverage purchases in remote Indigenous Australia: A stepped-wedge randomised controlled trial. *Lancet Public Health* **2017**, *2*, e82–e95. [CrossRef]

44. Popkin, B.M.; Hawkes, C. Sweetening of the global diet, particularly beverages: Patterns, trends, and policy responses. *Lancet Diabetes Endocrinol.* **2015**, *4*, 174–186. [CrossRef]

45. Imamura, F.; O'Connor, L.; Ye, Z.; Mursu, J.; Hayashino, Y.; Bhupathiraju, S.N.; Forouhi, N.G. Consumption of sugar sweetened beverages, artificially sweetened beverages, and fruit juice and incidence of type 2 diabetes: Systematic review, meta-analysis, and estimation of population attributable fraction. *Br. Med. J.* **2015**, *351*, h3576. [CrossRef] [PubMed]

46. Capewell, S.; Lloyd-Williams, F. Promotion of healthy food and beverage purchases: Are subsidies and consumer education sufficient? *Lancet Public Health* **2017**, *2*, e59–e60. [CrossRef]

47. World Health Organization. Fiscal Policies for Diet and Prevention of Noncommunicable Diseases. In *Proceedings of the Technical Meeting Report, 5–6 May 2015, Geneva, Switzerland*; World Health Organization: Geneva, Switzerland, 2016.

48. Ferguson, M.; O'Dea, K.; Chatfield, M.; Moodie, M.; Altman, J.; Brimblecombe, J. The comparative cost of food and beverages at remote Indigenous communities, Northern Territory, Australia. *Aust. N. Z. J. Public Health* **2016**, *40*, S21–S26. [CrossRef]

49. Hawkes, C. Sales promotion and food consumption. *Nutr. Rev.* **2009**, *67*, 333–342. [CrossRef] [PubMed]

50. Waterlander, W.; de Boer, M.; Schuit, A.; Seidell, J.; Steenhuis, I. Price discounts significantly enhance fruit and vegetable purchases when combined with nutrition education: A randomized controlled supermarket trial. *Am. J. Clin. Nutr.* **2013**, *97*, 886–895. [CrossRef] [PubMed]

51. Waterlander, W.E.; Ni Mhurchu, C.; Steenhuis, I. Effects of a price increase on purchases of sugar sweetened beverages. Results from a randomized controlled trial. *Appetite* **2014**, *78*, 32–39. [CrossRef] [PubMed]

52. Colchero, M.A.; Popkin, B.M.; Rivera, J.A.; Ng, S.W. Beverage purchases from stores in Mexico under the excise tax on sugar sweetened beverages: Observational study. *Br. Med. J.* **2016**, *352*, h6704. [CrossRef]

7

Food Insecurity and Hunger in Rich Countries—It is Time for Action against Inequality

Christina M. Pollard [1,*] and Sue Booth [2]

[1] Faculty of Health Science, School of Public Health, Curtin University, Perth 6845, Australia
[2] College of Medicine & Public Health, Flinders University, Adelaide 5000, Australia; sue.booth@flinders.edu.au
* Correspondence: C.Pollard@curtin.edu.au

Abstract: Household food insecurity is a serious public health concern in rich countries with developed economies closely associated with inequality. The prevalence of household food insecurity is relatively high in some developed countries, ranging from 8 to 20% of the population. Human rights approaches have the potential to address the structural causes, not just the symptoms of food insecurity. Despite most developed countries ratifying the Covenant on Economic, Social and Cultural Rights over 40 years ago, food insecurity rates suggest current social protections are inadequate. The contemporary framing of the solution to food insecurity in developed countries is that of diverting food waste to the hungry to meet the United Nations Sustainable Development Goals agenda (Goals 2 and 12.3). An estimated 60 million people or 7.2% of the population in high income countries used food banks in 2013. Although providing food assistance to those who are hungry is an important strategy, the current focus distracts attention away from the ineffectiveness of government policies in addressing the social determinants of food insecurity. Much of the action needed to improve household food security falls to actors outside the health sector. There is evidence of promising actions to address the social determinants of food insecurity in some developed countries. Learning from these, there is a strong case for government leadership, for action within and across government, and effective engagement with other sectors to deliver a coordinated, collaborative, and cooperative response to finding pathways out of food insecurity.

Keywords: food insecurity; hunger; developed countries; Sustainable Development Goals; social determinants; inequality; food banks

1. Introduction

Household food insecurity is a serious public health concern in rich countries with developed economies [1]. For example, in Australia, Canada, Europe, New Zealand, the United Kingdom, and the United States of America (US), improving household food and nutrition security is a public health priority. Food insecurity is costly, has wide-reaching consequences, and its effects extend beyond vulnerable populations. The two main ways of addressing food security in developed countries continue to be measures to respond to poverty including welfare entitlements and food relief [2]. As governments retreat from the issue, third sector organizations step in to deliver services to people in need, evidenced by the rapid proliferation of food banks and charitable food services. As expected, food assistance does little to address the underlying causes of food poverty and insecurity [3]. Clearly the response in developed countries is not working. There are tangible solutions to the problem, what is missing in many countries is the political will to fully acknowledge the problem and take the effective action.

Human rights-focused approaches have the potential to address the impact of government action or inaction, including the structural causes, not just the symptoms, of social inequities. The right to food is bound under international law in Article 25.1, *"Everyone has the right to a standard of living adequate for the health and well-being of himself and of his family, including food, clothing, housing and medical care and necessary social services, and the right to security in the event of unemployment, sickness, disability, widowhood, old age or other lack of livelihood in circumstances beyond his control."* p. 76 [4]. Enshrined in the International Covenant on Economic, Social and Cultural Rights (ICESCR) Article 11 [5] consenting nation states are obligated to respect, protect and fulfil their commitments, see General Commitment number 12 [5]. Adopted in 1966 [6] with entry into force in 1976, many developed countries have ratified ICESCR including: Australia (1975); Canada, United Kingdom, Great Britain, Northern Island (1976); Japan (1979); and Belgium (1983). The US is a notable exception, signing in 1977 but not yet ratified, and continues to express resistance towards economic and social rights [7].

Countries who are ratified are subject to investigations on their current situation by the Special Rapporteur on the Right to Food. Progress on the realisation of the right to food can be very slow, even in rich countries. Nearly 40 year after ratification, the 2012 Canadian review by the Special Rapporteur, found 57% of people living on social assistance were food insecure and concluded that Canadian cash transfers were insufficient for an adequate standard of living [8]. Although Canada's promotion of labour market participation as a strategy to overcome poverty was commended, it was recommended that their minimum wage legislation should be a 'living wage' [8]. Housing costs were noted as a key reason people were compelled to use food banks.

A sense of urgency to address food insecurity is implicit in the Global Sustainable Development Goals (SDG) which seek actions to realise human rights by 2030, and are determined to end poverty and hunger, in all their forms and dimensions . . . .. Goal 2 (2.1) has a target *"to end hunger and ensure access by all people, in particular the poor and people in vulnerable situations, including infants, to safe, nutritious and sufficient food all year round."* [9].

2. How You Define Food Insecurity Shapes the Response

How you define and measure a problem influences how you respond to it. Before effective action to address food insecurity can be taken, there is a need to agree on a definition of food security and understand its determinants. A clear definition provides the context for action and assists with identifying the desired outcomes. Since the early 1990s there have been numerous definitions of food insecurity with meanings and actions differing when applied at global, domestic, household, or individual levels. This paper refers to food and nutrition security at the household and individual level in rich countries.

The Committee on World Food Security in 2012, recognising that the response to food insecurity involved multidisciplinary actors who need to speak the same language, sought a standard definition. Food and nutrition security, existing *"when all people at all times have physical, social and economic access to food, which is safe and consumed in sufficient quantity and quality to meet their dietary needs and food preferences, and is supported by an environment of adequate sanitation, health services and care, allowing for a healthy and active life"* p. 8 [10] was adopted. Definitions change and reflect what is socially acceptable at the time. The 2012 definition encompassed some broader aspects of food insecurity, such as sanitation, health services, and care, but moved away from tenets which emphasise non-emergency provision [11], avoiding unorthodox procurement practices (scavenging, stealing, or other coping strategies), social justice, democratic decision making, community self-reliance [12], or providing diets rather than just food [11]. The determinants as well as the extent of the problem are important. Food insecurity is the therefore the limited or uncertain availability of nutritionally adequate or safe foods or limited or uncertain ability to acquire foods in socially acceptable ways [13].

The determinants of food and nutrition insecurity as well as the extent of the problem are important considerations when defining action. Between and within country differences are important considerations, including, but not limited to: geographical differences (e.g., urban versus rural); chronicity and severity levels; political, economic and social drivers; historical government positions; climate impact; and how these factors have changed over time.

3. The Framing of the Issue Determines the Response

The way a problem is framed, or publically portrayed, also shapes the way society responds. Framing food security issues in ways that resonate with the beliefs, priorities and needs of different audiences can mobilize support for action. Within country social inequalities, particularly poverty, lead to food insecurity [2], therefore it would make sense that the problem framing should be in terms of how to address social and economic inequity. Two main frames dominate the way developed countries define the problem of food insecurity and the way government and other key stakeholders' respond—societal benefit and food waste mitigation.

Societal benefit frames household food security in terms of how both individuals and society benefit when all members of society are food secure. Countries with high levels of food security benefit socially, economically, environmentally, and politically. The economic cost of food insecurity is not routinely reported in developed nations however estimates to date suggest they are substantial. Costs related to food insecurity in 2011 in the US were ~A$167.5 billion related to lost productivity, public education expenses, avoidable healthcare costs, and the cost of charity to keep families fed [14]. Food insecurity is associated with a range of physical and mental health issues which contribute significantly to healthcare costs, for example cardiovascular disease [15] and obesity [16]. There is a clear relationship between housing instability, food insecurity and access to health care amongst low income families [17]. Reducing food insecurity would see improvements in health, employment, productivity, and economic viability, and reductions in health care costs. This framing should inform arguments about the need for an urgent response to food insecurity in developed countries, as the cost of inaction is likely to be far more deleterious [14]. The complexity of social disadvantage contributing to poverty, through exposure to adversity throughout the life course and often across generations, should inform the responses to food insecurity [18,19].

Food waste mitigation, "*Waste not want not. Toward zero hunger. Food bank as a green solution to hunger*", is the contemporary framing used by the 2019 Global Foodbanking Network which frames foodbanks as the solution to hunger (SDG 2) and the environmental impact of food waste (SDG 12.3) [20]. Governments, the commercial sector, the voluntary sector, and social entrepreneurs are increasingly framing food waste diversion to the hungry as a social, economic, and environmental win:win:win [21]. There are significant economic, environmental, and social impacts of food surplus and waste, and countries need to ensure sustainable food systems to remain food secure [21]. The strongest solution to the problem is prevention that is, reducing food surplus at its source through holistic changes in the food system. The framing of the issue of food surplus and waste is currently focussed on recovery as the primary solution that is, reusing waste food for human consumption, an insufficient remedy for long term food insecurity and for food waste [21]. For example, in Australia and the UK, the voluntary sector partners with food businesses to divert food [2,22,23], and in France, food waste redistribution to charities is legislated [24]. Although these approaches may provide some food for relief agencies, unfortunately, the conflating of the two issues does not solve the fundamental and complex problems of either of them [23]. The problem of food surplus/waste distribution is the nature of the food distributed and the manner in which it is provided.

Framing food and nutrition security action within broad policy discourses (for example achieving the SDGs or economic and social policy reform) can generate commitment to act. The United Nation's World Health Organization and Food and Agriculture Organization Driving commitment for nutrition within the UN Decade of Action on Nutrition policy brief frames the argument that taking action on improving nutrition is a win-win option for many sectors and works to achieve at least 12 of the 17 SDGs. Designing frames to resonate with the people who can influence action is important [25].

Framing can be further enhanced to resonate with the people who influence action. For example, financial policy makers would likely be interested in societal benefits in terms of economic rationale (e.g., cost to health systems), civil society groups would be interested in 'the human right to adequate food and to freedom from hunger', and the vulnerability of children to malnutrition may resound with all audiences [25].

Reframing and focusing food insecurity to address the broader sustainable development issues of supporting human rights and sustainable development to create an equitable and prosperous society, will have much broader impacts than the current focus on redistributing food waste. For example, societal benefits in terms of economic rationale (e.g., cost to health systems, workforce productivity) would likely be of interest to financial policy makers; 'the human right to adequate food and to freedom from hunger' may inspire civil society groups; and the focus on vulnerability of children to malnutrition may resound with all audiences [25].

4. The Scale of the Problem of Food Insecurity

A double burden of malnutrition (high rates of undernutrition (including wasting, stunting, and micronutrient deficiencies) co-existing alongside overweight, obesity, and diet-related non-communicable diseases) is commonplace in many countries. In 2017, the absolute number of people affected by undernourishment or chronic food deprivation was estimated to be 821 million and 9 billion adults were overweight or obese. At the same time, 151 million children aged under 5 years were stunted and 38 million were either overweight or obese. Undernutrition contributes to 3.1 million (45% of total) deaths in children under five every year. The UN Decade of Action on Nutrition 2016–2025 (http://www.un.org/nutrition) aims to trigger intensified action to end hunger and eradicate all forms of malnutrition worldwide. Undernourishment, severe food insecurity, and malnutrition is more prevalent in developing economies, 90% of the worlds stunted children live in 36 countries with the highest level of chronic undernutrition. Taking action in these countries is clearly the highest priority to achieve the SDG [26].

5. How Big Is the Problem of Food Insecurity in Developed Countries?

"No Data, No Problem, No Action.", the title of a paper by Friel et al. (2009), captures the crux of the matter in terms of defining the problem of food insecurity in developed countries [27]. Relatively hidden in most developed countries, the population prevalence of food insecurity is largely unreported due to a lack of routine measurement and use of non-comparable measures. Food insecurity is closely associated with poverty and as some countries have no official government statistics, household food insecurity estimations are made using proxy measures such as national poverty lines (50 to 60% of median income) [28]. Estimated food insecurity prevalence is unexpectedly high in some rich countries, for example: Australia and Japan (21.7% of households, ~4.6 million people and 15.7%, ~19.8 million, respectively in 2012—based on 50–60% of the national poverty line); Canada (7.7%, ~1.9 million in 2007/8); the European Union (8.7% or 43.6 million when 27 countries are included); and the US (15% of the population, ~50 million) [28].

Canada and the US regularly monitor household food insecurity, while in other countries, such as the UK, it has been the rapid rise of food banks that has drawn attention to the issue [1]. Food insecurity monitoring using comparable measures should be a mandatory requirement across all countries as without the compulsory requirement national comparable estimates are at risk. Canada, who has monitored food insecurity since 2005, had some jurisdictions opt out of voluntary monitoring, undermining their ability to produce national estimates [29]. The Food and Agriculture Organization (FAO) of the United Nations supports the use of comparable measures of food insecurity to capture its magnitude, severity and causes [30]. The FAO supports an enabling environment for a rapid response to hunger through better data to: shape policies and programs; increase political commitment; support effective co-ordination and evidenced-based decision making. There is an urgent need for most developed countries to commit to using comparable measures and for most, significant effort is needed to meet this recommendation. This surveillance of within- and across-country food insecurity is crucial intelligence for the government and other sector's decision making regarding actions to address food insecurity, and a fundamental requirement for reporting against the SDGs.

6. The Responses to Food Insecurity

Most developed countries respond to food insecurity through the provision of food assistance delivered by the voluntary sector, with very limited government support [31]. Addressing the social determinants of food insecurity is the exception, for example, Norway's political agenda focuses on agricultural support, food pricing regulation, and universal social security [2]. Food assistance is usually in the form of food banks, pantries, parcels, and soup kitchens delivered by the voluntary or charitable sector. The US has embedded government funded food assistance programs: the Supplemental Nutrition Assistance Program (SNAP) of the Food Stamp Act of 1964, provided ~14% of Americans support for household food purchases at a cost of an estimated A$70 billion annually in 2018 [32]; the Special Supplemental Nutrition Program for Women, Infants and Children (WIC) serves 7 million participants a month at a cost of A$5.95 billion in 2016 [33].

Low cost food has been made available through food banks in the US since the late 1960s [34], which began opening in Europe 20 years later, and are now present in all Organisation for Economic Co-operation and Development (OECD) member states [31]. About 60 million people or 7.2% of high income country populations used them in 2013 [28]. The Global Foodbanking Network comprises over 800 food banks in 31 countries [19]. The proportion of the population accessing food banks is relatively high in some developed countries, for example, 12% of the US population (37 million people) in 2009 and 6% (19 million) of those living in the EU used foodbanks in 2011 [28]. It appears that food banks are now a permanent fixture in the response to food insecurity in developed countries, but at what cost?

Countries with relatively low public social spending have greater numbers of foodbank users. For example, the US has 12% of the population using foodbanks and spends 19.7% of Gross Domestic Product (GDP) on social expenditure whereas Belgium has ~1.9% total population using food banks and spent 29.6% of GDP on social expenditure in 2011 [28]. The rapid growth in food banks and public appeals for food donations or money for food suggest a normalisation of food aid in the UK [35] and other developed countries [36]. Despite food banks, food charity, and government programs, food insecurity is a growing problem in rich countries, so what is going wrong?

Each developed country has its own social protection systems or social welfare safety net which, due to reconstructions and cut backs to basic entitlements has meant that food banks have "*become secondary extensions of weakened social safety net*" p. 648 [37]. The inadequacy of developed countries' social protection systems is rendering people vulnerable to food insecurity, as demonstrated by increased food insecurity rates in these countries. In fact, "*Social protections systems, not the least unemployment and child benefits must be recalibrated to take into account the real cost of living and ensure adequate food for all, without compromising on other essentials*" p. X, the Special Rapporteur on the Right to Food [38]. Clearly, food banks can provide emergency food assistance but do not, in and of themselves, offer pathways out of food insecurity in developed nations [31].

The experience of being food insecure and seeking food assistance in rich countries can have negative impacts on the individual as it is traumatic, stressful, and detrimental to one's health and wellbeing [39,40]. In all societies, "*to be mentally healthy you must value and respect yourself*" p. 65 [41]. People who use food assistance in rich countries say they experience stigma, shame, and hopelessness [35,42–45]. Shame is a powerful emotion related to feeling foolish, stupid, ridiculous, inadequate, defective, incompetent, awkward, exposed, vulnerable, and insecure, based on seeing oneself negatively in the eyes of the other [46]. It is the inequality within rich countries that fosters feelings of inferiority, even before needing to seek food assistance. Independence is a core value in Western culture, people who need help to meet a basic need, such as food, are viewed as dependent and dependency is humiliating [47]. This is understandable as needing food assistance and the ways it is currently delivered is not considered socially acceptable, nor should it be in a wealthy country [48]. Another concern is that food banks and pantries strongly influence user's diets, yet are unable to support an adequate dietary intake [49,50]. Trying to address household food insecurity with community-based food interventions is not effective when solutions likely lie upstream in social protection policies [1].

7. What Should or Could Be Done and by Whom

A decade ago, the notion that 'equality is better for everyone' was eloquently expressed by Wilkinson and Pickett (2009) who asserted that to improve the quality of life in rich countries the focus must shift from building material standards and economic growth to finding ways to improve the psychological and social wellbeing of whole societies, essentially by reducing within country inequality [41].

When looking for what could or should be done to address food and nutrition security in developed countries, the discussion paper on addressing the social determinants of non-communicable diseases (NCD) provides a useful framework for multi-sectoral action outside the health sector [51]. Influenced by Friel et al.'s (2015) suggestions to address inequities in healthy eating [52], we adapted the framework for NCD action to one addressing food and nutrition security in developed countries, see Figure 1. Importantly, we have re-ordered the action focus based on potential to reduce food insecurity.

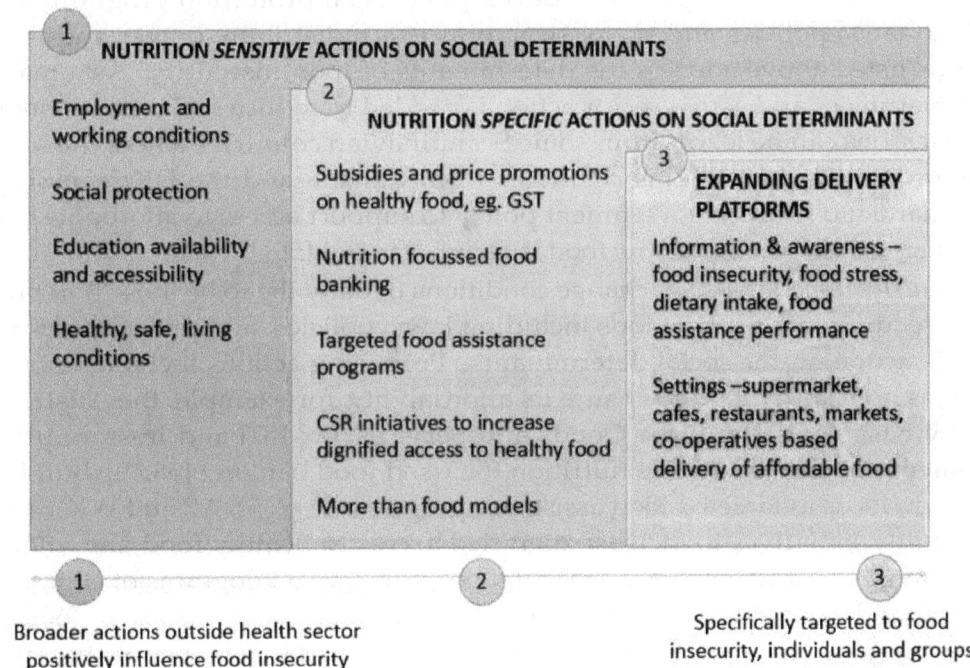

Figure 1. Typology of multi-sectoral actions on food and nutrition security (Adapted from Figure 8 p. 45 Discussion Paper Addressing the Social Determinants of Non-communicable Diseases [52]).

There is evidence to suggest some key actions to take to achieve the SDGs related to address food insecurity in developed countries. The prerequisites for action on the social determinants of food and nutrition security are high-level political commitment, governance mechanisms to facilitate and coordinate multi-sectoral responses, and robust structures for monitoring, evaluation, and accountability. As much of the required action needed to improve food and nutrition security is to be taken by actors outside the health sector, strong advocacy is needed to create cross-sector, cross-government engagement to build a shared understanding of the problem of food insecurity, outline potential actions, and delegations of responsibility. The initial advocacy focus to support the argument for cross-sector action for societal benefit, would include continuing to measure the problem and its impact and using this information to engage various sectors. There is likely to be benefit in high level government leadership bringing together key stakeholders for human development benefit, second to commercial interests. Fine-grained measurement, multilevel monitoring systems, action on the social and environmental determinants of health, and inclusive systems of governance are required to address food insecurity [27].

Political commitment to address nutrition can be created and strengthened over time through strategic action. Baker et al.'s (2018) review of factors that generated political commitment for nutrition action identified the following important drivers, irrespective of country: effective nutrition actor networks; strong leadership; civil society mobilisation; supportive political administrations; societal change and focusing events; cohesive and resonant framing; and robust data systems and available evidence [53]. Private sector interference was found to frequently undermine commitment in high-income countries.

Key actions to build food and nutrition security are in order of potential influence starting with food and nutrition sensitive, followed by food and nutrition specific actions, and lastly expanding delivery platforms. Some examples of promising actions are include:

(1) *Food and nutrition sensitive actions* include core business of non-health actors to address social determinants, including regulating employment and labour conditions, increasing access to education, challenging harmful gender norms, promoting a rights-enhancing legal environment, setting urban development policy or developing social protection programmes. Macro level changes to laws, policies and social structures can redistribute power and resources. All of the actions listed above address the determinants of food insecurity. As a matter of urgency, across government and across sector action is needed to reduce social and economic inequality. Valuable lessons can be learnt from some Scandinavian countries where the social protections systems promote equality [2] and studies from Canada and the UK focussing on reducing financial hardship [54,55]. Government policy to support access to affordable housing without compromising basic needs such as food is recommended [56].

(2) *Food and nutrition specific actions* change conditions of daily life to be those that provide food and nutrition security via interventions including laws, policies, and programmes whose primary purpose is action on the social determinants. Promising actions include: subsidies and price promotions on healthy food to ensure its affordability, for example, the Australian exemption of healthy basic foods from the Goods and Services Tax [57] and in-store price promotions; procurement policies promoting nutrition focussed food banking [58,59]; building support for the nutrition focus in targeted food assistance programs (e.g., SNAP and WIC); Corporate Social Responsibility initiatives to increase dignified access to healthy food and affordable food for all, for example, Lidl's 'Too Good to Waste' boxes selling 5 kilograms of slightly damaged but edible fruit and vegetables for just £1.50 [60]; 'More than food' models of food assistance that provide emergency relief with integrated support services to help people find pathways out of food insecurity [61,62]. Three key principles for the food service aspect of these models are: (1) a client-centred focus; (2) empowering individuals by fostering autonomy and enabling food choice in socially acceptable ways; and (3) providing opportunities for active involvement, social connection, and broader support [63].

(3) *Expanding delivery platforms* use settings to extend the reach of the health sector and extend the reach and impact of health-related information. This includes a focus on non-charitable food-service settings for example, supermarkets, cafes, restaurants, farmers markets, co-operatives, and social enterprise models to ensure affordable food is available to people at high risk of food insecurity in non-stigmatising ways. Government monitoring and surveillance systems, independent of the food industry and the charitable food sector should be developed to contribute country level information to inform appropriate actions. At a minimum these should include using standardised and robust measures of: household food and nutrition security that captures severity and prevalence and includes children (e.g., the United States Department of Agriculture (USDA)'s 18 item U.S. Household Food Security Survey Module where appropriate or part of the suite [64]); food related measures of financial stress (e.g., food stress [65]); routine measure of dietary intake, measured height and weight, and socioeconomic status; and food assistance services performance

indicators. Collectively these build information and intelligence systems to inform the delivery of targeted food insecurity interventions.

The impact of food insecurity is ultimately felt by the individual, the health system and all of society. Although not directly responsible for service delivery of the actions described above, the health sector is well placed to work with other sectors to support them to ensure effective responses to food insecurity. The three main priority actions of the health sector in developed countries to address food and nutrition insecurity are: (1) to provide the technical expertise (nutrition science, public health, food safety, and health promotion) to assist the development of food and nutrition policies to ensure interventions are nutritionally adequate and do not exacerbate health issues; (2) To contribute to the systematic monitoring and surveillance of the performance and outcomes of the comprehensive range of actions described above in terms of food security and other health outcomes; (3) Advocate on behalf of those who are rendered food insecure due to hardship and disadvantage for effective responses to food insecurity across government at all levels and stages of country development across the globe.

There is a key role for academia to provide the evidence base and independent voice to inform and evaluate policy and programs and to challenge existing paradigms and assumptions. The *International Journal of Environmental Research and Public Health* Special Issue on Addressing Food Insecurity in Developed Countries is a good example of how the research community can come together to provide evidence to guide policy and practice [66–86]. There are many opportunities for academics to partner with government, industry, and the third sector to translate research to practice to improve the lives of people rendered food insecure in rich nations.

The problem of food insecurity in developed countries is a growing problem with far reaching public health, social, and economic impacts. There will always be a need for food assistance to address emergency situations. But, this should not distract from the need to address the issue at its cause, in the words of Nelson Mandela, former President of South Africa, *"Overcoming poverty is not a gesture of charity. It is the protection of a fundamental human right, the right to dignity and a decent life."* We call for governments to initiate actions to address the social determinants of food insecurity and to lead a coordinated, collaborative, and cooperative response to finding pathways out of food insecurity guided by the expertise, enthusiasm, and commitment of the third sector and the voices of those who have had the experience.

Author Contributions: Conceptualization, C.M.P. and S.B; Writing—Original Draft Preparation, C.M.P. and S.B.; Writing—Review & Editing, C.M.P. and S.B.

References

1. Loopstra, R. Interventions to Address Household Food Insecurity in High-Income Countries. *Proc. Nutr. Soc.* **2018**, *77*, 270–281. [CrossRef]
2. Richards, C.; Kjærnes, U.; Vik, J. Food Security in Welfare Capitalism: Comparing Social Entitlements to Food in Australia and Norway. *J. Rural Stud.* **2016**, *43*, 61–70. [CrossRef]
3. Caraher, M.; Furey, S. *The Economics of Emergency Food Aid Provision. A Financial, Social and Cultural Perspective*, 1st ed.; Palgrave Pivot: London, UK, 2018.
4. General Assembly of the United Nations. Universal Declaration of Human Rights. In *Article 251 (United Nations) Resolution 217A*; General Assembly of the United Nations: Geneva, Switzerland, 1948.
5. Committee on Economic Social and Cultural Rights (CESCR). *General Comment No. 12: The Right to Adequate Food (Article 11)*; Committee on Economic Social and Cultural Rights (CESCR): Geneva, Switzerland, 1999.
6. United Nations. *Resolution Adopted by the General Assembly. 2200 (XXI). International Covenant on Economic, Social and Cultural Rights, International Covenant on Civil and Political Rights and Optional Protocolo the International Covenant on Civil and Political Rights. In A/RES/21/2200*; United Nations: Geneva, Switzerland, 1966.

7.   Piccard, A.M. The United States' Failure to Ratify the International Covenant on Economic, Social and Cultural Rights: Must the Poor be Always with Us? *Scholar* **2010**, *13*, 231.

8.   De Schutter, O. Report of the Special Rapporteur on the Right to Food, Addendum Mission to Canada*. In *A/HRC/22/50/Add1*; United Nations Human Rights Council: Geneva, Switzerland, 2012.

9.   Global Indicator Framework for the Sustainable Development Goals A/RES/71/313 E/CN.3/2018/2. Available online: unstats.un.org/sdgs/indicators/Global%20Indicator%20Framework%20after%20refinement_Eng.pdf (accessed on 10 April 2019).

10.   Committee on World Food Security. *Coming to Terms with Terminology*; Food and Agriculture Organization: Rome, Italy, 2012; pp. 1–26.

11.   Gottlieb, R.; Fisher, A. Community Food Security and Environmental Justice: Searching for a Common Discourse. *Agric. Hum. Values* **1996**, *13*, 23–32. [CrossRef]

12.   Bellows, A.C.; Hamm, M.W. US-Based Community Food Security: Influences, Practice, Debate. *Food Cult. Soc.* **2002**, *6*, 31–44.

13.   Olson, C.M.; Holben, D.H. Position of the American Dietetic Association: Domestic Food and Nutrition Security. *J. Am. Diet. Assoc.* **2002**, *102*, 1840–1847. [CrossRef]

14.   Shepard, D.S.; Setren, E.; Cooper, D. Hunger in America: Suffering We All Pay for. Center for American Progress. 2011, pp. 1–24. Available online: www.americanprogress.org/wp-content/uploads/issues/2011/10/pdf/hunger_paper.pdf (accessed on 10 April 2019).

15.   Seligman, H.K.; Laraia, B.A.; Kushel, M.B. Food Insecurity is Associated with Chronic Disease Among Low-Income NHANES Participants. *J. Nutr.* **2010**, *140*, 304–310. [CrossRef]

16.   Dinour, L.M.; Bergen, D.; Yeh, M.-C. The Food Insecurity–Obesity Paradox: A Review of the Literature and the Role Food Stamps may Play. *J. Am. Diet. Assoc.* **2007**, *107*, 1952–1961. [CrossRef] [PubMed]

17.   Miewald, C.; Ostry, A. A Warm Meal and a Bed: Intersections of Housing and Food Security in Vancouver's Downtown Eastside. *Hous. Stud.* **2014**, *29*, 709–729. [CrossRef]

18.   Chilton, M.; Knowles, M.; Bloom, S.L. The Intergenerational Circumstances of Household Food Insecurity and Adversity. *J. Hunger Environ. Nutr.* **2017**, *12*, 269–297. [CrossRef]

19.   Chilton, M.M.; Rabinowich, J.R.; Woolf, N.H. Very Low Food Security in the USA is Linked with Exposure to Violence. *Public Health Nutr.* **2014**, *17*, 73–82. [CrossRef] [PubMed]

20.   The Global FoodBanking Network. Waste Not Want Not. Toward Zero Hunger. Food Bank as a Green Solution to Hunger. 2019. Available online: www.foodbanking.org/wp-content/uploads/2019/03/GFN_WasteNot.pdf (accessed on 10 April 2019).

21.   Mourad, M. Recycling, Recovering and Preventing "Food Waste": Competing Solutions for Food Systems Sustainability in the United States and France. *J. Clean. Prod.* **2016**, *126*, 461–477. [CrossRef]

22.   Ruah Community Service. Registry Week 2016 Less Homeless Report. Perth: Ruah. 2016. Available online: https://view.publitas.com/ruah-community-services-1/registry-week-final-report-2016/page/1 (accessed on 10 April 2019).

23.   Caplan, P. Win-Win? Food Poverty, Food Aid and Food Surplus in the UK today. *Anthr. Today* **2017**, *33*, 17–22. [CrossRef]

24.   Angelique Chrisafis. French Law Forbids Food Waste by Supermarkets. Food Banks and Other Charities Welcome Law Making Large Shops Donate Unsold Food and Stop Spoiling Items to Deter Foragers. In The Guardian. Available online: www.theguardian.com/world/2016/feb/04/french-law-forbids-food-waste-by-supermarkets (accessed on 10 April 2019).

25.   World Health Organization and Food and Agriculture Organization of the United Nations. *Driving commitment for nutrition within the UN Decade of Action on Nutrition*; World Health Organization and Food and Agriculture Organization of the United Nations: Geneva, Switzerland, 2018; Available online: https://apps.who.int/iris/bitstream/handle/10665/274375/WHO-NMH-NHD-17.11-eng.pdf?ua=1 (accessed on 6 May 2019).

26.   FAO, IFAD, UNICEF, WFP, WHO. *The State of Food Security and Nutrition in the World 2018. Building Climate Resilience for Food Security and Nutrition*; FAO: Rome, Italy, 2018; Available online: https://reliefweb.int/report/world/state-food-security-and-nutrition-world-2018-building-climate-resilience-food-security (accessed on 6 May 2019).

27.   Friel, S.; Vlahov, D.; Buckley, R.M. No Data, No Problem, No Action: Addressing Urban Health Inequity in the 21st Century. *J. Urban Health* **2011**, *88*, 858–859. [CrossRef] [PubMed]

28. Gentilini, U. Banking on Food: The State of Food Banks in High-Income Countries. Institute of Development Studies, IDS Working Papers 2013, 1-18.CSP WORKING PAPER Number 008. Available online: www.ids.ac.uk/publications/banking-on-food-the-state-of-food-banks-in-high-income-countries/ (accessed on 10 April 2019).

29. PROOF Food Insecurity Policy Research. Monitoring Food Insecurity in Canada. Fact sheets. p. 2. Canada: PROOF; 2017:2. Available online: https://proof.utoronto.ca/wp-content/uploads/2016/06/monitoring-factsheet.pdf (accessed on 10 April 2019).

30. Food and Agriculture Organization of the United Nations. Information Systems for Food Insecurity and Nutrition. Available online: www.fao.org (accessed on 10 April 2019).

31. Riches, G. *Food Bank Nations: Poverty, Corporate Charity and the Right to Food*, 1st ed.; Routledge: London, UK, 2018.

32. Mozaffarian, D.; Liu, J.; Sy, S.; Huang, Y.; Rehm, C.; Lee, Y.; Wilde, P.; Abrahams-Gessel, S.; de Souza Veiga Jardim, T.; Gaziano, T. Cost-Effectiveness of Financial Incentives and Disincentives for Improving Food Purchases and Health through the US Supplemental Nutrition Assistance Program (SNAP): A Microsimulation Study. *PLoS Med* **2018**, *15*, e1002661. [CrossRef] [PubMed]

33. Carlson, S.; Neuberger, Z.; Rosenbaum, D. WIC Participation and Costs are Stable. Center on Budget and Policy Priorities 2017. Available online: www.cbpp.org/research/food-assistance/wic-participation-and-costs-are-stable (accessed on 10 April 2019).

34. Ghys, T. Taking Stock of the Ambiguous Role of Foodbanks in the Fight Against Poverty. *J. Poverty Soc. Justice* **2018**, *26*, 173–189. [CrossRef]

35. Purdam, K.; Garratt, E.A.; Esmail, A. Hungry? Food Insecurity, Social Stigma and Embarrassment in the UK. *Sociology* **2016**, *50*, 1072–1088. [CrossRef]

36. Tarasuk, V.; Eakin, J.M. Charitable Food Assistance as Symbolic Gesture: An Ethnographic Study of Food Banks in Ontario. *Soc. Sci. Med.* **2003**, *56*, 1505–1515. [CrossRef]

37. Riches, G. Food Banks and Food Security: Welfare Reform, Human Rights and Social Policy. Lessons from Canada? *Soc. Policy Adm.* **2002**, *36*, 648–663. [CrossRef]

38. Riches, G.; Silvasti, T. *First World Hunger Revisited Food Charity or the Right to Food?* 2nd ed.; Riches, G., Silvasti, T., Eds.; Palgrave Macmillan: Hampshire, UK, 2014.

39. Hecht, A.A.; Biehl, E.; Buzogany, S.; Neff, R. Using a Trauma-Informed Policy Approach to Create a Resilient Urban Food System. *Public Health Nutr.* **2018**, *21*, 1961–1970. [CrossRef]

40. Thompson, C.; Smith, D.; Cummins, S.J.S.S. Medicine: Understanding the Health and Wellbeing Challenges of the Food Banking System: A Qualitative Study of Food Bank Users, Providers and Referrers in London. *Soc. Sci. Med.* **2018**, *211*, 95–101. [CrossRef]

41. Wilkinson, R.; Pickett, K. *The Spirit Level. Why Equality is Better for Everyone*, 2nd ed.; Penguin Books: London, UK, 2010.

42. Middleton, G.; Mehta, K.; McNaughton, D.; Booth, S. The Experiences and Perceptions of Foodbank Amongst Users in High Income Countries: An international Scoping Review. *Appetite* **2018**, *120*, 698–708. [CrossRef]

43. Booth, S.; Begley, A.; Mackintosh, B.; Kerr, D.A.; Jancey, J.; Caraher, M.; Whelan, J.; Pollard, C.M. Gratitude, Resignation and the Desire for Dignity: Lived Experience of Food Charity Recipients and Their Recommendations for Improvement, Perth, Western Australia. *Public Health Nutr.* **2018**, *21*, 831–2841. [CrossRef]

44. Douglas, F.; MacKenzie, F.; Ejebu, O.-Z.; Whybrow, S.; Garcia, A.L.; McKenzie, L.; Ludbrook, A.; Dowler, E. "A Lot of People Are Struggling Privately. They Don't Know Where to Go or They're Not Sure of What to Do": Frontline Service Provider Perspectives of the Nature of Household Food Insecurity in Scotland. *Int. J. Environ. Res. Public Health* **2018**, *15*, 2738. [CrossRef] [PubMed]

45. Garthwaite, K. Stigma, Shame and 'People Like Us': An Ethnographic Study of Foodbank Use in the UK. *J. Poverty Soc. Justice* **2016**, *24*, 277–289. [CrossRef]

46. Scheff, T.J. Shame in Self and Society. *Symb. Interact.* **2003**, *26*, 239–262. [CrossRef]

47. Poppendieck, J. *Sweet Charity? Emergency Food and the End of Entitlement*, 1st ed.; Penguin Group: New York, NY, USA, 1998.

48. Silvasti, T. Participatory Alternatives for Food Charity? Finnish Development in an International Comparison. In *Participation, Marginalisation and Welfare Services—Concepts, Politics and Practice Across European Union Countries*, 1st ed.; Matthies, A.-L., Uggerhoj, L., Eds.; Ashgate: Farnham, UK, 2014; pp. 183–197.

49. Simmet, A.; Depa, J.; Tinnemann, P.; Stroebele-Benschop, N. The Nutritional Quality of Food Provided from Food Pantries: A Systematic Review of Existing Literature. *J. Acad. Nutr. Diet.* **2017**, *117*, 577–588. [CrossRef]

50. Simmet, A.; Depa, J.; Tinnemann, P.; Stroebele-Benschop, N. The Dietary Quality of Food Pantry Users: A Systematic Review of Existing Literature. *J. Acad. Nutr. Diet.* **2017**, *117*, 563–576. [CrossRef]

51. United Nations Development Programme. *Discussion Paper Addressing the Social Determinants of Non-communicable Diseases*; United Nations: New York, NY, USA, 2013; Available online: www.undp.org/content/dam/undp/library/hivaids/English/Discussion_Paper_Addressing_the_Social_Determinants_of_NCDs_UNDP_2013.pdf (accessed on 11 April 2019).

52. Friel, S.; Hattersley, L.; Ford, L.; O'Rourke, K. Addressing Inequities in healthy eating. *Health Promot. Int.* **2015**, *30*, ii77–ii88. [CrossRef] [PubMed]

53. Baker, P.; Hawkes, C.; Wingrove, K.; Demaio, A.R.; Parkhurst, J.; Thow, A.M.; Walls, H. What Drives Political Commitment for Nutrition? A Review and Framework Synthesis to Inform the United Nations Decade of Action on Nutrition. *BMJ Glob. Health* **2018**, *3*, e000485. [CrossRef] [PubMed]

54. Tarasuk, V. Implications of Basic Income Guarantee for Household Food Security. Northern Policy Institute Research Paper No. 24. 2017. Available online: https://proof.utoronto.ca/wp-content/uploads/2017/06/Paper-Tarasuk-BIG-EN-17.06.13-1712.pdf (accessed on 11 April 2019).

55. Loopstra, R.; Laylor, D. Financial Insecurity, Food Insecurity, and Disability: The Profile of People Receiving Emergency Food Assistance from The Trussell Trust Foodbank Network in Britain. June 2017. Available online: https://trusselltrust.org/wp-content/uploads/sites/2/2017/06/OU_Report_final_01_08_online.pdf (accessed on 11 April 2019).

56. Kirkpatrick, S.I.; Tarasuk, V. Housing Circumstances are Associated with Household Food Access among Low-Income Urban Families. *J. Urban Health* **2011**, *88*, 284–296. [CrossRef]

57. Landrigan, T.J.; Kerr, D.A.; Dhaliwal, S.S.; Savage, V.; Pollard, C.M. Removing the Australian Tax Exemption on Healthy Food Adds Food Stress to Families Vulnerable to Poor Nutrition. *Aust. New Zealand J. Public Health* **2017**, *41*, 591–597. [CrossRef] [PubMed]

58. Ross, M.; Campbell, E.C.; Webb, K.L. Recent Trends in the Nutritional Quality of Food Banks' Food and Beverage Inventory: Case Studies of Six California Food Banks. *J. Hunger Environ. Nutr.* **2013**, *8*, 294–309. [CrossRef]

59. Wetherill, M.S.; Williams, M.B.; White, K.C.; Li, J.; Vidrine, J.I.; Vidrine, D.J. Food Pantries as Partners in Population Health: Assessing Organizational and Personnel Readiness for Delivering Nutrition-Focused Charitable Food Assistance. *J. Hunger Environ. Nutr.* **2019**, *14*, 50–69. [CrossRef]

60. Too Good to Waste. Lidl UK. Available online: www.lidl.co.uk/en/Too-Good-To-Waste-15447.htm (accessed on 11 April 2019).

61. Martin, K.S.; Redelfs, A.; Wu, R.; Bogner, O.; Whigham, L. Offering More Than Food: Outcomes and Lessons Learned from a Fresh Start food pantry in Texas. *J. Hunger Environ. Nutr.* **2019**, *14*, 70–81. [CrossRef]

62. Martin, K.S.; Colantonio, A.G.; Picho, K.; Boyle, K.E. Self-Efficacy is Associated with Increased Food Security in Novel Food Pantry Program. *SSM Popul. Health* **2016**, *2*, 62–67. [CrossRef]

63. Booth, S.; Pollard, C.M.; Coveney, J.; Goodwin-Smith, I. 'Sustainable' Rather Than 'Subsistence' Food Assistance Solutions to Food Insecurity: South Australian Recipients' Perspectives on Traditional and Social Enterprise Models. *Int. J. Environ. Res. Public Health* **2018**, *21*, 2086. [CrossRef]

64. Food Security in the U.S Survey Tools. Available online: www.ers.usda.gov/topics/food-nutrition-assistance/food-security-in-the-us/survey-tools.aspx (accessed on 11 April 2019).

65. Landrigan, T.J.; Kerr, D.A.; Dhaliwal, S.S.; Pollard, C.M. Protocol for the Development of a Food Stress Index to Identify Households Most at Risk of Food Insecurity in Western Australia. *Int. J. Environ. Res. Public Health* **2018**, *16*, 79. [CrossRef]

66. Temple, J.B.; Russell, J. Food Insecurity among Older Aboriginal and Torres Strait Islanders. *Int. J. Environ. Res. Public Health* **2018**, *15*, 1766. [CrossRef] [PubMed]

67. Temple, J.B.; Booth, S.; Pollard, C.M. Social Assistance Payments and Food Insecurity in Australia: Evidence from the Household Expenditure Survey. *Int. J. Environ. Res. Public Health* **2019**, *16*, 455. [CrossRef]

68. Temple, J.B. The Association between Stressful Events and Food Insecurity: Cross-Sectional Evidence from Australia. *Int. J. Environ. Res. Public Health* **2018**, *15*, 2333. [CrossRef] [PubMed]

69. Simmet, A.; Tinnemann, P.; Stroebele-Benschop, N. The German Food Bank System and Its Users—A Cross-Sectional Study. *Int. J. Environ. Res. Public Health* **2018**, *15*, 1485. [CrossRef] [PubMed]

70. Salonen, A.S.; Ohisalo, M.; Laihiala, T. Undeserving, Disadvantaged, Disregarded: Three Viewpoints of Charity Food Aid Recipients in Finland. *Int. J. Environ. Res. Public Health* **2018**, *15*, 2896. [CrossRef]

71. Pollard, C.M.; Mackintosh, B.; Campbell, C.; Kerr, D.; Begley, A.; Jancey, J.; Caraher, M.; Berg, J.; Booth, S. Charitable Food Systems' Capacity to Address Food Insecurity: An Australian Capital City Audit. *Int. J. Environ. Res. Public Health* **2018**, *15*, 1249. [CrossRef] [PubMed]

72. McCarthy, L.; Chang, A.B.; Brimblecombe, J. Food Security Experiences of Aboriginal and Torres Strait Islander Families with Young Children in an Urban Setting: Influencing Factors and Coping Strategies. *Int. J. Environ. Res. Public Health* **2018**, *15*, 2649. [CrossRef] [PubMed]

73. Maynard, M.; Andrade, L.; Packull-McCormick, S.; Perlman, C.M.; Leos-Toro, C.; Kirkpatrick, S.I. Food Insecurity and Mental Health Among Females in High-Income Countries. *Int. J. Environ. Res. Public Health* **2018**, *15*, 1424. [CrossRef] [PubMed]

74. Mackay, S.; Buch, T.; Vandevijvere, S.; Goodwin, R.; Korohina, E.; Funaki-Tahifote, M.; Lee, A.; Swinburn, B. Cost and Affordability of Diets Modelled on Current Eating Patterns and on Dietary Guidelines, for New Zealand Total Population, Māori and Pacific Households. *Int. J. Environ. Res. Public Health* **2018**, *15*, 1255. [CrossRef] [PubMed]

75. Love, P.; Whelan, J.; Bell, C.; Grainger, F.; Russell, C.; Lewis, M.; Lee, A. Healthy Diets in Rural Victoria—Cheaper than Unhealthy Alternatives, yet Unaffordable. *Int. J. Environ. Res. Public Health* **2018**, *15*, 2469. [CrossRef]

76. Lee, A.; Lewis, M. Testing the Price of Healthy and Current Diets in Remote Aboriginal Communities to Improve Food Security: Development of the Aboriginal and Torres Strait Islander Healthy Diets Asap (Australian Standardised Affordability and Pricing) Methods. *Int. J. Environ. Res. Public Health* **2018**, *15*, 2912. [CrossRef]

77. Kleve, S.; Booth, S.; Davidson, Z.E.; Palermo, C. Walking the Food Security Tightrope—Exploring the Experiences of Low-To-Middle Income Melbourne Households. *Int. J. Environ. Res. Public Health* **2018**, *15*, 2206. [CrossRef]

78. Jessiman-Perreault, G.; McIntyre, L. Household Food Insecurity Narrows the Sex Gap in Five Adverse Mental Health Outcomes Among Canadian Adults. *Int. J. Environ. Res. Public Health* **2019**, *16*, 319. [CrossRef]

79. Gallegos, D.; Chilton, M.M. Re-Evaluating Expertise: Principles for Food and Nutrition Security Research, Advocacy and Solutions in High-Income Countries. *Int. J. Environ. Res. Public Health* **2019**, *16*, 561. [CrossRef] [PubMed]

80. Ferguson, M.; O'Dea, K.; Altman, J.; Moodie, M.; Brimblecombe, J. Health-Promoting Food Pricing Policies and Decision-Making in very Remote Aboriginal and Torres Strait Islander Community Stores in Australia. *Int. J. Environ. Res. Public Health* **2018**, *15*, 2908. [CrossRef] [PubMed]

81. Ejebu, O.-Z.; Whybrow, S.; Mckenzie, L.; Dowler, E.; Garcia, A.L.; Ludbrook, A.; Barton, K.L.; Wrieden, W.L.; Douglas, F. What Can Secondary Data Tell us about Household Food Insecurity in a High-Income Country Context? *Int. J. Environ. Res. Public Health* **2018**, *16*, 82. [CrossRef] [PubMed]

82. Daly, A.; Pollard, C.M.; Kerr, D.A.; Binns, C.W.; Caraher, M.; Phillips, M. Using Cross-Sectional Data to Identify and Quantify the Relative Importance of Factors Associated with and Leading to Food Insecurity. *Int. J. Environ. Res. Public Health* **2018**, *15*, 2620. [CrossRef] [PubMed]

83. Clay, L.A.; Papas, M.A.; Gill, K.B.; Abramson, D.M. Factors Associated with Continued Food Insecurity among Households Recovering from Hurricane Katrina. *Int. J. Environ. Res. Public Health* **2018**, *15*, 1647. [CrossRef] [PubMed]

84. Carrillo-Álvarez, E.; Penne, T.; Boeckx, H.; Storms, B.; Goedemé, T. Food Reference Budgets as a Potential Policy Tool to Address Food Insecurity: Lessons Learned from a Pilot Study in 26 European Countries. *Int. J. Environ. Res. Public Health* **2018**, *16*, 32. [CrossRef] [PubMed]

85. Brown, C.; Laws, C.; Leonard, D.; Campbell, S.; Merone, L.; Hammond, M.; Thompson, K.; Canuto, K.; Brimblecombe, J. Healthy Choice Rewards: A Feasibility Trial of Incentives to Influence Consumer Food Choices in a Remote Australian Aboriginal Community. *Int. J. Environ. Res. Public Health* **2019**, *16*, 112. [CrossRef]

86. Becerra, M.B.; Mshigeni, S.K.; Becerra, B.J. The Overlooked Burden of Food Insecurity among Asian Americans: Results from the California Health Interview Survey. *Int. J. Environ. Res. Public Health* **2018**, *15*, 1684. [CrossRef]

8

Factors Associated with Continued Food Insecurity among Households Recovering from Hurricane Katrina

Lauren A. Clay [1,3,4,]* **ⓘ**, **Mia A. Papas** [2], **Kimberly B. Gill** [3] **and David M. Abramson** [4]

[1] Health Services Administration, D'Youville College, Buffalo, NY 14201, USA
[2] Christiana Care Health System, Value Institute, Wilmington, DE 19899, USA; mia.papas@christianacare.org
[3] Disaster Research Center, University of Delaware, Newark, DE 19716, USA; kgill@udel.edu
[4] College of Global Public Health, New York University, New York, NY 10012, USA;
  david.abramson@nyu.edu
* Correspondence: clayl@dyc.edu

Abstract: In 2010, 14.5% of US households experienced food insecurity, which adversely impacts health. Some groups are at increased risk for food insecurity, such as female-headed households, and those same groups are often also at increased risk for disaster exposure and the negative consequences that come with exposure. Little research has been done on food insecurity post-disaster. The present study investigates long-term food insecurity among households heavily impacted by Hurricane Katrina. A sample of 683 households participating in the Gulf Coast Child and Family Health Study were examined using a generalized estimation model to determine protective and risk factors for food insecurity during long-term recovery. Higher income (Odds Ratio (OR) 0.84, 95% Confidence Interval (CI) 0.77, 0.91), having a partner (OR 0.93; 95% CI 0.89, 0.97), or "other" race were found to be protective against food insecurity over a five-year period following disaster exposure. Low social support (OR 1.14; 95% CI 1.08, 1.20), poor physical health (OR 1.08; 95% CI 1.03, 1.13) or mental health (OR 1.13; 95% CI 1.09, 1.18), and female sex (OR 1.05; 95% CI 1.01, 1.10) were risk factors. Policies and programs that increase access to food supplies among high-risk groups are needed to reduce the negative health impacts of disasters.

Keywords: food insecurity; disaster; family health; Hurricane Katrina; mental health; physical health; social support

1. Introduction

In 2010, 14.5 percent of households in the United States experienced food insecurity, an increase from 11.0 percent in 2005 and 10.9 percent in 2006. Furthermore, 9.8 percent of households with children experienced food insecurity at some point during 2010, affecting 3.9 million households [1].

Food insecurity is higher than the national average for households with children, headed by a single adult, with low income, in rural or urban areas, for minorities, and those residing in the South region of the US [1,2]. The United States Department of Agriculture (USDA) reports that food insecurity is three times more prevalent in single-female-headed households compared to households headed by married couples [3,4]. Furthermore, food insecurity is more than twice as likely in households headed by Hispanic or Black individuals than those households headed by non-Hispanic whites [2]. Food insecurity in the South in 2010 was 10.4 percent, higher than the West (9.4 percent), Midwest (8.1 percent) and Northeast (7.7 percent) regions [1]. In addition to socio-economic factors, a caregiver with poor physical and mental health, disability, weaker social ties and emotional support, and changes in housing or income stability are risk factors for child food insecurity [5–9].

Many research studies have demonstrated that children in food insecure households are at risk for adverse physical and mental health consequences, such as behavioral problems, lower educational achievement, psychosocial dysfunction, depressive symptoms, suicidal symptoms, anxiety, and chronic health conditions [10–16]. A recent literature review completed by Gunderson and colleagues found that food-insecure children are more likely to experience "anemia, lower nutrient intake, cognitive problems, higher levels of aggression and anxiety, poorer general health, poorer oral health, and higher risk of being hospitalized, having asthma, having some birth defects, or experiencing behavioral problems" [17].

Even though there are a number of assistance programs to increase nutritious food intake among those at risk, such as the Special Supplemental Feeding Program for Women, Infant, and Children (WIC), the Supplemental Nutrition Assistance Program (SNAP), and the National School Lunch Program (NSLP), food insecurity remains high in the United States, due at least in part to the lack of understanding about the causes of food insecurity and lack of evidence for effective policy and program solutions [17]. Gaps in research on food insecurity remain. While research shows that disability influences food security, for example, little research has investigated how disability is associated with food insecurity risk. Many studies of risk and protective factors use nationally representative samples in the United States; little research has focused on overlooked groups or special populations outside of traditional demographic groups. Policy solutions are likely to look different for specific populations, such as those that have experienced a significant disaster event. Long-term data collection has also been called for to better understand how food insecurity changes over time, as well as studies that incorporate qualitative methods and the voices of children to more fully tell the story of food insecurity in the U.S. [17–19].

Few studies have focused on food insecurity post-disaster in the United States. Programs have been implemented to aid food-insecure populations after disaster, such as modifications to allowable purchases for Supplemental Nutrition Assistance Program (SNAP) beneficiaries after Superstorm Sandy in New Jersey so families were able to repurchase lost food supplies [20], however little is understood about those that are living on the cusp of food insecurity that may be pushed into insecurity due to the disruption of a disaster or other change in circumstance, such as changes in housing or decline in mothers' mental health [9].

We know that vulnerability to disaster exposure and negative consequences vary based on resource access, age, physical ability, sex, race and ethnicity, and living conditions [21–23]. We also know that single women, single mothers, and caregivers, in addition to experiencing increased risk of food insecurity, are also more vulnerable following disasters [3,4,24], and race, ethnicity, disability, functional and access needs, and mental health contribute to decreased disaster preparedness and may impede or slow disaster recovery [25–31]. Following disaster exposure, resources are lost, including material (personal property), social (social support), and neighborhood-based resources due to relocation, and food insecurity is common or the odds of food insecurity increase [32–36]. Resource loss contributes to psychological distress, such as anxiety, depression, and post-traumatic stress disorder (PTSD) [33,34,37]. This loops back to the influence of caretaker mental health on child food security.

Factors contributing to food insecurity and disaster risk are complex, and the impact from each influences health outcomes. However, few studies have explored food insecurity in a post-disaster setting. In summary, prior research has established the impact of food insecurity on health and well-being, the noted risk factor of changes in housing and economic circumstance on food insecurity risk, the need for longitudinal study of food insecurity, and the evidence of increased food insecurity risk post-Hurricane Katrina. Given this, the present study examines long-term food insecurity in a sample of households heavily impacted by Hurricane Katrina, taking into account resource loss and demographic characteristics.

2. Materials and Methods

2.1. Sample and Data Collection

Households were surveyed as part of the Gulf Coast Child and Family Health (G-CAFH) Study, a longitudinal study of household disaster recovery following Hurricane Katrina in Louisiana and Mississippi. Households were recruited in 2006 and participated in an annual follow up. Households were randomly sampled from census blocks classified by Federal Emergency Management Agency (FEMA) assessments as moderately to extensively damaged, and from FEMA subsidized housing. The current analysis examined data from households that participated in waves two, three, and four of the G-CAFH Study. Wave two was collected between May and July 2007 ($n = 803$), wave three was collected between June and August 2008 ($n = 777$), and wave four was collected between October 2009 and March 2010 ($n = 844$), resulting in a four-year observation period for 683 households. A bias analysis conducted by the G-CAFH Study team demonstrated that there are no significant differences due to attrition between the cohort at wave one and at wave four. Additional information on study design and methodology has been published elsewhere [38,39].

2.2. Measures

Food insecurity was assessed in waves two, three, and four of the study by asking participants to think about their basic needs over the past three to six months. In wave two, respondents were asked to report on the past six months, "How well has your need for food for the household been met?" (not met, somewhat met, or met completely), and in waves three and four, respondents were asked, "In the past three months, how often it has happened there was not enough money in the household for food that you (the family) should have?" (never, once in a while, fairly often, or very often). Respondents were classified as food insecure in each wave if they answered that the need was not met or they fairly or very often did not have enough money in the household for food. The United States Department of Agriculture defines food insecurity as "a household-level economic and social condition of limited or uncertain access to adequate food [40]." The G-CAFH study questions are intended to capture social and economic limitations to access adequate food. Although not validated against the USDA measure for food insecurity, these questions provide a starting point to understand food insecurity in a disaster-affected population.

Social support was assessed by asking respondents if they had someone they could count on for everyday favors, such as borrowing a little money, to care for you if you were confined to a bed for several weeks, to lend you money for a medical emergency, to talk to about family relationship troubles, or to help you find housing if you had to move. Respondents were categorized as having low social support if they responded yes to fewer than two of these statements.

Physical and mental health were self-reported by respondents using the Short Form (SF)-12 Health Survey [41]. The Mental Component Score (MCS) and Physical Component Score (PCS) were computed. A PCS score of less than 45 was classified as Physical Health Distress, and an MCS score of less than 42 was classified as Mental Health Distress, consistent with past research [41,42]. Respondents were classified as having a disability if they responded "disabled" when reporting on characteristics of the household.

Demographic variables included in this analysis included income (<$10 K, $10–20 K, $20–35 K, $35–50 K, >$50 K), age (18–34, 35–49, 50–65, 66+), race and ethnicity (Black, White, Latino, other), and sex (male, female) and were self-reported by G-CAFH participants.

2.3. Statistical Analysis

Generalized estimating equations were used to determine bivariate associations between each exposure variable and our outcome over time. In addition, this longitudinal modeling strategy was employed to examine multivariate associations between exposures and food insecurity after adjustment for confounding. Models utilized wave of data collection as the family variable and study identification number as the link variable. Generalized estimating equations enable analysis of repeated measures over time and take into account the dependent structure of the data, given within-person correlation. The benefits of this approach include accounting for within-subject and within-group correlation and accommodating inconsistent intervals between data points [43]. Factors that were independently associated with food insecurity over time were included in a multivariate longitudinal model that utilized a generalized estimating equation. Stata 13 version 1 was used for analyses (StataCorp LP, College Station, TX, USA) [44].

3. Results

Table 1 presents demographic characteristics of the sample ($n = 683$) at each wave. Changes in age, sex, partnership status, and race/ethnicity composition over time were assessed, and findings show there was stability in characteristics over the three time periods (all p-values for change >0.05). The sample was 51.5 percent Black, 43 percent White and 2.7 percent Latino. Over 60% of respondents were female. Changes in employment status, income level, and number of moves since Hurricane Katrina were statistically significant over the three waves of data collection. Employment dropped in the fourth wave of follow up, and income and number of moves increased over time.

Table 1. Sample Characteristics and significance of change over time.

Sample Characteristics	Wave 2 (2007)	Wave 3 (2008)	Wave 4 (2009–2010)
	n (within col %)	n (within col %)	n (within col %)
Employed (20+ h per week) **	335 (45.6)	349 (45.5)	328 (40.0)
Partnered (married, living as married)	341 (42.5)	344 (44.5)	372 (44.2)
Income *			
<$10 K	274 (34.3)	224 (29.1)	241 (28.7)
$10–20 K	258 (32.3)	214 (27.8)	265 (31.5)
$20–35 K	126 (15.8)	157 (20.39)	149 (17.7)
$35–50 K	71 (8.9)	88 (11.4)	87 (10.3)
>$50 K	58 (7.3)	68 (8.8)	84 (10.0)
Don't know/refused	12 (1.5)	19 (2.5)	15 (1.8)
Age			
18–34	154 (19.2)	129 (16.7)	142 (16.8)
35–49	272 (34.0)	266 (34.4)	272 (32.2)
50–65	271 (33.8)	271 (35.0)	305 (36.1)
66+	104 (13.0)	108 (14.0)	125 (14.8)
Number of moves since Katrina [Mean (SD)] ***	3.79 (2.00)	3.81 (2.04)	4.59 (2.95)
Race/Ethnicity			
Black	420 (51.5)		
White	351 (43.0)		
Latino	22 (2.7)	Constant variables	
Other	23 (2.8)		
Sex			
Male	305 (39.3)		
Female	471 (60.7)		

* $p < 0.05$, ** $p < 0.01$, *** $p < 0.001$.

Food insecurity, disability, mental health, and social support prevalence in the study sample changed significantly over time (Table 2). Food insecurity ranged from 30.4 percent in wave two to 20.1 percent in wave three. In wave four, food insecurity prevalence increased slightly to 23.1 percent. Disability prevalence increased with each subsequent wave of data collection, from 13.4 percent in wave two to 20.5 percent in wave four. Poor mental health and low social support prevalence decreased with each subsequent wave of data collection (47.9 to 38.5 and 24.2 to 15.3 percent, respectively).

Table 2. Sample Health Characteristics and significance of change over time ˆ.

Health Characteristics	Wave 2	Wave 3	Wave 4
	n (within col %)	*n* (within col %)	*n* (within col %)
Food insecurity ***	244 (30.4)	163 (21.0)	194 (23.1)
Disabled ***	98 (13.4)	121 (15.8)	173 (20.5)
Poor physical health	405 (50.7)	397 (51.2)	435 (51.7)
Poor mental health ***	383 (47.9)	300 (38.7)	324 (38.5)
Low social support ***	186 (24.2)	129 (18.4)	125 (15.3)

*** $p < 0.001$. ˆ *p*-values from chi2 statistic reported for at least one difference between waves.

Examination of bivariate associations among health, demographic characteristics, and the outcome food insecurity indicated employment, partnership, income, older age (66+), and white race are statistically significant and inversely associated with food insecurity, while female sex, moves since Katrina, disability, poor physical and mental health, and low social support were statistically significant and positively associated with food insecurity (Table 3).

Table 3. Bivariate association between demographic characteristics and health status with food insecurity over time ˆ.

Demographic and Health Characteristics	Beta Coefficient	Standard Error
Employed (20+ h per week) ***	−0.08	0.02
Partnered (married, living as married) ***	−0.10	0.02
Income (<$10 K)		
$10–20 K **	−0.06	0.02
$20–35 K ***	−0.16	0.03
$35–50 K ***	−0.24	0.03
>$50 K ***	−0.30	0.03
Don't know/refused	−0.11	0.06
Age (18–34)		
35–49	0.02	0.03
50–65	−0.03	0.03
66+ **	−0.11	0.04
Race/Ethnicity (Black)		
White **	−0.06	0.02
Latino	0.07	0.07
Other	−0.12	0.07
Sex (Male)		
Female ***	0.08	0.02
Moves since Katrina *	0.01	0.004
Disabled ***	0.13	0.02
Poor physical health ***	0.10	0.02
Poor mental health ***	0.17	0.02
Low social support ***	0.17	0.02

* $p < 0.05$, ** $p < 0.01$, *** $p < 0.001$. ˆ xtgee models run for each independent variable and the dichotomous outcome food insecurity.

These factors were included in a generalized estimation equation model for panel data to determine associations with food insecurity two to five years after initial exposure to Hurricane Katrina (Table 4). Respondents who reported having a partner (OR 0.93; 95% CI 0.89, 0.97), higher income ($35–50 K OR 0.89; 0.83, 0.96; >$50 K OR 0.84; 0.77, 0.91), and being White (OR 0.95; 0.91, 1.10) or "other" race (OR 0.84; 0.73, 0.97) were less likely to report food insecurity over a five-year time frame post-disaster. Respondents who were female (OR 1.05; 1.01, 1.10), reported poor physical health (OR 1.08; 1.03, 1.13) or mental health (OR 1.13; 1.09, 1.18), or low social support (OR 1.14; 1.08, 1.20) were more likely to report food insecurity over time.

Table 4. Odds of reporting food insecurity by demographic and health characteristics of respondents over time.

Demographic and Health Characteristics	Odds Ratio	95% CI
Employed (20+ h per week)	1.00	(0.94, 1.04)
Partnered (married, living as married) *	0.93	(0.89, 0.97)
Income (<$10 K)		
$10–20 K	0.99	(0.94, 1.04)
$20–35 K **	0.92	(0.86, 0.98)
$35–50 K **	0.89	(0.83, 0.96)
>$50 K ***	0.84	(0.77, 0.91)
Don't know/refused	1.01	(0.85, 1.19)
Age (18–34)		
35–49	1.03	(0.97, 1.10)
50–65	0.96	(0.90, 1.02)
66+	0.90	(0.83, 0.98)
Race/Ethnicity (Black)		
White *	0.95	(0.91, 0.99)
Latino	1.06	(0.93, 1.21)
Other *	0.84	(0.73, 0.97)
Sex (Male)		
Female *	1.05	(1.01, 1.10)
Moves since Katrina	1.01	(0.997, 1.01)
Disabled ^	1.06	(1.00, 1.13)
Poor physical health **	1.08	(1.03, 1.13)
Poor mental health ***	1.13	(1.09, 1.18)
Low social support ***	1.14	(1.08, 1.20)

* $p < 0.05$, ** $p < 0.01$, *** $p < 0.001$. ^ $p = 0.05$.

4. Discussion

According to the USDA, average food insecurity prevalence in 2007–2009 in Louisiana and Mississippi was 10.0 percent and 17.1 percent, respectively [45]. We would expect baseline rates of food insecurity in this sample to be similar. We found food insecurity prevalence was 30.4, 21.0, and 23.1 percent in waves two, three, and four of data collection in the present sample, much higher than average state prevalence rates over a similar time frame. However, caution is warranted in comparing food insecurity rates from our study to the National average, since a standardized, validated measure of food insecurity was not included in the G-CAFH study, as the purpose of the study was to more broadly understand child and family health during long-term disaster recovery and it was not focused specifically on food insecurity. However, the high rate of food access issues described in this population make it increasingly important to examine the food environment post-disaster as it is not well understood, and there is little in the literature on the impact of disasters on those families that experience food insecurity during the year or may be living on the edge, and the disruption due to a disaster creates greater household strain.

In this sample of households heavily impacted by Hurricane Katrina, being female, having poor physical and mental health, and low social support were risk factors for food insecurity during long-term disaster recovery, and having a partner, greater income, and being non-Hispanic white or "other" race were protective against food insecurity. This is consistent with food insecurity research that demonstrates that female-headed households, individuals with poor physical or mental health, decline in mothers' physical or mental health and weaker social ties and emotional support are associated with increased food insecurity [3–5,8,9]. It is also consistent with the disaster literature that shows that certain populations are more vulnerable to increased disaster risk and adverse consequences following disasters, such as those with poor physical or mental health, women, and individuals with low social support [21,22,24,28–30,34]

The research question and analyses were planned after data collection was completed for waves one through four of the G-CAFH study, therefore the limitations of secondary analysis apply to the present investigation. There was no pre-event data on food insecurity prevalence for this sample due to the unpredictable nature of disasters, therefore we were not able to determine whether food insecurity was a pre-existing issue for families recovering from Hurricane Katrina or a new situation. For this analysis, the inconsistent wording of the food insecurity question may have resulted in different interpretations by the study participants from wave one to waves two and three. Data on this cohort, however, provide a number of distinct benefits that contribute to the existing literature. It was noted earlier that much of the food insecurity research has been conducted with nationally representative samples [17]. This investigation examined a sample of households heavily impacted by a disaster, and starts to tell the story of household food insecurity in a new population. Another strength of this study is in showing a picture of longer-term recovery and food insecurity through a longitudinal study design, which are costly and rare in the disaster literature [46,47]. The study was also carefully designed and executed to enable longitudinal analysis on a cohort, with an 87.6 percent retention rate at wave four of data collection.

To improve disaster outcomes and reduce recovery time, efforts to mitigate, prepare for, and respond to disasters should focus on engagement with vulnerable groups, such as those with physical and mental health distress, female-headed households, and socially isolated populations, to ensure adequate food access and availability. Following disasters, transportation lines may be interrupted, causing access issues for people with physical disabilities and mobility impairments. Further compounding access issues, supply chains may be interrupted, reducing the availability of foods in some areas following disasters [48,49]. Individuals with low social support may lack people to rely on for rides or other help to access foods. For individuals with poor mental health, the additional stress of the disaster experience may exacerbate conditions and result in lower self-efficacy and reduced functioning.

To reduce food insecurity during long-term recovery from disasters, programs and policies should be implemented to increase access to financial support for food or to ensure access to food supplies. One example of such an intervention is the re-issuance of SNAP or WIC benefits to replace spoiled or soiled food supplies and the expansion of benefits to include prepared foods, to enable families living without kitchen facilities to use benefits for meals, as was done following Superstorm Sandy in New Jersey to meet community needs [20]. Systematically adjusting these programs and making the policy known to the end user may reduce uncertainty following disasters and increase utilization. Furthermore, programs that are targeted to reach single-headed, female-headed, low-income, and minority households during non-disaster times with information about securing food in a disaster may reduce vulnerability. Such programs might include educational sessions on food provisions and programs following disasters, facilitation of neighborhood block or community based bulk purchasing of non-perishable foods, or availability of disaster preparedness kits including non-perishable foods through food banks or other food programs. Communicating and building a rapport with community organizations and high risk populations in non-disaster times may also enable more effective post-disaster communication about resources, programs, and services available to affected households. Additional research is needed to determine the effectiveness of policy interventions, such as the re-issued SNAP benefits, for reducing food insecurity post-disaster.

It is also interesting to note that number of moves post-Katrina was not a statistically significant predictor of food insecurity during long-term recovery. The food insecurity literature shows that a change in housing or income stability increases the risk of food insecurity [9]. The present study includes a sample of households heavily impacted by Hurricane Katrina, with families moving an average of 4.59 times at five years post-Katrina. However, in the present analysis, this was not associated with increased food insecurity risk. Additional research on households experiencing food and housing insecurity post-disaster is needed to better understand this circumstance.

This sample was part of a longitudinal study of child and family health following Hurricane Katrina, a group of households heavily impacted or displaced by Hurricane Katrina. This analysis is only a first step towards understanding food insecurity in a post-disaster setting among displaced families, but is not generalizable to all disaster affected populations or the general U.S. population. Additional research is needed on a representative sample of households impacted by disaster and in other geographic locations and hazard types.

5. Conclusions

Populations at increased risk for food insecurity also experience increased disaster risk and consequences. Disaster managers and public health practitioners working in these two spheres may be able to find synergy in non-disaster times, as well as when preparing for, responding to, and supporting recovery from disasters. Mitigation of food insecurity in the absence of a disaster may increase resilience to disasters for vulnerable households. Additional research on the experience of households that are food insecure at times during the year and those living with marginal food security, where exposure to a disaster leads them to have low or very low food security, is needed to better understand the health impacts of disaster and how to better meet the needs of this population. A better understanding of the role of housing disruption in a post-disaster setting is also needed to inform policies and programs to mitigate food insecurity for families recovering from disaster.

Author Contributions: Conceptualization, L.A.C., M.A.P., K.B.G., D.M.A.; Methodology, L.A.C., M.A.P., D.M.A.; Formal Analysis, L.A.C., M.A.P.; Investigation, L.A.C., M.A.P., K.B.G., D.M.A.; Data Curation, L.A.C., D.M.A.; Writing—Original Draft Preparation, L.A.C., M.A.P.; Writing—Review & Editing, L.A.C., M.A.P., K.B.G., D.M.A.

Acknowledgments: The authors would like to acknowledge the original research team that conducted the Gulf Coast Child and Family Health Study at the National Center for Disaster Preparedness, the Children's Health Fund for funding the research, and the families that participated in the study for generously sharing their experiences in Hurricane Katrina so that we may learn about and work to improve the disaster recovery process.

References

1. Coleman-Jensen, A.; Nord, M.; Andrews, M.; Carlson, S. *Household Food Security in the United States in 2011;* ERR-141, United States Department of Agriculture, Economic Research Service: Washington, DC, USA, September 2012.

2. Nord, M.; Andrews, M.; Carlson, S. *Household Food Security in the United States, 2008;* ERR-83, United States Department of Agriculture, Economic Research Service: Washington, DC, USA, November 2009.

3. Hill, S.A. Cultural images and the health of African American women. *Gender Soc.* **2009**, *23*, 733–746. [CrossRef]

4. Schulz, A.J.; Mullings, L. *Gender, Race, Class, and Health: Intersectional Approaches;* Jossey-Bass: San Francisco, CA, USA, 2006.

5. Kaushal, N. *Income and Food Insecurity: New Evidence from the Fragile Families and Child Wellbeing Study*; Columbia University: New York, NY, USA, 2013.

6. Balistreri, K. *Family Structure, Work Patterns and Time Allocations: Potential Mechanisms of Food Insecurity among Children*; University of Kentucky Center for Poverty Research Discussion Paper Series, DP2012-07; Available online: http://www.ukcpr.org/Publications/DP2012-07.pdf (accessed on 3 May 2018).

7. Noonan, K.; Corman, H.; Reichman, N.E. Effects of Maternal Depression on Family Food Insecurity. *Econ. Hum. Biol.* **2016**, *22*, 201–215. [CrossRef] [PubMed]

8. Anderson, P.M.; Butcher, K.; Hoynes, H.; Schanzenbach, D.W. Beyond Income: What Else Predicts Very Low Food Security among Children? *South. Econ. J.* **2016**, *82*, 1078–1105. [CrossRef]

9. Jacknowitz, A.; Morrisey, T. *Food Insecurity across the First Five Years: Triggers of Onset and Exit*; University of Kentucky Center for Poverty Research Discussion Paper Series, DP2012-08; Available online: http://www.ukcpr.org/Publications/DP2012-08.pdf (accessed on 3 May 2018).

10. Bronte-Tinkew, J.; Zaslow, M.; Capps, R.; Horowitz, A.; McNamara, M. Food insecurity works through depression, parenting, and infant feeding to influence overweight and health in toddlers. *J. Nutr.* **2007**, *137*, 2160–2165. [CrossRef] [PubMed]

11. Casey, P.H.; Szeto, K.L.; Robbins, J.M.; Stuff, J.E.; Connell, C.; Gossett, J.M.; Simpson, P.M. Child health-related quality of life and household food security. *Arch. Pediatr. Adolesc. Med.* **2005**, *159*, 51–56. [CrossRef] [PubMed]

12. Jyoti, D.F.; Frongillo, E.A.; Jones, S.J. Food insecurity affects school children's academic performance, weight gain, and social skills. *J. Nutr.* **2005**, *135*, 2831–2839. [CrossRef] [PubMed]

13. Winicki, J.; Jemison, K. Food insecurity and hunger in the kindergarten classroom: Its effect on learning and growth. *Contemp. Econ. Policy* **2003**, *21*, 145–157. [CrossRef]

14. Kleinman, R.E.; Murphy, J.M.; Little, M.; Pagano, M.; Wehler, C.A.; Regal, K.; Jellinek, M.S. Hunger in children in the United States: Potential behavioral and emotional correlates. *Pediatrics* **1998**, *101*, e3. [CrossRef] [PubMed]

15. Weinreb, L.; Wehler, C.; Perloff, J.; Scott, R.; Hosmer, D.; Sagor, L.; Gundersen, C. Hunger: Its impact on children's health and mental health. *Pediatrics* **2002**, *110*, e41. [CrossRef] [PubMed]

16. Whitaker, R.C.; Phillips, S.M.; Orzol, S.M. Food insecurity and the risks of depression and anxiety in mothers and behavior problems in their preschool-aged children. *Pediatrics* **2006**, *118*, e859–e868. [CrossRef] [PubMed]

17. Gundersen, C.; Ziliak, J.P. Childhood food insecurity in the US: Trends, causes, and policy options. *Future Child.* **2014**, *24*, 1–19. [CrossRef]

18. Huang, J.; Guo, B.; Kim, Y. Food insecurity and disability: Do economic resources matter? *Soc. Sci. Res.* **2010**, *39*, 111–124. [CrossRef]

19. Coleman-Jensen, A.; Nord, M.; Singh, A. *Household Food Security in the United States in 2012*; ERR-155; United States Department of Agriculture, Economic Research Service: Washington, DC, USA, September 2013.

20. USDA Offers Food Assistance to Those Affected by Hurricane Sandy. Available online: https://www.fns.usda.gov/pressrelease/2012/034012 (accessed on 10 May 2018).

21. Comfort, L.; Wisner, B.; Cutter, S.; Pulwarty, R.; Hewitt, K.; Oliver-Smith, A.; Wiener, J.; Fordham, M.; Peacock, W.; Krimgold, F. Reframing disaster policy: The global evolution of vulnerable communities. *Environ. Hazards* **1999**, *1*, 39–44.

22. Wisner, B.; Blaikie, P.; Cannon, T.; Davis, I. *At Risk: Natural Hazards, People's Vulnerability and Disasters*, 2nd ed.; Psychology Press: New York, NY, USA, 2004.

23. Klinenberg, E. *Heat Wave. A Social Autopsy of Disaster in Chicago*; The University of Chicago Press: Chicago, IL, USA, 2002.

24. Enarson, E.; Fothergill, A.; Peek, L. Gender and disaster: Foundations and directions. In *Handbook of Disaster Research*; Rodríguez, H., Quarantelli, E.L., Dynes, R., Eds.; Springer: New York, NY, USA, 2007; pp. 130–146.

25. Ablah, E.; Konda, K.; Kelley, C.L. Factors Predicting Individual Emergency Preparedness: A Multi-state Analysis of 2006 BRFSS Data. *Biosecur. Bioterror.* **2009**, *7*, 317–330. [CrossRef] [PubMed]

26. Bethel, J.W.; Foreman, A.N.; Burke, S.C. Disaster preparedness among medically vulnerable populations. *Am. J. Prev. Med.* **2011**, *40*, 139–143. [CrossRef] [PubMed]

27. Eisenman, D.P.; Zhou, Q.; Ong, M.; Asch, S.; Glik, D.; Long, A. Variations in disaster preparedness by mental health, perceived general health, and disability status. *Disaster Med. Public Health Prep.* **2009**, *3*, 33–41. [CrossRef] [PubMed]

28. Bolin, R.; Jackson, M.; Crist, A. Gender inequality, vulnerability, and disaster: Issues in theory and research. In *The Gendered Terrain of Disaster: Through Women's Eyes*; Enarson, E., Hearn Morrow, B., Eds.; Praeger: Westport, CT, USA, 1998; pp. 27–44.

29. Fothergill, A.; Maestas, E.G.; Darlington, J.D. Race, ethnicity and disasters in the United States: A review of the literature. *Disasters* **1999**, *23*, 156–173. [CrossRef] [PubMed]

30. Phillips, B.D. *Disaster Recovery*; Taylor and Francis: Boca Raton, FL, USA, 2009.

31. Clay, L.A.; Goetschius, J.B.; Papas, M.A.; Kendra, J. Influence of Mental Health on Disaster Preparedness: Findings from the Behavioral Risk Factor Surveillance System, 2007–2009. *J. Homel. Secur. Emerg. Manag.* **2014**. [CrossRef]

32. Hobfoll, S.E. Conservation of resources: A new attempt at conceptualizing stress. *Am. Psychol.* **1989**, *44*, 513–524. [CrossRef] [PubMed]

33. Freedy, J.R.; Shaw, D.L.; Jarrell, M.P.; Masters, C.R. Towards an Understanding of the Psychological Impact of Natural Disasters: An Application of the Conservation Resources Stress Model. *J. Trauma. Stress* **1992**, *5*, 441–454. [CrossRef]

34. Zwiebach, L.; Rhodes, J.; Roemer, L. Resource loss, resource gain, and mental health among survivors of Hurricane Katrina. *J. Trauma. Stress* **2010**, *23*, 751–758. [CrossRef] [PubMed]

35. Clay, L.A.; Papas, M.; Gill, K.; Abramson, D. Food Insecurity during Long-term Recovery from Hurricane Katrina: A Longitudinal Analysis. *Ann. Epidemiol.* **2017**, *27*, 527–528. [CrossRef]

36. Hutson, R.A.; Trzcinski, E.; Kolbe, A.R. Features of child food insecurity after the 2010 Haiti earthquake: Results from longitudinal random survey of households. *PLoS ONE* **2014**, *9*, e104497. [CrossRef] [PubMed]

37. Arata, C.M.; Picou, J.S.; Johnson, G.D.; McNally, T.S. Coping with technological disaster: An application of the conservation of resources model to the Exxon Valdez oil spill. *J. Trauma. Stress* **2000**, *13*, 23–39. [CrossRef] [PubMed]

38. Abramson, D.M.; Stehling-Ariza, T.; Park, Y.S.; Gruber, D.; Wilson, C.; Sury, J.; Banister, A.N. *Second Wind: The Impact of Hurricane Gustav on Children and Families Who Survived Katrina*; Columbia University: New York, NY, USA, 2009.

39. Abramson, D.M.; Stehling-Ariza, T.; Park, Y.S.; Walsh, L.; Culp, D. Measuring Individual Disaster Recovery: A Socioecological Framework. *Disaster Med. Public Health Prep.* **2010**, *4*, S46. [CrossRef] [PubMed]

40. United States Department of Agriculture, Definitions of Food Insecurity. 2017. Available online: https://www.ers.usda.gov/topics/food-nutrition-assistance/food-security-in-the-us/definitions-of-food-security/ (accessed on 10 May 2018).

41. Ware, J.E., Jr.; Kosinski, M.; Keller, S.D. A 12-Item Short-Form Health Survey: Construction of scales and preliminary tests of reliability and validity. *Med. Care* **1996**, *34*, 220–233. [CrossRef] [PubMed]

42. Abramson, D.; Stehling-Ariza, T.; Garfield, R.; Redlener, I. Prevalence and predictors of mental health distress post-Katrina: Findings from the Gulf Coast Child and Family Health Study. *Disaster Med. Public Health Prep.* **2008**, *2*, 77–86. [CrossRef] [PubMed]

43. Fitzmaurice, G.M.; Laird, N.M.; Ware, J.H. *Applied Longitudinal Analysis*, 2nd ed.; Wiley-Interscience: Hoboken, NJ, USA, 2011.

44. StataCorp. *Stata Statistical Software*; StataCorp: College Station, TX, USA, 2013.

45. Nord, M.; Coleman-Jensen, A.; Andrews, M.; Carlson, S. *Household Food Security in the United States, 2009*; ERR-108; United States Department of Agriculture, Economic Research Service: Washington, DC, USA, November 2010.

46. Riad, J.K.; Norris, F.H. The influence of relocation on the environmental, social, and psychological stress experienced by disaster victims. *Environ. Behav.* **1996**, *28*, 163–182. [CrossRef]

47. Shrubsole, D. *Natural Disasters and Public Health Issues: A Review of the Literature with a Focus on the Recovery Period*; ICLR Research Paper Series; Institute for Catastrophic Loss Reduction: Toronto, ON, Canada, 1999.

48. Holguín-Veras, J.; Pérez, N.; Ukkusuri, S.; Wachtendorf, T.; Brown, B. Emergency logistics issues affecting the response to Katrina: A synthesis and preliminary suggestions for improvement. *Transp. Res. Rec.* **2007**, *2022*, 76–82. [CrossRef]

49. Holguín-Veras, J.; Jaller, M.; Van Wassenhove, L.N.; Pérez, N.; Wachtendorf, T. On the unique features of post-disaster humanitarian logistics. *J. Oper. Manag.* **2012**, *30*, 494–506. [CrossRef]

9

Protocol for the Development of a Food Stress Index to Identify Households Most at Risk of Food Insecurity in Western Australia

Timothy J. Landrigan *⬤, Deborah A. Kerr⬤, Satvinder S. Dhaliwal and Christina M. Pollard⬤

School of Public Health, Curtin University, Kent Street, GPO Box U1987, Perth 6845, Australia;
D.Kerr@curtin.edu.au (D.A.K.); S.Dhaliwal@curtin.edu.au (S.S.D.); C.Pollard@curtin.edu.au (C.M.P.)
* Correspondence: timothy.landrigan@postgrad.curtin.edu.au

Abstract: Food stress, a similar concept to housing stress, occurs when a household needs to spend more than 25% of their disposable income on food. Households at risk of food stress are vulnerable to food insecurity as a result of inadequate income. A Food Stress Index (FSI) identifies at-risk households, in a particular geographic area, using a range of variables to create a single indicator. Candidate variables were identified using a multi-dimensional framework consisting of household demographics, household income, household expenses, financial stress indicators, food security, food affordability and food availability. The candidate variables were expressed as proportions, of either persons or households, in a geographic area. Principal Component Analysis was used to determine the final variables which resulted in a final set of weighted raw scores. These scores were then scaled to produce the index scores for the Food Stress Index for Western Australia. The results were compared with the Australian Bureau of Statistics' Socio-Economic Indexes for Areas to determine suitability. The Food Stress Index was found to be a suitable indicator of the relative risk of food stress in Western Australian households. The FSI adds specificity to indices of relative disadvantage specifically related to food insecurity and provides a useful tool for prioritising policy and other responses to this important public health issue.

Keywords: food insecurity; food stress; food affordability

---

1. Introduction

The different Socio-Economic Indexes for Areas (SEIFA) developed by the Australian Bureau of Statistics (ABS) measure various aspects of socio-economic status. The four different indexes measure relative socio-economic disadvantage (IRSD), relative socio-economic advantage or disadvantage (IRSAD), education and occupation (IEO), and economic resources (IER) [1], however, none of those indexes provide a suitable measure of food insecurity or food stress. The variables used in constructing these indexes are wider socio-economic measures and don't relate specifically to food insecurity. In order to measure food insecurity, these indexes need to be used in conjunction with other data such as food costs to provide an indication of the impact of socio-economic status and food costs on health [2–6].

The concept of a Food Stress Index (FSI) is to provide a simple indication of the potential for food stress of households in a particular geographic location which may be postcode, Statistical Area, Local Government Area or another region. It is a single index that encompasses all aspects of food insecurity to provide information about the likelihood households in a geographic area are suffering food stress.

Housing stress is usually defined as occurring for those households who spend more than 30% of their income on housing costs, whether that is rent or mortgage [7]. This is particularly critical for those households whose income is in the 1st or 2nd quintile. Housing affordability relates to a household's or a person's ability to pay for their housing. The impacts of housing stress are widespread as this impacts a household's spending patterns and has wider effects on the economy as a whole.

Food stress is a similar concept to housing stress and occurs when a household needs to spend more than 25% of their disposable income on food [8]. Australian research has shown that welfare-dependent and low-income households are suffering food stress [9–11]. Between 2008 and 2012, this food inequality has risen in Australia [12].

Households at risk of food stress are vulnerable to food insecurity as a result of inadequate income. Food security is "when all people, at all times, have physical and economic access to sufficient, safe and nutritious food to meet their dietary needs and food preferences for an active and healthy life." [13]. The 2011–2012 Australian Health Survey (AHS) found that four per cent of all Australian households 'ran out of food in the last 12 months and couldn't afford to buy more', increasing to seven per cent of households in the most disadvantaged areas, compared to only one per cent in the least disadvantaged areas. The prevalence was higher among Aboriginal and Torres Strait Islander households with 22% overall and 31% of those households in remote areas running out of food in the previous year [14]. Research looking at the relationship between food security status and multiple socio-demographic variables found that 36% of survey participants had low or very low food security [15].

The United States Department of Agriculture has a Food Security Survey Module (FSSM) [16,17] that is run every two years to measure levels of food security in the United States. In Australia the only routine food security measure is the single-item question on the AHS which does not effectively measure levels of food insecurity [18]. There is no measure, equivalent to the USDA FSSM, that allows routine monitoring of the prevalence of food insecurity at a population level in Australia with the only research to date being undertaken in small geographic areas using small samples [15,18].

Food affordability is defined as the amount of money a household spends on food, relative to income of that household. It is of greater concern for lower income households as they spend a greater proportion of their income on food [19]. Food affordability impacts not only the wider economy through the impacts on spending patterns, but also on health by affecting the ability to purchase healthy and nutritious food [20,21]. While some household expenses are fixed (e.g., rent or utility expenses), the food budget is changeable and can be cut back if needed with nutrition consequences [22]. If one household expense increases (e.g., an increase in rent) then this will impact on that household's food affordability leading to additional stress on the food budget; i.e., food stress. As a household becomes food stressed, they become vulnerable to food insecurity as they have less available income to meet their dietary needs.

The Food Stress Index is designed as a single measure, using currently available data without the need for additional and expensive surveillance, that ranks geographic areas based on the likelihood that households in those areas are food stressed. The FSI is not a measure of food insecurity as not every household in geographic areas at high risk of food stress would be food insecure; the FSI shows particular geographic areas where households would be more vulnerable to food insecurity. A FSI could be used to measure the impact food affordability has on chronic disease such as diabetes and cardiovascular disease. It could also be used to highlight areas or households in need of food relief.

2. Materials and Methods

2.1. Developing a Food Stress Index

The methodology used to create the Food Stress Index is similar methodology to that used to develop the Australian Bureau of Statistics' SEIFA [1] index. The FSI is a weighted combination of select variables that results in a score that can be used to rank areas according to the likelihood of food stress in each area. The index is assigned to areas and reflects the characteristics of the households of people living in an area.

Starting with a broad list of potential or candidate variables covering all aspects of food stress and socio-economic indicators, Principal Component Analysis [23] was used to reduce these variables to a single index which indicates the likelihood households in the selected geographic area are suffering food stress. Low index scores indicate less likelihood of food stress while high index scores indicate more likelihood of food stress. The methodology is discussed in detail below.

2.2. The List of Candidate Variables

In order to encapsulate various aspects of food affordability and food stress a wide range of candidate variables were considered when constructing the Food Stress Index. This resulted in an initial set of over 50 candidate variables from eight different datasets from existing surveys. The framework for the selection of variables was based around the following dimensions:

- Household demographics
- Household income
- Household expenses
- Financial stress
- Food affordability
- Geographic information.

Table 1 outlines the dimensions and candidate variables that were considered when developing the index. At this stage, no consideration was made to the availability of the data, only what variables ideally would be suitable when constructing a Food Stress Index. Final decisions on the availability and suitability of the candidate variables were made in the next step.

Table 1. Candidate variables for a Food Stress Index.

Dimensions	Description of Measure	Description of Candidate Variables	Data Source
Household demographics	Proportion households by family composition	Couple families with children under 15 Single parent families with children under 15 Couple families with no children under 15 Single parent families with no children under 15	ABS: 2016 Census, Datapacks, General Community Profile, Western Australia [24]
Aboriginal and Torres Strait Islander Peoples	Proportion of Aboriginal and Torres Strait Islander households	Indigenous status	ABS: 2016 Census, Datapacks, General Community Profile, Western Australia [24]
Household income	Income quintiles of household	Proportion of households in the lowest income quintile Proportion of households in the highest income quintile	ABS: 2016 Census, Tablebuilder, Counting Persons, Place of Enumeration, Equivalised Total Household Income (weekly) [24]
Household expenses	Proportion of income used for household expenses (excluding food)	Housing costs (rent/mortgage) Transport Utilities Education	ABS: Household Expenditure Survey [25]
Financial stress indicators	A measure of whether households may be experiencing economic hardship, based on how many of the financial stress indicators a household experiences.	Financial stress experiences (e.g., unable to raise funds for an emergency, unable to pay bills on time) Missing out experiences (e.g., could not afford a holiday for at least a week, could not afford a special meal once a week)	ABS: Household Expenditure Survey [25]
Food affordability and access	Food affordability for the household. Access to food for the household.	Proportion of income required to purchase a healthy meal plan. Number of supermarkets within geographic area as an indication of access to affordable food.	2013 Food Access and Cost Survey [26]

The initial set of candidate variables was reduced before constructing the final index. When reducing the variables to a more manageable set, consideration was made of the suitability of each variable, and the potential to match variables by the selected geography, in this case the ABS' geographic classification of Statistical Area 2. This meant that variables that were not available on the same geographic basis for the respective households were not considered further. It is anticipated that the index will be regularly updated, and it was important that data was available from within the last five years to maintain relevance. Census data met both of these considerations and was the preferred source of data. In the case of the Food Access and Cost Survey (FACS) [26], the most recent data was from 2013 and the 2016 Census of Population and Housing [24] was used for all other variables.

From the list of variables in Table 1, household expense variables and financial stress indicators weren't available within the five-year period, or at the desired geography for this work. The sources for these variables are irregular surveys run by the ABS; as a result these variables were excluded from the Food Stress Index.

2.3. Description of Variables Used

The variables relate to persons, families or households and were expressed as a proportion of units in an area with the specified characteristic. Each of the dimensions is discussed below.

2.3.1. Household Demographics

Household composition, including family size, the number of parents and the age of any children provides a good indicator of household size, income and expenses. A single parent household with children under the age of 15 will have more difficulty earning income and meeting weekly expenses as they are generally able to only work on a part-time or casual basis due to child care commitments [27]. Single parent households also have to spend a greater proportion of their income to purchase a healthy meal plan [19].

The 2016 Australian Census shows that 45% of families were families with two parents and children while 38% of families were couples without children, and 16% were single parent families [24]. Using this information, the variables selected to demonstrate most, and least likelihood of food stress are the proportions of single parent or two parent households, with or without children under 15, within the selected geographic area.

2.3.2. Indigenous Status

The Indigenous status of a household provides a strong indicator of whether or not that household is likely to suffer from food stress. There are high unemployment rates and low income among Aboriginal and Torres Strait Islander peoples as well as significant disparities in health status between Aboriginal and Torres Strait Islander peoples and other Australians [28]. The proportion of Indigenous households from the 2016 Census was used.

2.3.3. Household Income

Income is an important indicator of the likelihood of food stress with households in the lowest income quintiles needing to spend a higher proportion of the income on food than those households in the highest income quintiles [19]. The income variable used was the Equivalised Total Household Income variable from the 2016 Census. Equivalised household income is household income which has been adjusted by an 'equivalence scale' based on the number of adults and children in the household [1].

Low income was defined as the proportion of households in the first quintile of the equivalised household income distribution; i.e., those households earning between $1 and $25,999 per year. These households represent those most likely to suffer food stress. The households least likely to suffer food stress were defined as those in the top income quintile, earning more than $78,000 per year.

2.3.4. Food Affordability

Food costs, as measured by the proportion of income required to purchase a healthy meal plan for a household, vary depending on the income of the household. Households that need to spend more than 25% of their income on food are suffering food stress [8] and the proportion of income required provides the strongest indicator of food stress.

Data from the 2013 FACS [26] was used to estimate food affordability; i.e., the proportion of income required to purchase a healthy meal plan for households of different compositions and incomes.

2.3.5. Geographic Information

Most of the data was taken from ABS datasets so each of the variables was available on ABS geography and Statistical Area 2 (SA2) was used as the base geography. Data from the FACS was also available by SA2s. Various SA2s were excluded from the list of SA2s because of the type of area (e.g., national parks, airports and industrial areas) or there was insufficient data (i.e., two or more variables unavailable). When the invalid areas were removed, 228 SA2s remained of the 253 SA2s in Western Australia. Data from the 2013 FACS was only available for 76 SA2s so the Food Stress Index was created for these SA2s.

2.4. Reduced Set of Variables

The final set of 13 variables selected is shown in Table 2.

Table 2. Reduced set of variables used to construct the Food Stress Index.

Dimensions	Description
Household demographics	Proportion of couple families with no children under 15 Proportion of couple families with children under 15 Proportion of one parent families with no children under 15 Proportion of one parent families with children under 15
Aboriginal and Torres Strait Islander Peoples	Proportion of Aboriginal and Torres Strait Islander households
Household income	Proportion of households in the lowest equivalised household income quintile (i.e., less than $500 per week) Proportion of households in the highest equivalised household income quintile (i.e., more than $1499 per week)
Food affordability	Proportion of income required to buy healthy food–couple family on welfare income Proportion of income required to buy healthy food–couple family on low income Proportion of income required to buy healthy food–couple family on average income Proportion of income required to buy healthy food–one parent family on welfare income Proportion of income required to buy healthy food–one parent family on low income Proportion of income required to buy healthy food–one parent family on average income

Once the initial variables were identified, Principal Component Analysis (PCA) [23] was used to create the Food Stress Index. The PCA technique summarises a number of correlated variables into a set of new uncorrelated components to allow for easier analysis. By removing correlated variables, the technique reduces the number of variables to a set that summarises the information and enables easier analysis. The PCA process results in a set of weighted raw scores that can then be scaled to produce the index scores for the Food Stress Index.

2.4.1. Create Proportions for the List of Initial Variables

Each variable was created as a proportion of units within the selected geography. For household composition, this was the proportion of families within the area. For the household income and Indigenous status variables, the proportion of households was used. For the food affordability variables, the proportion of income was used.

Each variable was then standardised to a mean of 0 and a standard deviation of 1 using R [29].

2.4.2. Create Correlation Matrix

The correlation matrix was calculated, and highly correlated variables were removed to avoid over-representation of food stress. When two variables measuring conceptually similar aspects of food affordability or food stress had a correlation coefficient of 0.8 in absolute value, one of them was removed.

2.4.3. Conduct Initial PCA

Next, Principal Component Analysis was conducted on the reduced set of variables to obtain the loadings for each variable on the first principal component. Any variables with resulting loadings less than 0.3 were removed on the grounds they were not strong enough to indicate food stress. The PCA step was then repeated until there were no variables with loadings less than 0.3 in absolute value. This resulted in a reduced set of variables, with at least one variable in each of the dimensions covering the food stress and food affordability measures.

2.5. Calculate and Scale the Index

Once there was a reduced set of variables, the final step was to calculate the final index. For each SA2, each standardised variable was multiplied by its weight, then summed across all variables. The weight was obtained by dividing the loading for each variable by the square root of the eigenvalue. In order to ensure that low scores indicate least likely to suffer food stress, and high scores indicate most likely to suffer food stress, the sign (positive or negative) for each indicator was set accordingly. That is, indicators of high food stress were given positive signs and indicators of low food stress were given negative signs.

This resulted in scores for each SA2. See the formula below.

$$Z_{SA2} = \sum_{j=1}^{p} \frac{L_j}{\sqrt{\lambda}} \times v_{j,SA2}$$

where

Z_{SA2} = raw score for the SA2
$v_{j,SA2}$ = standardised variable of the j-th variable for the SA2
L_j = loading for the j-th variable
λ = eigenvalue of the principal component
p = total number of variables in the index

To create a meaningful index, the scores were scaled with a mean of 1000 and standard deviation of 100 to create a new set of scores ranking the SA2s in order from least likely to suffer food stress to most likely to suffer food stress.

3. Results

The Food Stress Index was created for 76 SA2s in Western Australia. The scores ranged from 873.5 for North Perth (which is in the most advantaged SEIFA quintile), to 1400.4 for Halls Creek (in the most disadvantaged SEIFA quintile). This meant that households in the inner Perth suburb of North Perth are the least likely to suffer food stress in Western Australia and households in the remote north-west town of Halls Creek are most likely to suffer food stress. Table 3 shows the SA2s in each quintile of the Food Stress Index.

Table 3. Food Stress Index for Statistical Areas in Western Australia by quintile, ranging from 1 (least likelihood of food stress) to 5 (most likelihood of food stress).

Food Stress Index Quintile	Western Australia Statistical Areas
1	Applecross—Ardross, Ashburton, Baldivis, Booragoon, Greenwood—Warwick, Innaloo—Doubleview, Karratha, Mount Hawthorn—Leederville, Murdoch—Kardinya, Newman, North Perth, Ocean Reef, Subiaco—Shenton Park, Success—Hammond Park, Wembley—West Leederville—Glendalough, Wembley Downs—Churchlands—Woodlands
2	Australind—Leschenault, Belmont—Ascot—Redcliffe, Bentley—Wilson—St James, Byford, Carramar, Coolbellup, Craigie—Beldon, Eaton—Pelican Point, Esperance Region, Kalgoorlie, Margaret River, Murray, Rivervale—Kewdale—Cloverdale, South Bunbury—Bunbury, Thornlie
3	Albany, Augusta, Busselton, Capel, Denmark, East Bunbury—Glen Iris, Esperance, Geraldton—North, Gingin—Dandaragan, Gnowangerup, Harvey, Maddington—Orange Grove—Martin, Manjimup, Pinjarra, Rockingham
4	Alexander Heights—Koondoola, Beckenham—Kenwick—Langford, Bridgetown—Boyup Brook, Broome, Dowerin, Exmouth, Kambalda—Coolgardie—Norseman, Kulin, Merredin, Moora, Mukinbudin, Narrogin, Northam, Pemberton, Roebourne
5	Armadale—Wungong—Brookdale, Calista, Carnarvon, Cooloongup, Derby—West Kimberley, East Pilbara, Geraldton, Girrawheen, Gosnells, Halls Creek, Kununurra, Leinster—Leonora, Meekatharra, Parmelia—Orelia, Plantagenet, Roebuck

The Food Stress Index scores were compared with SEIFA Index of Relative Socio-economic Advantage and Disadvantage (IRSAD) for consistency. For example, the IRSAD for Mt Hawthorn/Leederville falls in the tenth decile, meaning persons living there are most advantaged. This aligns well with the Food Stress Index for Mt Hawthorn/Leederville which falls in the first decile, meaning persons living there have the least likelihood of food stress. To test the suitability of the FSI, a Spearman's correlation was run to determine the relationship between the Food Stress Index and the IRSAD index. There was a strong, negative correlation with the IRSAD index ($r = -0.89$, $p < 0.001$).

4. Discussion

The Food Stress Index provides a measure of the likelihood that households in a geographic area are vulnerable to food stress. When applied to Statistical Area 2 (SA2), households in the more remote areas of Western Australia are most likely to suffer food stress (e.g., East Pilbara, Halls Creek, Kununurra). Households in Perth metropolitan areas are least likely to suffer from food stress (e.g., North Perth, Mount Hawthorn and Ocean Reef). The FSI provides more information on food security than the widely used SEIFA which measures socioeconomic status. For example, although Ashburton is in a remote part of Western Australia and is in the third quintile for SEIFA, the FSI takes into account the high proportion of households in Ashburton that are in the highest income quintile and the low proportion of single parent families, resulting in a low Food Stress Index. Similarly, within the Perth metropolitan area, households in Girrawheen, are more likely to suffer food stress due the high proportion of households in the lowest income quintile and the high proportion of Indigenous households.

One of the limitations of this research was that some of the candidate variables (i.e., household expense and financial stress data) were not available at the required level of detail when the analysis was undertaken. Although this data wasn't included it was still possible to construct a suitable index with the available data. Further research is planned to determine the implications of including this data if it becomes available.

5. Conclusions

The Food Stress Index, the first of its kind in Australia, is a suitable indicator of the risk of food stress in Western Australian households. It incorporates a range of variables to measure food stress including food costs, household composition and household incomes. Further research is needed to develop the FSI methodology for smaller geographic areas such as Statistical Area 1 (SA1) to be more representative of households. Population weighted averages of the SA1s would be used to construct indexes for larger geographies. The FSI could be applied to all Australian households, providing a useful tool for national food security. The FSI can be used for to highlight areas where households are more likely to be food stressed and more vulnerable to food insecurity. Policy and intervention planning can then better target services to where they are needed.

Author Contributions: T.J.L. conceived the study and undertook the analysis. T.J.L. and C.M.P. authored the original manuscript. All authors read and approved the final manuscript. T.J.L. undertook this work as part of his Doctor of Philosophy.

Acknowledgments: T.J.L. is supported through an Australian Government Research Training Program Scholarship.

References

1. ABS. Census of Population and Housing: Socio-Economic Indexes for Areas (SEIFA). Available online: http://www.abs.gov.au/websitedbs/censushome.nsf/home/seifa (accessed on 18 June 2018).

2. Backholer, K.; Spencer, E.; Gearon, E.; Magliano, D.J.; McNaughton, S.A.; Shaw, J.E.; Peeters, A. The association between socio-economic position and diet quality in Australian adults. *Public Health Nutr.* **2016**, *19*, 477–485. [CrossRef] [PubMed]

3. Barosh, L.; Friel, S.; Engelhardt, K.; Chan, L. The cost of a healthy and sustainable diet—Who can afford it? *Aust. N. Z. J. Public Health* **2014**, *38*, 7–12. [CrossRef] [PubMed]

4. Brimblecombe, J.; Ferguson, M.; Liberato, S.C.; Ball, K.; Moodie, M.L.; Magnus, A.; Miles, E.; Leach, A.J.; Chatfield, M.D.; Ni Mhurchu, C.; et al. Stores Healthy Options Project in Remote Indigenous Communities (SHOP@RIC): A protocol of a randomised trial promoting healthy food and beverage purchases through price discounts and in-store nutrition education. *BMC Public Health* **2013**, *13*, 744. [CrossRef] [PubMed]

5. Godrich, S.; Lo, J.; Davies, C.; Darby, J.; Devine, A. Prevalence and socio-demographic predictors of food insecurity among regional and remote Western Australian children. *Aust. N. Z. J. Public Health* **2017**, *41*, 585–590. [CrossRef] [PubMed]

6. Palermo, C.; McCartan, J.; Kleve, S.; Sinha, K.; Shiell, A. A longitudinal study of the cost of food in Victoria influenced by geography and nutritional quality. *Aust. N. Z. J. Public Health* **2016**, *40*, 270–273. [CrossRef] [PubMed]

7. Yates, J.; Gabriel, M. *Housing Affordability in Australia*; Australian Housing and Urban Research Institute: Melbourne, Australia, 2006.

8. Ward, P.R.; Coveney, J.; Verity, F.; Carter, P.; Schilling, M. Cost and affordability of healthy food in rural South Australia. *Rural Remote Health* **2012**, *12*, 1938. [PubMed]

9. Ward, P.R.; Verity, F.; Carter, P.; Tsourtos, G.; Coveney, J.; Wong, K.C. Food stress in Adelaide: The relationship between low income and the affordability of healthy food. *J. Environ. Public Health* **2013**, *2013*, 968078. [CrossRef] [PubMed]

10. Williams, P.; Hull, A.; Kontos, M. Trends in affordability of the Illawarra healthy food basket 2000–2007. *Nutr. Diet.* **2009**, *66*, 27–32. [CrossRef]

11. Wong, K.C.; Coveney, J.; Ward, P.; Muller, R.; Carter, P.; Verity, F.; Tsourtos, G. Availability, affordability and quality of a healthy food basket in Adelaide, South Australia. *Nutr. Diet.* **2011**, *68*, 8–14. [CrossRef]

12. Pollard, C.; Begley, A.; Landrigan, T. The Rise of Food Inequality in Australia. In *Food Poverty and Insecurity: International Food Inequalities*; Caraher, M., Coveney, J., Eds.; Springer International Publishing: Cham, Switzerland, 2016; pp. 89–103.

13. FAO. Rome Declaration on World Food Security. 1996. Available online: http://www.fao.org/docrep/003/w3613e/w3613e00.htm (accessed on 13 September 2018).

14. ABS. Australian Aboriginal and Torres Strait Islander Health Survey: Nutrition Results—Food and Nutrients. Available online: http://www.abs.gov.au/AUSSTATS/abs@.nsf/Lookup/4727.0.55.005Main+Features12012-13?OpenDocument (accessed on 14 March 2018).

15. Butcher, L.M.; O'Sullivan, T.A.; Ryan, M.M.; Lo, J.; Devine, A. Utilising a multi-item questionnaire to assess household food security in Australia. *Health Promot. J. Austr.* **2018**. [CrossRef] [PubMed]

16. Bickel, G.; Nord, M.; Price, C.; Hamilton, W.; Cook, J. *Guide to Measuring Household Food Security, Revised 2000*; U.S. Department of Agriculture, Food and Nutrition Service: Alexandria, VA, USA, 2000.

17. Coleman-Jensen, A.; Rabbitt, M.P.; Gregory, C.A.; Singh, A. *Household Food Security in the United States, 2017*; ERR-256; U.S. Department of Agriculture, Economic Research Service: Alexandria, VA, USA, 2018.

18. McKechnie, R.; Turrell, G.; Giskes, K.; Gallegos, D. Single-item measure of food insecurity used in the National Health Survey may underestimate prevalence in Australia. *Aust. N. Z. J. Public Health* **2018**, *42*, 389–395. [CrossRef] [PubMed]

19. Landrigan, T.J.; Kerr, D.A.; Dhaliwal, S.S.; Savage, V.; Pollard, C.M. Removing the Australian tax exemption on healthy food adds food stress to families vulnerable to poor nutrition. *Aust. N. Z. J. Public Health* **2017**, *41*, 591–597. [CrossRef] [PubMed]

20. Booth, S.; Smith, A. Food security and poverty in Australia-challenges for dietitians. *Aust. J. Nutr. Diet.* **2001**, *58*, 150–156.

21. Lee, A.; Mhurchu, C.N.; Sacks, G.; Swinburn, B.; Snowdon, W.; Vandevijvere, S.; Hawkes, C.; L'Abbé, M.; Rayner, M.; Sanders, D.; et al. Monitoring the price and affordability of foods and diets globally. *Obes. Rev.* **2013**, *14*, 82–95. [CrossRef] [PubMed]

22. Lloyd, S.; Lawton, J.; Caraher, M.; Singh, G.; Horsley, K.; Mussa, F. A tale of two localities. *Health Educ. J.* **2010**, *70*, 48–56. [CrossRef]

23. Joliffe, I.T. *Principal Component Analysis*, 2nd ed.; Springer: New York, NY, USA, 2002.

24. ABS. Census of Population and Housing. Available online: http://www.abs.gov.au/websitedbs/censushome.nsf/home/data?opendocument#from-banner=LN (accessed on 31 May 2018).

25. ABS. Household Expenditure Survey, Australia. Available online: http://www.abs.gov.au/AUSSTATS/abs@.nsf/mf/6530.0 (accessed on 22 May 2018).

26. Pollard, C.; Savage, V.; Landrigan, T.J.; Hanbury, A.; Kerr, D.A. Food Access and Cost Survey Western Australia. 2013. Available online: https://ww2.health.wa.gov.au/~{}/media/Files/Corporate/Reports%20and%20publications/Chronic%20Disease/Food-Access-and-Cost-Survey-Report-2013-Report.pdf (accessed on 13 September 2018).

27. Western Australian Council of Social Service Inc. *2017 Cost of Living Report*; Western Australian Council of Social Service Inc.: West Perth, Australia, 2017.

28. AHMAC. *Aboriginal and Torres Strait Islander Health Performance Framework Report 2006*; AHMAC: Canberra, Australia, 2006.

29. R Core Team. *R: A Language and Environment for Statistical Computing*; R Foundation for Statistical Computing: Vienna, Austria, 2014.

10

You can't Find Healthy Food in the Bush: Poor Accessibility, Availability and Adequacy of Food in Rural Australia

Jill Whelan [1,*] , Lynne Millar [2,3] , Colin Bell [1] , Cherie Russell [4] , Felicity Grainger [4], Steven Allender [5] and Penelope Love [4,6]

[1]   School of Medicine, Global Obesity Centre, Deakin University, Geelong 3220, Australia;
      colin.bell@deakin.edu.au
[2]   Australian Health Policy Collaboration, Victoria University, Melbourne 3000, Australia;
      lynne.millar@vu.edu.au
[3]   Australian Institute for Musculoskeletal Science (AIMSS), The University of Melbourne and Western Health,
      St Albans 3021, Australia
[4]   School of Exercise and Nutrition Sciences, Deakin University, Geelong 3220, Australia;
      caru@deakin.edu.au (C.R.); fgrainge@deakin.edu.au (F.G.); penny.love@deakin.edu.au (P.L.)
[5]   School of Health and Social Development, Global Obesity Centre, Deakin University,
      Geelong 3220, Australia; steven.allender@deakin.edu.au
[6]   Institute for Physical Activity and Nutrition (IPAN), Deakin University, Geelong 3220, Australia
*   Correspondence: jill.whelan@deakin.edu.au

Abstract: In high-income countries, obesity disproportionately affects those from disadvantaged and rural areas. Poor diet is a modifiable risk factor for obesity and the food environment a primary driver of poor diet. In rural and disadvantaged communities, it is harder to access affordable and nutritious food, affecting both food insecurity and the health of rural residents. This paper aims to describe the food environment in a rural Australian community (approx. 7000 km^2 in size) to inform the development of community-relevant food supply interventions. We conducted a census audit of the food environment (ground truthing) of a local government area (LGA). We used the Nutrition Environment Measurement tools (NEMS-S and NEMS-R) to identify availability of a range of food and non-alcoholic beverages, the relative price of a healthy compared to a less healthy option of a similar food type (e.g., bread), the quality of fresh produce and any in-store nutrition promotion. Thirty-eight food retail outlets operated at the time of our study and all were included, 11 food stores (NEMS-S) and 27 food service outlets (NEMS-R). The mean NEMS-S score for all food stores was 21/54 points (39%) and mean NEMS-R score for all food service outlets was 3/23 points (13%); indicative of limited healthier options at relatively higher prices. It is difficult to buy healthy food beyond the supermarkets and one (of seven) cafés across the LGA. Residents demonstrate strong loyalty to local food outlets, providing scope to work with this existing infrastructure to positively impact poor diet and improve food security.

Keywords: rural; food supply; food security; obesity

1. Introduction

Globally, obesity is a leading cause of chronic disease and premature death [1]. In low and middle-income countries, it impacts the wealthy, shifting to the rural poor as the country's economy develops [1,2]. In high income countries, such as Australia, it impacts everyone but disproportionately affects those from more disadvantaged and rural areas [2]. Consequently, rural residents in Australia have higher rates of obesity and are more likely to die early from concomitant conditions including diabetes, heart disease and other chronic diseases [2,3].

Internationally and within Australia, poor diet has been identified as a leading modifiable risk factor contributing to the high burden of disease and obesity [3,4], and there is some evidence that the food environment is related to healthiness of diet among adults [5] and children [6]. These reviews highlight the lack of consistency in measurements of these associations which is to be expected in this emerging field but, nonetheless, some relationships are evident.

Some studies have identified that neighbourhoods without supermarkets have more diet-related health outcomes such as obesity and chronic disease [7]. In rural and/or disadvantaged communities, it is harder than in urban environments to access affordable and nutritious foods [8,9]. Availability varies as it is potentially constrained by the long distance required to travel to food stores [10], and limitations to fresh food supply delivery and increased prices occur with greater distance from the key metropolitan centres [11]. A consequence of these food supply constraints is that rural residents, and rural food retailers, in order to reduce the risk of waste, tend to purchase longer shelf-life foods [12], many of which may be less nutritious than the fresh options. Rural areas have a higher proportion of general stores to larger supermarkets compared to urban areas, providing fewer healthy options at higher prices and unpredictable quality [13,14]. These differences are most commonly attributed to limited transportation, storage and economies of scale for food distribution to rural areas [15].

Many rural areas experience diminishing population sizes, which reduces financial viability leading to the consolidation or closure of food stores [16,17]. With poor access to healthy food within close proximity, rural residents are reliant on transportation (public or private), incurring additional costs, and they frequently are forced to shop outside their local area, a phenomenon known as 'out-shopping' [17]. Out-shopping creates a vicious cycle for rural economies as revenue shifts to outside enterprises, and local businesses struggle to provide sufficient variety at low cost to attract and retain customers [17], adding further to rural economic decline. General stores, and 'take-away' food outlets, located in close proximity to residents, often with extended operating hours, may become the main source of food for rural communities [18], particularly those with limited mobility.

The food environment is defined as the "accessibility, availability and adequacy of food within a community or region" [19] and comprises three sub-environments: community, organizational and consumer. The community food environment (number, type, location and accessibility of retail food outlets); the organizational food environment (type and availability of healthy food within settings, such as workplaces, schools and at home); and the consumer food environment (price, promotion, placement, nutrition information, quality and availability of healthy food within retail food outlets) [19,20].

Importantly, food environment research should be considered alongside the concept of food insecurity, where people are unable to obtain a nutritious diet through socially acceptable means on a regular basis [21]. Within rural Australia, causes of food insecurity are discussed within five domains, these are: 1. access (economic and physical access to food), 2. inadequate supply (availability), 3. affordability, 4. inappropriate use of food (food safety, food preparation, nutritional status) and 5. trade policy [9]. Within this paper, we concentrate on three of these domains: access, supply/availability and affordability of food insecurity. The NEMS-S and NEMS-R tools are designed to collect data on food availability and access and do not aim to collect data on available food relief services, such as food pantries and community meals programs. The focus of this study is on the food and beverages stocked within retail food outlets in the area with a view to understanding access and availability of quality food produce at an affordable price. Whilst it might be expected that food insecurity would be linked with under-weight, research indicates that obesity is most prevalent amongst those at highest risk of food insecurity [22,23]. Other broad reaching health effects that have been identified in the literature include, disturbed sleep patterns, maternal depression, type 2 diabetes, anaemia poorer child health and higher rates of hospitalisation linked with poor infant feeding practices. Lifelong impacts include learning difficulties and adverse developmental outcomes [3].

These two major public health issues of obesity and food security should therefore be considered simultaneously, using local food environment data to inform positive environmental changes to enhance health.

Food environment interventions have the potential to improve population level diet quality in an equitable manner by ensuring an affordable, high quality food supply [24], and Glanz et al. argue that community and consumer food sub-environments should be given particular attention as they have the potential to promote and impact healthier choices at the point of purchase [20]. Measurement of community and consumer food environments is problematic, however, a recent review of retail food environment measures has provided some direction [25] by identifying the most common store types as supermarkets, grocery stores, convenience and corner stores. These store types are commonly categorized by number of registers [26,27] or sum of aisle length [28]. The review [25] also identified the two most frequently internationally used measures as the USDA's Thrifty Food Plan tool, developed to identify food and beverage purchases to meet minimum USA healthy diet requirements [29]; and the Nutrition Environment Measurement Survey for Stores (NEMS-S) which assesses the nutrition environment more broadly based on availability, price and quality [30]. NEMS-S is one of a suite of nutrition environment measurement tools that have been assessed for interrater reliability, test-re-test reliability and face and criterion validity; and adapted for use in several studies [30]. The NEMS-R tool comprises an observational checklist of 25 items [31] and is designed to assess the availability of healthier food and beverages on main and children's menus. In Australia, studies of food environments have focused on availability and access in urban settings and remote Indigenous communities, with most exploring food pricing [32].

Where nutrition environment measurement tools have been used in rural settings, either internationally or in Australia, they have presented with limitations to efficacy in these settings. For example, studies of food pricing commonly rely on a 'healthy food basket' conceptualization [33], where data include prices of a pre-defined list of 'healthy' foods in quantities representative of various household units, thereby enabling comparison across regions and over time [12]. However, exclusion of generic brands [34], exclusion of stores that contain fewer than 90% of the 44 items, and lack of quality assessment of fresh produce limit its usefulness and applicability in rural and remote areas.

While the definition of food environments is clear, and there is growing awareness of the need to intervene, less is known about the true disparity in the healthfulness of food environments in rural compared to urban areas. There is a paucity of evidence of the quality of rural food environments generally [15] and in Australian non-Indigenous communities specifically. The aim of this paper is to describe the food environment in a rural Australian community for use in future development of community-relevant food supply interventions.

2. Methods

2.1. Design

Census audit of rural food environment using the NEMS-S [30] and NEMS-R tools [31].

2.2. Context

This study took place in a rural, remote local government area (LGA) within Australia, as part of a broader community-wide obesity prevention study. Within the study, community stakeholders identified the local food supply as a determinant of unhealthy weight. Data published in 2014 show the LGA experienced a very poor chronic disease risk profile and above average adult prevalence of overweight and obesity at around 15% above the state average at that time. Concomitant health behaviours were of concern with high sugar sweetened beverage per capita consumption almost twice the state average and higher than average take-away meal consumption [35]. Located 350 km from the nearest capital city, the LGA has a total population of approximately 7000 people spread across approximately 7000 km^2 comprising farming land and several rural and remote towns with populations ranging from between 150 and 2302 people. The predominant crops include various grains and legumes which are be 'shipped out' for processing [36]. Within Australia there are four major chain supermarkets, and the smallest of these has a presence within this community.

2.3. Selection of Retail Food Outlets

We used the categories in Table 1 to define retail food outlets. These were adapted to the rural Australian context from Glanz et al. [20] and Innes-Hughes [26].

Table 1. Categorization of retail food stores and food service outlets.

Food Stores	Food Service
Supermarket—sells food products and other items, large scale, may open for extended hours on most days of the week. (Register numbers: 1 to 5)	Restaurants Sit-down—order and pay at table, table service, food eaten at outlet e.g.,: traditional restaurants
General—sells food products and other items, small scale, typically in a small town. General stores generally have reduced hours and usually are not open on weekends.	Fast-casual—order and pay at counter, may have table service, food eaten at outlet or taken away e.g.,: hotels (pubs) and cafés
Convenience stores (North American)—extended hours, stocking a limited range of household goods and groceries.	Fast-food—order, pay and served food at counter, quick service, food usually eaten away from outlet e.g.,: take-aways and bakeries

Thirty-nine retail food outlets were identified across the LGA using the community directory available on the LGA website. 'Ground truthing' (physically viewing and recording of outlets) identified that an additional four outlets had opened, and that three outlets had closed. Two petrol stations were excluded, as their food supply was extremely limited. All food outlets operating at the time of the study that met the definitions outlined in Table 1 were included (n = 38).

2.4. Selection of Food Environment Measurement Tools

We used the Nutrition Environment Measures Survey for Stores (NEMS-S) and Restaurants (NEMS-R) due to their validated status and peer-reviewed evidence of use in a variety of settings. NEMS-S scored high on reliability; percent agreement (92–100%), inter-rater reliability kappas (0.84–1.00) and test-retest (0.73–1.00) [30]. NEMS-R also scored generally high on inter-rater reliability, kappas mostly greater than 0.80 (0.27–0.97); percent agreement (77.6–99.5%), and test-retest: most kappa values greater than 0.80 (0.46–1.0) [31]. Scoring of the NEMS-S tool was based on the published scoring tool [30] and NEMS-R was scored using the revised scoring system provided in 2011 [37].

2.5. Nutrition Environment Measures Survey for Stores (NEMS-S)

The original, American-based, NEMS-S tool [30] includes 11 indicator food categories: milk, fruit, vegetables, ground/minced beef, hot dogs, frozen dinners, baked goods, beverages—diet soft drink and fruit juice, bread, chips, breakfast cereal. These food categories reflected the fat and calories of a typical diet and those most recommended for healthful eating at the time the tool was developed (2007) [30]. The following modifications were made to the NEMS-S tool for the Australian context. Measures were converted from imperial to metric, and chicken (skin on and skin off) was substituted for hotdogs (being a more commonly available and consumed food in Australia). Australian reference brands were used, and Australian seasonal fruit and vegetables were included. Common breakfast cereal and bakery options were also included. Due to the importance of calcium rich foods in the Australian Guide to Healthy Eating [38], data were collected on the availability and price comparisons of cheese and yoghurt, however, these were not included in the NEMS scoring protocol to allow comparison with previous studies.

The modified NEMS-S tool was piloted in three rural community retail food outlets to test for face validity. Our modified tool maintained the 11 categories as per the NEMS-S scoring tool with a maximum possible score of 54, (availability: maximum 30, pricing: maximum 18 and quality: maximum 6 (as fruit and vegetables only included)). Between one and three points were awarded for availability depending on product type and the number of varieties available. Affordability is assessed through comparative pricing. The price of food was scored comparatively with two points being awarded if the price of better nutrient profile food was cheaper than the regular varieties. Quality was scored as 'acceptable' or 'unacceptable' based on the appearance of the majority of a given type of fruits or vegetables; an unacceptable rating was applied if the produce was 'clearly bruised, old looking, over-ripe, or spotted' [30] (p. 284). As per the NEMS scoring protocol, a quality score of 1 was awarded if 25–49% of the produce met an acceptable standard, 2 points were awarded if between 50–74% of the produce was acceptable and 3 points awarded if 75% or more of the produce was 'acceptable'. An overall score combining all three dimensions was calculated. A higher score obtained in the NEMS-S tool equates to a healthier food environment.

2.6. Nutrition Environment Measures Survey for Restaurants (NEMS-R)

NEMS-R comprises a menu review and observational visit, (and if required, an interview with restaurant staff) to review the 25 items assessed for availability of healthier food and beverages on menus. Points are awarded for healthier options, for example: low fat dressings, whole grain breads, baked rather than fried foods, among others [31]. Factors that support or challenge healthy eating are measured and further points are awarded for signage/promotions, nutrition information and notations on menus. Points are deducted for unhealthy promotions such as super-sizing, all-you-can-eat offers, and unhealthy combo-meal deals [31]. Possible NEMS-R scores range from −5 to 23 (for establishments without a specific children's menu) and −8 to 32 (for establishments with a children's menu) [39].

Minor modifications to language were required to ensure NEMS-R was relevant to the Australian context. The term 'entree' in USA generally means main course and in Australia it means a smaller first course, therefore all references to entrée were removed and replaced with the Australian language of 'main course'. The size of the meal was captured through the retention of the question related to reduced-size portions offered on menu. NEMS-R collects data on 'low carb promotions' which was the 'diet fad' of choice at the time the tool was developed (2007). Instead we collected data on any 'diet fads' outside the Australian Guide to Healthy Eating (AGHE), such as raw foods or paleo diets that were popular at the time of data collection (2017). We also modified milk to include all lower fat milk options, typically 2% fat milk in Australia, (NEMS: 1% or non-fat). We administered the NEMS-R tool on all food service outlets in the study LGA. As there are no fast food chain outlets in the study LGA to enable a comparison between small family owned businesses and large chain store food outlets we administered the NEMS-R on a neighbouring large fast-food chain outlet. As per NEMS-S we pilot tested the modified NEMS-R for face validity. A higher score on NEMS-R also indicates a healthier food environment.

2.7. Data Collection

Prior to data collection, JW and PL undertook online NEMS training [40], then provided face-to-face training to CR and FG. Data were collected over four days from 19 to 22 June 2017. Retail food outlets were not informed of the assessment ahead of time, permission was obtained on entering the premises. Store owners were advised of the purpose of the study on entering the premises. Most of the data could be collected without interaction with the staff of the food premises. Where interaction was required, food retailers freely shared the required information.

All researchers conducted an initial NEMS-S and NEMS-R survey together and thereafter worked in pairs to ensure consistency between scoring. Test-retest reliability was performed on a 5% sample (n = 2/38) as per NEMS protocol. The results indicated a high level of test-retest reliability with NEMS-R kappa of 0.825 and NEMS-S kappa of 0.781. Surveys took between 20 and 60 min to complete dependent on the size of the outlet. Data were recorded using hard copy survey sheets and then entered into the relevant NEMS-S or NEMS-R Excel spreadsheet. A random sample of 25% of data entries was assessed for accuracy. No errors were found in this cross check. Ethical approval for this study was obtained through Deakin University [HEAG-H 80_2016].

2.8. Data Analysis

Data were prepared using NEMS Excel spreadsheets and the NEMS scoring system [30,37,39] and STATA release 15 [41]. Primary outcome measures were: availability, price and quality of healthy foods compared across store types (supermarkets and general stores), food service (restaurants, fast casual—hotels, fast casual—cafes, fast food), and geographic locations to identify if cost, availability, promotions, healthiness and quality of food varied across the LGA. Food was classified into the core food groups of the Australian Guide to Healthy Eating to determine if the foods recommended were available and if they were more or less expensive than unhealthier foods. Descriptive statistics on the availability of the Australian core food groups and discretionary foods were reported. For NEMS-S data, t-tests were used to compare the availability, price, quality of food between type of store (supermarket or general store) and separate linear regressions were used to compare the availability, price, quality between communities (north, central, south). For all statistics, p-values < 0.05 were deemed statistically significant.

Published studies appear to have applied different scoring protocols, therefore, we have converted our NEMS scores to percentage figures to enable comparison with other studies using these tools. In keeping with NEMS tools a higher percentage indicates a food environment more conducive to healthy eating.

3. Results

The exploration of the community food environment found a total of 38 outlets, all of which are included in the data analysis (100% RR), with 11 being food stores and 27 food service outlets (sit-down n = 13, fast-casual n = 7, fast food n = 7).

3.1. Food Stores

Of the 11 food stores, five were supermarkets and six were general stores. Table 2 shows the maximum possible score and mean scores for each of the three sub-categories of availability, price and quality for stores overall and by type of food store (the higher the score, the healthier the food environment). A total mean score of 21.0 (SD 4.6) out of a possible 54 points was obtained for the LGA as a whole. The overall NEM-S score was significantly higher for supermarkets (mean = 24.8, SD 2.6) than general stores (mean = 17.8 SD 3.2; t(2,9) = 3.9, $p < 0.05$) as was the availability of healthy foods score (supermarkets (mean = 21.4, SD 3.0); general stores (mean = 12.0, SD 3.0; t(2,9) = 5.2, $p < 0.05$).

Table 2. NEMS-S Food Stores Scores for all stores, grocery stores and general stores and p values resulting from t-tests between store type.

		All Food Stores (n = 11)		Supermarkets (n = 5)		General Stores (n = 6)		p
	Max	Mean	SD	Mean	SD	Mean	SD	
Availability	30	16.3	5.7	21.4	3.0	12.0	3.0	$p < 0.05$
Price	18	1.1	1.0	1.2	1.1	1.0	1.1	NS *
Quality	6	4.6	2.1	5.4	1.3	4.0	2.5	NS *
Total Score	54	21.0	4.6	24.8	2.6	17.8	3.2	$p < 0.05$

* NS—Non-significant at $p \geq 0.05$.

Table 3 compares the mean NEMS-S scores for stores in the north (n = 3), central (n = 5) and south (n = 3) of the LGA. The mean NEMS-S score was highest in the central area at 24.8 (44%) where the two largest supermarkets were located. There were no statistically significant differences on any category between areas.

Table 3. NEMS-S score means from stores in the northern, central, and southern areas of the rural local government area.

Food Stores (n = 11)		North (n = 3)		Central (n = 5)		South (n = 3)	
	Max	Mean	SD	Mean	SD	Mean	SD
Availability	30	14.0	5.2	19.0	8.7	17.3	2.5
Price	18	1.2	1.1	1.3	1.2	0.7	1.2
Quality	6	4.8	1.6	6.0	0.0	3.0	3.0
Total Score	54	20.0	4.4	24.0	4.6	19.7	5.1

A breakdown of the availability of healthier choices and price differential across the Australian core food groups is shown in Appendix A. In most, but not all cases regardless of store types, healthier choices were more expensive and less available.

All supermarkets and general stores sold reduced fat milk. The price comparisons showed the price of reduced fat milk was more expensive than full fat milk in all stores. Low fat cheese and/or low fat yoghurt was only available in 27% of food stores and, where it was available' low fat options were more expensive than full fat. Wholegrain bread was available in all stores and more expensive than white bread in 27% of stores. Overall, healthier varieties of cereals (including rice, pasta, grains) were more expensive 60% of the time compared to their healthier counterparts. Low fat minced beef (ground beef) was available at two food stores across the Shire; at one of these it was more expensive than full fat minced beef and the other store stocked only low-fat minced beef so no price comparison was possible. The remaining nine stores stocked full fat varieties only. All five supermarkets and four of the six general stores stocked a wide variety of fruit and vegetables (10 or more). None of the food stores displayed any healthy eating promotions at the time of the surveys.

3.2. Food Service Outlets

Twenty-eight food service outlets were surveyed however, one café closed before collection of follow-up information and was excluded from the study (n = 27). All food service outlets were independent stores, with no fast food chain outlets in this rural community. Table 4 describes the type of food service establishment, number of outlets, explanation of the categorization, the mean and standard deviation NEMS-R score.

Table 4. Types and number of food service outlets across the Local Government Area and a comparison fast food chain outlet with their mean NEMS-R Scores and their scores as a percentage of the maximum NEMS-R Score (−5 to 23).

Food Service	Number of Outlets	NEMS-R SCORE		% of Max NEMS-R SCORE (−5 to 23)
	N	Mean	SD	%
Fast Casual: Hotels/pubs/restaurant	13	1.8	1.6	7.8
Fast Casual: Café	7	7.0	5.6	30.0
Fast Food: Take-aways	5	2.0	2.9	8.7
Fast Food: Bakeries	2	4.0	0.7	17.4
Total	27	3.0	4.0	13.0
Comparison	1	10.0	0.0	43.0

The mean NEMS-R score was low at 3 (SD 4.0) out of a possible 23, (excluding children's menu) [39] across the LGA. Nine of the 27 food service outlets offered a children's menu, eight of these scored two points, one scored five points (possible scoring range −3 to 9). One fast food outlet received a negative score indicating that the store sold almost exclusively unhealthy foods and encouraged over-consumption by promoting up-selling through 'meals deals' that comprise fried foods and sugar sweetened beverages at a price cheaper than purchasing items individually. Aside from one café in the central area scoring 17, no other food service outlet scored higher than eight. NEMS-R scoring of a comparison neighbouring fast food chain store, that predominately sold fried food, scored 10. Table 5 shows comparisons between different areas of the LGA, with the central area having a slightly better food environment as scored on NEMS-R.

Table 5. NEMS-R score means for the north, central and south of the Local Government Area.

	Score Range	NORTH			CENTRAL			SOUTH		
Number of outlets	27	9			13			5		
		MEAN	SD	% *	MEAN	SD	%	MEAN	SD	%
NEMS-R score	−8–32	2.0	1.0	6%	4.0	5.0	12%	3.0	3.0	9%

* percentage score calculated as a % mean of maximum possible score.

There was no statistically significant difference between these geographic boundaries or between types of outlets and the mean total. Table 6 reports NEMS-R according to food service outlet and compares means across the three measures of availability, facilitators and barriers to healthy eating. Means scores across hotels, cafes, fast food and bakeries were all low (maximum possible scores, means and standard deviations shown in the table). There were no statistically significant differences between these store types, though café's in general scored higher than hotels/pubs. Health promoting practices, as defined by NEMS-R, include signage/promotions, nutrition information/notations on menus, and reduced portion sizes.

Table 6. NEMS-R scores by type of food service outlet and health promoting practices.

Type of Outlet		Total		Hotels/Pubs/ Restaurant *		Cafes		Fast Food		Bakeries	
Outlets (n (%))		27 (100)		13 (48.1)		7 (25.9)		5 (18.5)		2 (7.4)	
NEMS-R items	Possible Score (A score closer to the maximum possible score indicates a healthier food environment.)	M	SD	M	SD	M	SD	M	SD	M	SD
Availability of healthy choices	0–15	2.8	2.5	1.4	1.4	5.3	3.1	2.6	1.5	3.5	0.7
Facilitators of healthy eating	0–8	0.4	1.4	0.2	0.4	1.1	2.6	−1.0	1.4	0.0	0.0
Barriers to healthy eating	−5–0	−0.3	0.8	0.0	0.0	−0.3	0.8	−1.0	1.4	0.0	0.0

* The scores of the one restaurant were combined with hotels/pubs to preserve anonymity.

The most frequent practice observed was the provision of diet soda (100% of food service outlets), and low fat milk (about two thirds of food service outlets) with two using it as the default option in hot and cold drinks. Across the area, 23% of food service outlets offered at least one main meal designated as 'healthy' according to NEMS-R standards. Fried, french fry-style potato chips were served at the majority (88%) of food service outlets. About a third (37%) offered a children's menu, from which one menu item met the NEMS-R definition of 'healthy' and two menu items included a healthy side as per published definition [31]. About a quarter (23%) offered unprocessed fruit for sale, 15% had non-fried vegetables identified on their menus. Across all food service outlets, just under half had wholemeal bread available, and just over half offered 100% fruit juice. Nutritional information and healthy menu items were identified in only one food service outlet. Bottled water was available for sale at all food service outlets, with some offering free tap water. Data on the collection of freely available tap water was not a component of the NEMS-R tool.

4. Discussion

The aim of this study was to describe the food environment in a rural Australian community in order to inform future community-relevant food supply interventions. We provide a comprehensive account of the community and consumer food environments in this LGA. The findings provide evidence that major changes to the food environment are needed for healthy foods to be available equitably to all community members. Food stores scored poorly on food availability and comparative pricing. Among food stores, healthier options were more expensive than their unhealthy alternative, and we observed variable quality of fresh fruit and vegetables. The availability of food service outlets (n = 27) was more predominant than food stores (n = 11), with the majority (n = 26) receiving low scores indicating healthy choices of prepared food were generally difficult to obtain across this LGA.

While NEMS tools have been used internationally across a variety of settings including rural environments [42,43], many have adapted the tool to local context thereby limiting direct comparability of these findings with our study. There are also no similar studies within Australia either measuring the food environment of a whole rural LGA or using the NEMS tools to undertake a comprehensive food environment audit.

4.1. Food Stores

Generally smaller store sizes have been correlated with lower NEMS-S scores and fewer healthy foods than larger supermarkets [44]. In our study, there was no statistically significant difference in the comparative pricing score between supermarkets and general stores, this may be due to a number of reasons. Firstly, both scores for comparative pricing (healthy vs. unhealthy price of a similar product), were very poor (1.2 and 1.0 respectively out of a possible 18 points); secondly, the small number of stores across the LGA limits statistical analysis, thirdly all supermarkets were small in size with the largest one having five registers, the smallest just one register, this limits the stock they can carry and may constrain their bargaining power in regards to food supply logistics to obtain healthy choices at a reasonable price. We consider the lack of variability in the quality score to be related to the quality scoring systems within the NEMS protocol where an 85% score translates to 100% on analysis. We consider some of our stores were over-scored on quality due to this protocol.

Our findings are consistent with studies that have identified rural areas typically have smaller and fewer supermarkets which equates to less variety, poorer quality and higher prices than in urban areas [7,43,45]. In Australia, four major supermarket chains exist, only the smallest of these was present in this community, all food stores in this LGA would be considered small in an urban context. In comparison with international studies, our food store environment score (39%) is lower than scores obtained in rural USA (around 60%) [7,42]. Our very low score indicates a food environment that is not conducive to healthy eating. However it also provides a baseline environment score and potential opportunity for food supply interventions to make a big impact on the availability of healthy choices.

Transport services to remote Indigenous communities are cited as barriers to a healthier food supply [46]. We contend that non-Indigenous rural and remote areas, locally and internationally, experience similar issues and all may benefit from food stores working together to negotiate lower freight costs [9], thereby, increasing supply and lowering prices. In the shorter term, interventions supported by food store owners show potential to improve healthier choices, these include: taste tests, free samples of healthier choices and communication interventions [47], also nutrition-style shelf labelling has been shown to be effective at nudging healthier choices [48].

Food store owners perceive that barriers to purchasing, stocking and promoting healthy food include consumer preferences for high fat, high sugar and low prices, along with lower wholesale availability of healthy food [47]. Within a small, low income, low profit-margin community, a useful strategy may be to provide financial incentives to healthy food procurement [8]. All interventions should not only focus on store proximity but availability of healthy choices [49]. Given that rural residents typically demonstrate strong loyalty to local food stores [50], these stores are well placed to positively impact dietary choices.

4.2. Food Service Outlets

Across the study area there are no major chain fast food outlets but 27 independent locally owned pubs, fast food outlets and cafes, with the majority of these providing inexpensive readily available high fat foods. Although the methodology differed, our findings are consistent with the Australian study by Innes-Hughes et al. (2012) [26] where take-away outlets in each town offered very few healthy foods, and high fat choices dominated menus.

Consistent with Pereira [43] we found the most widespread 'healthier practice' within food service outlets to be the availability of diet soda (100% in our study c.f. 80%). Healthy menu item availability was low with less than 30% of venues offering even one healthy choice (as defined by NEMS) [42,43]. The one food service outlet that scored well (74%) applies the State Government Healthy Choices Guidelines [51] supporting product promotion, placement and healthy meal deals. Other than this higher score, we observed that our comparison fast food chain outlet scored better than most of the food service outlets within the LGA, mainly due to the signage used rather than the health of the food on offer.

Our very low baseline restaurant score of 3 (SD 4.0) is indicative of an urgent need to intervene with multiple opportunities to improve the healthiness of food offerings within food service outlets [50]. Martinez-Donate (2015) [42] reported improved NEMS-R scores post introduction of a suite of strategies to promote healthier choices, including point-of-purchase labelling and promotions of healthier items. Children's menus could be improved through the introduction of healthy sides as default and reducing serving sizes [52]. Changing to healthier oils in takeaway outlets has been shown to reduce saturated fat intake in previous studies [53] and given the pervasiveness of deep fried food in the study area, a reduction in the use of unhealthy fats may be a useful first step in conjunction with the broader systemic changes required.

4.3. NEMS Tools for a Rural Australian Context

We identified limitations with the NEMS tools in the Australian rural context. With regards to NEMS-S, we considered the quality score protocol often created an over-statement of actual produce quality. Where we assigned a score of 75%, this was equated to 100% score in the overall score. In regards to NEMS-R we considered a smaller portion at a cheaper price should have been awarded a score. We also consider ready access to free tap water should receive additional points. We have some concerns about the importance placed on nutritional promotion given the example of our comparison store, which scored better than most stores, despite the mainly unhealthy food offerings.

4.4. Strengths

To our knowledge, this study is the first in Australia to apply the validated NEMS tools including all food stores across a single local government area, and is one of very few examining the food environment in a rural Australian context. Our study used ground-truthing to provide an accurate representation of the current food environment at a given point in time.

4.5. Limitations

By only collecting data within the LGA geographical borders, out-shopping to larger towns has not been accounted for. In this study there was no comparison group. The study was conducted at a single point in time so does not necessarily provide data on usual food availability, quality or pricing. One might expect seasonality would contribute to variation of produce, or variations in days of the week, which may be influenced by supplier drop off or residents' weekly shops. This study was limited to the rural, Australian context in which it was conducted, thus application of the results may not be appropriate for or applicable to other contexts. Also food environments can change rapidly, as evidenced in this and similar studies by businesses closing during the time of the audit [7].

5. Conclusions

Our findings showed that the healthfulness of the food environment for this remote local government area of rural Victoria is poor. Healthy options, nutrition information and nutrition promotion are not available at most food stores across the LGA.

Outside a supermarket it is very difficult to purchase healthy food in this rural community, made more challenging by the fact that supermarkets are often a significant distance from residents' homes. Given that food environments are a key determinant of obesity [54] and rural loyalty to local business [49], the current predominately unhealthy food environment provides scope to work with food retailers and consumers to ensure healthier options are more visible, available and affordable. This may enable consumers to make healthier choices and thereby impact positively on the health of this community.

Successful interventions have utilised multipronged strategies to improve both food supply and customer demand [8]. We consider it a priority to affect the food environment as a frontline intervention before embarking on, or alongside, any individual behaviour change strategies to ensure healthy food choices are available when consumers seek to choose these.

6. Recommendations

More research is required to explore the relationship between the food environment and food security in rural Australia and with health of those who reside there.

Author Contributions: Conceptualization, J.W., C.B. and P.L.; Data curation, J.W., C.R., F.G. and P.L.; Formal analysis, J.W., L.M., C.R., F.G. and P.L.; Funding acquisition, J.W.; Investigation, J.W. and P.L.; Methodology, J.W. and P.L.; Project administration, J.W. and P.L.; Resources, J.W. and P.L.; Supervision, J.W., L.M., C.B., S.A. and P.L.; Writing—original draft, J.W., L.M., C.B., C.R. and P.L.; Writing—review & editing, J.W., L.M., C.B., C.R., F.G., S.A. and P.L.

Acknowledgments: Thanks to the local food stores for allowing us to collect this information.

Appendix A

Table A1. Availability of more healthful options, and pricing features for supermarkets and general stores, across the local government area, 2017.

Core Food Group (AGHE ref)	Total N = 11	Super-Markets N = 5	General Stores N = 6
Availability of healthier breakfast cereal > 2 varieties	9	5	4
n (%) cost healthy cereal < unhealthy	5	3	2
Whole grain bread availability	10	5	5
>2 varieties whole wheat bread	8	5	3
Price same for both	7	4	3
Price higher for whole wheat	3	1	2

Table A1. *Cont.*

Core Food Group (AGHE ref)	Total N = 11	Super-Markets N = 5	General Stores N = 6
DAIRY OR ALTERNATIVES			
Low-fat/skim **milk** available	11	5	6
Price Higher for low-fat/skim milk	11	5	6
Low-fat **cheese** available	3	3	0
Price Same for both	2	2	0
Price Higher for low-fat	1	1	
Low fat Yoghurt availability	3	3	0
Price Lower for lowest-fat	1	1	0
Price Same for both	1	1	0
Price Higher for low-fat	1	1	
FRESH FRUIT AVAILABILITY—NUMBER OF VARIETIES			
<5 varieties	1		1
5–9 varieties	3		3
10 varieties	7	5	2
FRESH VEGETABLES AVAILABILITY—NUMBER OF VARIETIES			
5–9 varieties	2	0	2
10 varieties	9	5	4
MEAT OR MEAT ALTERNATIVES			
Low-fat mince availability (beef or turkey)	2	2	0
Higher price for lean meat	1	1	
Chicken availability—skinless breast	5	4	1
Price Higher for skinless	3	3	
Legumes available (could also be classified as vegetables)	10	5	5
Eggs available	10	5	5
DISCRETIONARY FOODS			
Healthier snack alternatives to chips (e.g., Grain Waves) (Baked alternative to fried potato crisps)	4	4	0
Chips- Price- (Fried potato crisps)			
Price Lower for Grain Waves than Smiths Chips	0	0	0
Price Higher for Grain Waves than Smiths Chips	4	4	
Healthier dry biscuits available (e.g., water crackers)	11	5	6
Price Lower for water crackers than BBQ shapes (Savoury crackers)	10	5	5
Diet soft drinks available	10	5	5
Same price for both	10	5	5
100% Juice Availability-	9	5	4
Lower for 100% juice (2 L)	1	1	
Same for both	1		1
Higher for 100% juice (2 L)	4	2	2

References

1. Roberto, C.A.; Swinburn, B.; Hawkes, C.; Huang, T.T.K.; Costa, S.A.; Ashe, M.; Zwicker, L.; Cawley, J.H.; Brownell, K.D. Patchy progress on obesity prevention: Emerging examples, entrenched barriers, and new thinking. *Lancet* **2015**, *385*, 2400–2409. [CrossRef]
2. Australian Institute of Health and Welfare. *Australian Burden of Disease Study: Impact and Causes of Illness and Death in Australia 2011.S Bod 4*; AIHW, Ed.; Australian Institute of Health and Welfare: Canberra, Australia, 2016.
3. Swinburn, B.A.; Sacks, G.; Hall, K.D.; McPherson, K.; Finegood, D.T.; Moodie, M.L.; Gortmaker, S.L. The global obesity pandemic: Shaped by global drivers and local environments. *Lancet* **2011**, *378*, 804–814. [CrossRef]
4. Forouzanfar, M.H.; Alexander, L.; Anderson, H.R.; Bachman, V.F.; Biryukov, S.; Brauer, M.; Burnett, R.; Casey, D.; Coates, M.M.; Cohen, A.; et al. Global, regional, and national comparative risk assessment of 79 behavioural, environmental and occupational, and metabolic risks or clusters of risks in 188 countries, 1990–2013: A systematic analysis for the global burden of disease study 2013. *Lancet* **2015**, *386*, 2287–2323. [CrossRef]
5. Rahmanian, E.; Gasevic, D.; Vukmirovich, I.; Lear, S.A. The association between the built environment and dietary intake-a systematic review. *Asia Pac. J. Clin. Nutr.* **2014**, *23*, 183–196. [PubMed]
6. Engler-Stringer, R.; Le, H.; Gerrard, A.; Muhajarine, N. The community and consumer food environment and children's diet: A systematic review. *BMC Public Health* **2014**, *14*, 522. [CrossRef] [PubMed]
7. Vilaro, M.; Barnett, T. The rural food environment: A survey of food price, availability, and quality in a rural Florida community. *Food Public Health* **2013**, *3*, 111–118. [CrossRef]
8. Gittelsohn, J.; Rowan, M.; Gadhoke, P. Interventions in small food stores to change the food environment, improve diet, and reduce risk of chronic disease. *Prev. Chronic Dis.* **2012**, *9*. [CrossRef]
9. National Rural Health Alliance. *Food Security and Health in Rural and Remote Australia*; Australian Government: Rural Industries Research and Development Corporation: Canberra, Australia, 2016.
10. Health Canada. *Measuring the Food Environment in Canada*; Ministry of Health: Ottawa, ON, Canada, 2013.
11. Lebel, A.; Noreau, D.; Tremblay, L.; Oberlé, C.; Girard-Gadreau, M.; Duguay, M.; Block, J.P. Identifying rural food deserts: Methodological considerations for food environment interventions. *Can. J. Public Health* **2016**, *107*, 5353. [CrossRef] [PubMed]
12. Palermo, C.; McCartan, J.; Kleve, S.; Sinha, K.; Shiell, A. A longitudinal study of the cost of food in Victoria influenced by geography and nutritional quality. *Aust. N. Z. J. Public Health* **2016**, *40*, 270–273. [CrossRef] [PubMed]
13. Vilaro, M.; Barnett, T. The rural food environment: A survey of food price, availability, and quality in a rural florida community. *Food Public Health* **2013**, *3*, 10–5923.
14. Hardin-Fanning, F.; Rayens, M.K. Food cost disparities in rural communities. *Health Promot. Pract.* **2015**, *16*, 383–3911. [CrossRef] [PubMed]
15. Lenardson, J.D.; Hansen, A.Y.; Hartley, D. Rural and remote food environments and obesity. *Curr. Obes. Rep.* **2015**, *4*, 46–53. [CrossRef] [PubMed]
16. Byker Shanks, C.; Ahmed, S.; Smith, T.; Houghtaling, B.; Jenkins, M.; Margetts, M.; Schultz, D.; Stephens, L. Availability, price, and quality of fruits and vegetables in 12 rural Montana counties, 2014. *Prev. Chronic Dis.* **2015**, *12*, E128. [CrossRef] [PubMed]
17. Bardenhagen, C.J.; Pinard, C.A.; Pirog, R.; Yaroch, A.L. Characterizing rural food access in remote areas. *J. Commun. Health* **2017**, *42*, 1008–1019. [CrossRef] [PubMed]
18. Gantner, L.A.; Olson, C.M.; Frongillo, E.A.; Wells, N.M. Prevalence of nontraditional food stores and distance to healthy foods in a rural food environment. *J. Hunger Environ. Nutr.* **2011**, *6*, 279–293. [CrossRef]
19. Rideout, K.; Mah, C.; Minaker, L. *Food Environments: An Introduction for Public Health Practice*; National Collaborating Centre for Environmental Health British Columbia Centre for Disease Control: Vancouver, BC, Canada, 2015.
20. Glanz, K.; Sallis, J.F.; Saelens, B.E.; Frank, L.D. Healthy nutrition environments: Concepts and measures. *Am. J. Health Promot.* **2005**, *19*, 330–333. [CrossRef] [PubMed]
21. Rychetnik, L.; Webb, K.; Story, L.; Katz, T. *Food Security Options Paper: A Planning Framework and Menu of Options for Policy and Practice Intervention*; Nutrition Centre for Population Health: Sydney, Australia, 2003.

22. Burns, C. *A Review of the Literature Describing the Link between Poverty, Food Insecurity and Obesity with Specific Reference to Australia*; VicHealth: Melbourne, Australia, 2004.

23. Dhurandhar, E.J. The food-insecurity obesity paradox: A resource scarcity hypothesis. *Physiol. Behav.* **2016**, *162*, 88–92. [CrossRef] [PubMed]

24. Backholer, K.; Spencer, E.; Gearon, E.; Magliano, D.J.; McNaughton, S.A.; Shaw, J.E.; Peeters, A. The association between socio-economic position and diet quality in Australian adults. *Public Health Nutr.* **2016**, *19*, 477–485. [CrossRef] [PubMed]

25. Glanz, K.; Johnson, L.; Yaroch, A.L.; Phillips, M.; Ayala, G.X.; Davis, E.L. Measures of retail food store environments and sales: Review and implications for healthy eating initiatives. *J. Nutr. Educ. Behav.* **2016**, *48*, 280–288. [CrossRef] [PubMed]

26. Innes-Hughes, C.; Boylan, S.; King, L.A.; Lobb, E. Measuring the food environment in three rural towns in new south wales, Australia. *Health Promot. J. Aust.* **2012**, *23*, 129–133. [CrossRef]

27. Krukowski, R.A.; West, D.S.; Harvey-Berino, J.; Prewitt, T.E. Neighborhood impact on healthy food availability and pricing in food stores. *J. Commun. Health* **2010**, *35*, 315–320. [CrossRef] [PubMed]

28. Cameron, A.J. The shelf space and strategic placement of healthy and discretionary foods in urban, urban-fringe and rural/non-metropolitan Australian supermarkets. *Public Health Nutr.* **2018**, *21*, 593–600. [CrossRef] [PubMed]

29. United States Department of Agriculture. USDA Food Plans: Cost of Food. Available online: https://www.cnpp.usda.gov/USDAFoodPlansCostofFood (accessed on 22 July 2018).

30. Glanz, K.; Sallis, J.F.; Saelens, B.E.; Frank, L.D. Nutrition environment measures survey in stores (NEMS-S): Development and evaluation. *Am. J. Prev. Med.* **2007**, *32*, 273–281. [CrossRef] [PubMed]

31. Saelens, B.E.; Glanz, K.; Sallis, J.F.; Frank, L.D. Nutrition environment measures study in restaurants (NEMS-R): Development and evaluation. *Am. J. Prev. Med.* **2007**, *32*, 282–289. [CrossRef] [PubMed]

32. Hector, D.; Boylan, S.; Lee, A. *Healthy Food Environment Scoping Review*; PANORG: Sydney, Australia, 2016.

33. Palermo, C.; Wilson, A. Development of a healthy food basket for Victoria. *Aust. N. Z. J. Public Health* **2007**, *31*, 360–363. [CrossRef] [PubMed]

34. Chapman, K.; Innes-Hughes, C.; Goldsbury, D.; Kelly, B.; Bauman, A.; Allman-Farinelli, M. A comparison of the cost of generic and branded food products in Australian supermarkets. *Public Health Nutr.* **2013**, *16*, 894–900. [CrossRef] [PubMed]

35. Department of Health and Human Services. *Victorian Population Health Survey 2014: Modifiable Risk Factors Contributing to Chronic Disease*; Department of Health and Human Services, Ed.; State Government of Victoria: Melbourne, Australia, 2016.

36. Australian Bureau of Statistics. Data by Region. Available online: http://stat.abs.gov.au/itt/r.jsp?databyregion#/ (accessed on 25 July 2018).

37. Saelens, B.; Glanz, K.; Sallis, J.; Frank, L. NEMS-R Scoring Systems Dimensions. Available online: http://www.med.upenn.edu/nems/measures.shtml (accessed on 22 July 2018).

38. National Health and Medical Research Council. *Australian Guide to Healthy Eating*; NHMRC, Ed.; National Health and Medical Research Council: Canberra, Australia, 2013.

39. NEMS-R Scoring Systems Dimensions. Available online: https://www.med.upenn.edu/nems/measures.shtml (accessed on 20 July 2018).

40. University of Pennsylvania. NEMS Online Training. Available online: http://www.med.upenn.edu/nems/onlinetraining.shtml (accessed on 16 May 2018).

41. StataCorp. *Statacorp Stata Statistical Software: Release*, version 15; StataCorp: College Station, TX, USA, 2017.

42. Martínez-Donate, A.P.; Riggall, A.J.; Meinen, A.M.; Malecki, K.; Escaron, A.L.; Hall, B.; Menzies, A.; Garske, G.; Nieto, F.J.; Nitzke, S. Evaluation of a pilot healthy eating intervention in restaurants and food stores of a rural community: A randomized community trial. *BMC Public Health* **2015**, *15*, 136. [CrossRef] [PubMed]

43. Pereira, R.F.; Sidebottom, A.C.; Boucher, J.L.; Lindberg, R.; Werner, R. Assessing the food environment of a rural community: Baseline findings from the heart of new Ulm project, Minnesota, 2010–2011. *Prev. Chronic Dis.* **2014**, *11*. [CrossRef] [PubMed]

44. Cauchi, D.; Pliakas, T.; Knai, C. Food environments in Malta: Associations with store size and area-level deprivation. *Food Policy* **2017**, *71*, 39–47. [CrossRef]

45. Ghosh-Dastidar, M.; Hunter, G.; Collins, R.L.; Zenk, S.N.; Cummins, S.; Beckman, R.; Nugroho, A.K.; Sloan, J.C.; Dubowitz, T. Does opening a supermarket in a food desert change the food environment? *Health Place* **2017**, *46*, 249–256. [CrossRef] [PubMed]

46. National Rural Health Alliance. *Freight Improvement Toolkit—Getting Quality Healthy Food to Remote Indigenous Communities*; National Rural Health Alliance: Canberra, Australia, 2007.

47. Kim, M.; Budd, N.; Batorsky, B.; Krubiner, C.; Manchikanti, S.; Waldrop, G.; Trude, A.; Gittelsohn, J. Barriers to and facilitators of stocking healthy food options: Viewpoints of Baltimore city small storeowners. *Eco. Food Nutr.* **2017**, *56*, 17–30. [CrossRef] [PubMed]

48. Cameron, A.; Charlton, E.; Ngan, W.; Sacks, G. A systematic review of the effectiveness of supermarket-based interventions involving product, promotion, or place on the healthiness of consumer purchases. *Curr. Nutr. Rep.* **2016**, *5*, 129–138. [CrossRef]

49. Marshall, D.; Dawson, J.; Nisbet, L. Food access in remote rural places: Consumer accounts of food shopping. *Reg. Stud.* **2018**, *52*, 133–144. [CrossRef]

50. Cannuscio, C.C.; Tappe, K.; Hillier, A.; Buttenheim, A.; Karpyn, A.; Glanz, K. Urban food environments and residents' shopping behaviors. *Am. J. Prev. Med.* **2013**, *45*, 606–614. [CrossRef] [PubMed]

51. Healthy Eating Advisory Service. The Healthy Choices Framework. Available online: https://heas.health.vic.gov.au/sites/default/files/HEAS-healthy-choices-framework.pdf (accessed on 24 June 2018).

52. Ayala, G.X.; Castro, I.A.; Pickrel, J.L.; Williams, C.B.; Lin, S.-F.; Madanat, H.; Jun, H.-J.; Zive, M. A restaurant-based intervention to promote sales of healthy children's menu items: The kids' choice restaurant program cluster randomized trial. *BMC Public Health* **2016**, *16*, 250. [CrossRef] [PubMed]

53. Simmons, A.; Sanigorski, A.M.; Cuttler, R.; Brennan, M.; Kremer, P.; Mathews, L.; Swinburn, B. *Nutrition and Physical Activity in Children and Adolescents: Report 6: Lessons Learned from Colac's be Active Eat Well Project (2002-6)*; Department of Human Services Victoria, Melbourne, Vic.: Melbourne, Australia, 2009. Available online: http://dro.deakin.edu.au/view/DU:30021654 (accessed on 24 June 2018).

54. Butland, B.; Jebb, S.; Kopelman, P.; McPherson, K.; Thomas, S.; Mardell, J.; Parry, V. *Foresight: Tackling Obesities—Future Choices Project Report*; Government Office of Science: London, UK, 2007.

Healthy Choice Rewards: A Feasibility Trial of Incentives to Influence Consumer Food Choices in a Remote Australian Aboriginal Community

Clare Brown [1,*], Cara Laws [1], Dympna Leonard [2], Sandy Campbell [3], Lea Merone [1], Melinda Hammond [1], Kani Thompson [1], Karla Canuto [1,4] and Julie Brimblecombe [5]

[1] Apunipima Cape York Health Council, 4870 Cairns, Australia; cara.laws@apunipima.org.au (C.L.); lea.merone@apunipima.org.au (L.M.); melinda.hammond@apunipima.org.au (M.H.); kani.thompson@apunipima.org.au (K.T.); karla.canuto@jcu.edu.au (K.C.)

[2] Australian Institute of Tropical Health and Medicine, College of Public Health Medical and Veterinary Sciences, James Cook University, 4870 Cairns, Australia; dympna.leonard@jcu.edu.au

[3] Centre for Indigenous Health Equity Research, Central Queensland University, 4870 Cairns, Australia; s.campbell@cqu.edu.au

[4] Wardliparingga Aboriginal Health, South Australian Health and Medical Research Institute, 5001 Adelaide, Australia

[5] Department of Nutrition, Dietetics and Food, Monash University, 3168 Melbourne, Australia; julie.brimblecombe@monash.edu

* Correspondence: clare.brown@apunipima.org.au

Abstract: Poor diet including inadequate fruit and vegetable consumption is a major contributor to the global burden of disease. Aboriginal and Torres Strait Islander Australians experience a disproportionate level of preventable chronic disease and successful strategies to support Aboriginal and Torres Strait Islander people living in remote areas to consume more fruit and vegetables can help address health disadvantage. Healthy Choice Rewards was a mixed methods study to investigate the feasibility of a monetary incentive: store vouchers, to promote fruit and vegetable purchasing in a remote Australian Aboriginal community. Multiple challenges were identified in implementation, including limited nutrition workforce. Challenges related to the community store included frequent store closures and amended trading times, staffing issues and poor infrastructure to support fruit and vegetable promotion. No statistically significant increases in fruit or vegetable purchases were observed in the short time frame of this study. Despite this, community members reported high acceptability of the program, especially for women with children. Optimal implementation including, sufficient time and funding resources, with consideration of the most vulnerable could go some way to addressing inequities in food affordability for remote community residents.

Keywords: Aboriginal and Torres Strait Islander; remote; community store; fruit and vegetables; incentive; subsidy; food security; nutrition; diet

1. Introduction

Food security is a major global issue [1]. Strategies to achieve physical and economic access to sufficient, safe and nutritious food are important for all and this is especially important for Indigenous Peoples who often experience the most severe economic and health disparities [2]. Australia is a wealthy country but high levels of food insecurity have been documented for Aboriginal and Torres Strait Islander people compared to other Australians (22% versus. 3.7%) [3]. In Australia, food insecurity is highest among Aboriginal and Torres Strait Islander people living in remote locations (31%) compared to non-remote (20%) [3].

The life expectancy gap of 10–11 years between Aboriginal and Torres Strait Islander people and non-Indigenous Australians is well known [4]. Recent national survey reports indicate that Aboriginal and Torres Strait Islander people consume a diet that is relatively poor compared to other Australians, with lower intakes of fruit and vegetables and higher intakes of sugar sweetened beverages and nutritionally poor foods [3]. Chronic diseases, much of which are diet-related were responsible for 70% of the gap in health between Aboriginal and Torres Strait Islanders and non-Indigenous Australians in 2011 [5]. Contributing to this are the higher rates of overweight and obesity, cardiovascular disease, chronic kidney disease and type two diabetes [4].

Many factors influence the nutritional status of Aboriginal and Torres Strait islander people, including socioeconomic disadvantage and other historical, social, environmental and geographical factors [6–8]. Healthy foods in remote Aboriginal and Torres Strait Islander communities cost more than urban areas [9–11]. The 2016 Census shows the median household weekly income in the remote region of interest is AUD $987 for a mean household size of 3.8 people [12]. This is 70% of the median state of Queensland household income of AUD $1402 per week with a lower average household size of 2.6 people [12]. On this lower income, remote area residents in Queensland pay 41% more for fruit and 12% more for vegetables compared with Queenslanders living in urban areas [9]. Research has shown that when food choices are made under budget constraints, consumer purchasing behaviour is driven by maximising energy value for money (dollars per megajoule), resulting in the purchase of fewer nutrient rich foods such as fruit and vegetables and more nutrient poor, energy dense foods [13,14].

There is a well-established link between increased fruit and vegetable consumption and improved health outcomes [15]; consequently, increasing consumption of fruit and vegetables has been identified as an important measure to achieve health gains nationally [16]. In addition to improved health, it has been estimated that if vegetable consumption in Australia was 10% higher, government expenditure on health care could be reduced by AUD $100 million annually [17]. If all Australians met the recommended daily intake of vegetables this saving would increase nine fold [17]. The potential savings are likely to be more pronounced for Aboriginal and Torres Strait Islander people living in remote areas due to the higher burden of disease experienced and the high costs of delivering remote health services.

In the context of increasing health care costs and government budget cuts threatening progress in the prevention of chronic disease [18], it is important to investigate cost effective measures to address health disadvantage for Aboriginal and Torres Strait Islander people living in remote communities and provide clear recommendations for policy makers. There is a growing body of research demonstrating the potential for food price changes to influence diet quality and drive positive population health gains [19–24]. Government policy options in pricing strategies include unhealthy food taxation, healthy food subsidies and price discount schemes to promote healthy food environments [25,26]. In Australia, two large supermarket price discount randomised controlled trials have recently been completed, both showing the effectiveness of price discounts on fruit and vegetable purchasing [22,23]. One of these projects, the Stores Healthy Options at Remote Indigenous Communities (SHOP@RIC) was implemented in 20 remote communities in Northern Territory and achieved a 12.7% increase in purchases of fruit and vegetables [22].

Strategies to make fruit and vegetables more accessible to Aboriginal and Torres Strait Islander families living in remote communities have the potential to reduce health inequality and subsequent health care costs. Here we report on a feasibility trial of a monetary incentive to promote fruit and vegetable purchasing in one remote community. To our knowledge, the effectiveness of immediately rewarding healthy purchasing behaviours has not yet been explored in a remote Aboriginal and Torres Strait Islander community context.

2. Materials and Methods

2.1. Setting

Apunipima Cape York Health Council (Apunipima) community nutrition project staff conducted a study in 2015 to assess the feasibility of implementing a fruit and vegetable incentive in a very remote Australian community store in far north Queensland, located around 2500 km from the nearest major city. This remote community has approximately 1400 residents with most (90.4%) identifying as Aboriginal and/or Torres Strait Islander [27]. The community experiences low levels of formal education, low income, reliance on social security payments and high dependency ratios [27]. While the people of this community value traditional foods and traditional food systems, the community store is the main source of food for residents for their daily needs. The next nearest grocery store is 200 km away; a three hour drive by dirt road.

2.2. Design

A mixed methods approach was used and included collection of qualitative data using semi-structured interviews, participant observation, a weekly electronic survey on store and wider community contextual information and a quantitative assessment of store sales data. Feasibility of the intervention was assessed in terms of acceptability, voucher uptake, implementation issues and impact on fruit and vegetable sales. All customers of the store were eligible to participate. Study implementation was led by Apunipima community nutrition staff.

2.3. Healthy Choice Rewards Program

The Healthy Choice Rewards (HCR) program offered community store customers an incentive of a fruit and vegetable voucher to the value of AUD $10 each time a set minimum amount was spent on fruit and vegetables. Store staff participated in semi-structured interviews prior to the study to inform the reward system design and determine what supports would need to be in place for implementation. Two phases of the minimal amount spent were trialed: phase one required a AUD $20 spend on fresh fruit and vegetables to receive a AUD $10 HCR voucher to be redeemed on the date of purchase; phase two required a AUD $15 spend on fresh fruit and vegetables to receive a AUD $10 HCR voucher to be redeemed within three days. Frozen, tinned and dried fruit and vegetables were not included as part of the minimum spend as they could not be easily distinguished in the store's electronic grocery management system. The vouchers were redeemable for fresh, frozen, tinned or dried fruit and vegetables and excluded tinned fruit in syrup and frozen potato chips and wedges. Vegetable packs valued at AUD $10 were available for sale. The store was reimbursed for the value of any vouchers used.

The incentive was available for 32 weeks; phase one ran for 15 weeks, followed immediately by phase two for 17 weeks. The HCR vouchers appeared as black and white plain text print outs at the end of customer store dockets. The reward offer was promoted in English and local language using posters, flyers, radio advertisements and electronic register screen displays at the store.

Project staff visited the community monthly during the intervention period to promote HCR. During the visits they delivered healthy cooking demonstrations, distributed healthy recipe flyers, spoke with community members on how to utilise the offer and assisted store staff in merchandising the fruit and vegetable display. Between visits the project team provided weekly phone and email support to the store manager to maintain program promotion and assist with processing the vouchers.

2.4. Data Collection

To determine the feasibility of the HCR program the primary outcome measures included: acceptability of the voucher incentive to customers and store staff, voucher uptake and redemption and identification of the opportunities and challenges of implementation. A secondary measure included per capita total fruit and vegetable intake derived from store sales purchasing data.

2.4.1. Acceptability

Following completion of both phases of the intervention, we invited store staff and store customers (community members) to provide feedback through semi-structured face-to-face interviews (customer or staff satisfaction interviews). Demographics on age, gender, Aboriginal and Torres Strait Islander status, and employment were collected. Project staff (one of whom is a Torres Strait Islander woman) with training and experience interviewing Aboriginal and Torres Strait Islander community members conducted the interviews. To promote the feedback opportunities to the community, the team engaged in local activities including performing a healthy cooking demonstration and organising a group fishing trip with a healthy lunch. All customer and store staff interviewees ($n = 34$) received a fruit and vegetable voucher to the value of AUD $10 to acknowledge their time contributed. In addition to the customer satisfaction interviews conducted at the completion of the program, four customer interviews were conducted during phase one to inform intervention changes for phase two.

2.4.2. Voucher Uptake

Weekly HCR voucher redemption data were collected using the stores' electronic point of sale system.

2.4.3. Implementation

Interview data was also used to assess implementation issues. Project staff also routinely recorded observational data with hand written notes on their regular community visits.

2.4.4. Fruit and Vegetable Sales

Electronic point-of sale data including product description, unit weight, number of units sold, and dollar value were collected weekly for all food and drink sales for the duration of the project period and the same time-period in the previous year. A purpose built weekly electronic survey used in the SHOP@RIC trial [22] collected descriptive data from the store manager on potential factors influencing usual food and drink purchasing such as population movements, community events and activities, frequency of food delivery to the store and retail management practices. This data collection aimed to contextualise store sales data and account for community-level factors that may have influenced purchasing behaviours during the intervention.

2.5. Data Analysis

2.5.1. Acceptability and Implementation

Interview data and project observations were collated in Excel. Two project staff members independently coded interview responses and grouped these into emerging themes. Apunipima staff members who had research experience reviewed the coding results and resolved inconsistencies by consensus.

2.5.2. Voucher Uptake

To evaluate HCR voucher uptake, we compared the number of vouchers issued and number of vouchers redeemed across both program phases.

2.5.3. Fruit and Vegetable Sales

A pre-post point-of-sale analysis of purchasing was completed by Menzies School of Health Research in January 2016. Weekly point-of-sale data were uploaded to a purpose-built Microsoft Access database and coded into relevant food groups. Aggregated weekly point-of-sale data for the 32 week study period were compared to the same time-period in the previous year, to account for seasonal variation. Per capita daily fruit and vegetable consumption for the community was estimated by dividing the average sales for the study period by 32 weeks × 7 days and the usual population estimates obtained from 2011 Australian Bureau of Statistics national census data. The average per capita daily amounts of fruit and vegetables purchased were converted from weights measured in grams to average number of serves using Australian Dietary Guideline definitions for standard fruit and vegetable weights (i.e., 150 g per serve for fruit and 75 g per serve for vegetables) [16]. Statistical analysis was performed using the paired t-test technique to compare sales in phase 1 and phase 2 with the baseline time-periods in the previous year. p Values of less than 0.05 were considered statistically significant. Contextual factors were uploaded into an Access Database and frequency of occurrence was graphed on a weekly timescale and considered against the results reported from the purchase data to identify potential variables impacting store sales and to assist interpretation of the impact of the incentive on the outcome measures.

2.6. Ethical Approval

James Cook University Human Research Ethics Committee (HREC H5938) and the combined Northern Territory Department of Health and Menzies School of Health research Human Research Ethics Committee (HREC 2014-2313) granted ethical approval for the study.

3. Results

3.1. Acceptability

A total of 28 post program customer satisfaction interviews were completed. The majority of customers interviewed identified as Aboriginal and/or Torres Strait Islander people (82.1%) and were women (71.4%). Additionally, 68% of responders reported being employed at the time of the interview. Of those interviewed, more women that were employed than not employed reported using the HCR voucher. All respondents reported they would like the offer to continue and 61% of respondents indicated that HCR encouraged their family to consume more fruit and vegetables. All store staff interviewed following the completion of the project ($n = 6$) reported they wanted the offer to occur again. Community members identified that healthy eating was important for health but there were many challenges and competing priorities to eat a healthy and nutritious diet. They also provided suggestions for improving the program.

3.1.1. Community Perceptions of Healthy Eating

Healthy eating was viewed as important for participants and HCR was seen as a valuable program as it promoted healthy food choices, as one grandmother said, "It's important, it is very important. Kids need to eat healthy. We don't want to see our kids wither away, we want them to have a healthy choice"

The HCR program was also seen as a good reminder to consume fruit and vegetables, "Like you remind kids, 'don't do that', it's good to remind us Aboriginal people to eat more fruits and vegetables because sometimes we forget" [Female Elder].

Healthy eating was seen as especially important for women with children or young families, as one female participant responded, "Being healthy is especially important for kids to grow strong, good clean blood for [to prevent] anaemia ... [it is] good for people with plenty of children, good for their health".

3.1.2. Challenges and Competing Priorities to Consume a Healthy Diet

Community members described facing many challenges to healthy eating including high food costs and limited available money to spend on healthy food, as one participant described, "It's expensive here, there is hardly enough money to buy food".

Although the HCR program was valued and seen to encourage fruit and vegetable consumption, it was not enough to alleviate the high cost of food as one respondent indicated, "It was really good. It encourages people to get more fruit and vegetables. AUD $10 doesn't get you much, but it's good".

While another participant reported, "AUD $10 only gets you two or three fruit and vegetables because of costings of the shop".

Other reported challenges to consuming healthy eating included limited access to health hardware such as no fridge to store food at home, limited availability of fresh produce and concerns over quality of this produce by the time it arrives in the community. It was also noted that community members have increasing dependency on takeaway foods rather than preparing homemade meals. Another concern was that children are now preferring the taste of sweet discretionary foods from the store rather than traditional bush foods.

Some responders also reported that healthy eating was not a priority for everyone, for example there may be other competing priorities based on social factors that are viewed as more important or there may be basic challenges such as the inability to shop for groceries. This was particularly thought to be the case for people with little money, those who did not live at one fixed address (living between multiple houses), those relying on meals provided by family (such as the frail elderly) and even people who struggled with addictions such as alcohol, drugs or gambling.

3.1.3. Suggestions for Improving the HCR Program

Feedback from the customer interviews suggested that future incentives may be more effective if the reward system was tailored specifically for women with children and used electronic store loyalty cards instead of paper-based vouchers. Other recommendations from the interviews included: increased flexibility of redemption parameters, more support from store staff (such as explaining the voucher and helping determine AUD $10 worth of fruit and vegetables so it is more convenient for the customer), offering higher incentives and strengthening promotion through increased community involvement. Store staff observed an increase in customer interest in HCR following promotion by the visiting nutrition team and noted that customers reported that uptake of the incentive could have been be improved with greater promotion.

3.2. Voucher Uptake

Voucher redemption rates averaged 28.6% (95% CI: 26, 31) for the duration of the study. A total of 2150 vouchers were issued and 632 redeemed. Redemption rates were higher during phase two of the study compared to phase one, averaging 30% (95% CI: 30, 31) and 27% (95% CI: 21, 32) respectively. The highest redemption rate (44%) was recorded on a week when project staff were at the store performing cooking demonstrations raising awareness about the project and assisting with merchandising of fresh produce.

3.3. Implementation

Four of the six staff interviewed reported having issues with the reward offer and required more support to run the offer. Issues identified by store staff included: being unsure of how to process the voucher in the store electronic grocery management system; having too many customers at once to help other customers claim their voucher; limited time to prepare the AUD $10 fruit and vegetable packs for customers to redeem; customers complaining of losing their receipts and customers refusing the voucher as it meant they needed to queue up a second time to redeem their reward.

Several challenges that impacted on project implementation at the store level were observed by project staff including store infrastructure issues; support for store staff to run the offer; and support for store managers to promote fresh produce. Fresh produce displays were impacted by transport issues; infrastructure issues, such as limited equipment to display produce; the hot climate affecting the temperature control of open display refrigeration units; and store air-conditioning and refrigeration units often breaking down. Supporting store staff proved challenging due to a shortage of trained and experienced staff; high turnover and low attendance among store staff; variable expertise among store management in merchandising of fresh produce and limited capacity of Community and Store Nutritionists to provide sufficient support to store staff. In addition, due to issues impacting the community during the study period such as community unrest, forced store closures and amended trading hours were reported on 23 out of 32 weeks.

Implementation of the project was strengthened by the existing rapport of project staff with community and regular presence in the community; strong partnerships with industry and the research sector; and support from community, local Council and the Store Group to implement the project.

3.4. Fruit and Vegetable Sales

The voucher incentive was not successful in increasing fruit and vegetable store sales during the study period compared to sales for the same time period in the previous year. In fact, despite including voucher purchases, a 7% reduction in total fruit sales was observed between the two periods, decreasing from 41 to 38 g/person/day (0.27 to 0.25 serves/person/per day), $p = 0.01$. Non-significant reductions in sales of vegetables and overall food and drink sales were also observed.

4. Discussion

This feasibility study describes a monetary incentive strategy to promote fruit and vegetable consumption in a remote Aboriginal community in Australia. While we were unsuccessful in increasing fruit and vegetable purchases during the intervention period, qualitative data indicates that there was a high level of acceptability of the program by community members. This study also highlights the many challenges to be considered in implementing food subsidy strategies to improve nutritional health in the remote community context.

The HCR project was completed in 2015 as part of implementing a key objective of the Cape York Food and Nutrition Strategy—to ensure equitable food affordability, availability and access comparable to urban Australia [28]. This project therefore works towards addressing the high costs of nutritious foods in remote Aboriginal and Torres Strait Islander communities; a known barrier to healthy eating.

Although the project staff made frequent trips to the community, store staff and management identified the need for more support. Furthermore, interview data suggested that voucher uptake could have been improved with strengthened promotion. These findings are consistent with other studies demonstrating that consumers need to be made aware of promotional offers [29]. Limited funding for this project and limited community nutrition workforce on the ground restricted promotion efforts. Sufficient resource allocation for promotion and nutrition workforce should be prioritised in future programs. Additionally, interview data indicated that the paper-based voucher system was not always well understood by customers and was reported to be a barrier to participation and could have therefore influenced voucher uptake. An electronic store loyalty card system was recommended by stakeholders as a preferred alternative. This option was explored in the early phases of study, however, the cost of implementing the system with such limited funding was prohibitive but should be considered in any future interventions.

Women who were employed were most likely to report using the HCR in customer satisfaction interviews. Qualitative data indicated that healthy eating was considered by community members to be more of a priority for women with children or young families. Given that improving access to nutritious food for at-risk mothers, infants and children is a key priority of the 2013–2023 National Aboriginal and Torres Strait Islander Health Plan [30], these findings warrant further investigation. If a reward incentive or subsidy were to be targeted towards smaller population subgroups such as women with children, an individual or household level measure of food and drink purchasing would be needed rather than store population level purchasing data.

This study provided information of fruit and vegetable consumption data for this community which differ from other information sources. Average fruit and vegetables sales were estimated to be equivalent to 0.25 serves/person/day for fruit and 0.92 serves/person/day for vegetables during the study period. These results are lower than self-reported data from the 2012–2013 National Aboriginal and Torres Strait Islander Nutrition and Physical Activity Survey (NATSINPAS) which reported

Aboriginal and Torres Strait Islander people living in remote areas across Australia consume on average 0.9 serves of fruit and 1.7 serves of vegetables per day [31]. The NATSINPAS combines results from remote and very remote areas and includes fruit and vegetable components from mixed food sources (such as lasagna), which will likely result in a higher reported intake [31]. While observed differences may also be the result of the different methodology used, a recent comparison of dietary estimates from the very remote sample of the NATSINPAS to food and beverage purchase data from 20 remote Northern Territory community stores suggests over-reporting of fruit and vegetable consumption with self-reporting data [32]. A strength of using sales data is that in a very remote community where there is only one food retail store it provides an objective proxy of population diet [32,33]. For this study, the closest alternative food retail store is 200 km away from the community. Our results are more consistent with a Northern Territory study which reported an average of 0.3–0.7 serves of fruit and 1.1–2.1 serves of vegetables sold per person per day across three remote Aboriginal communities [34].

The limitations of this study are that it was conducted in one remote community only and for a short time period, with limited staffing. These factors reflect the currently limited resources available for nutrition promotion in this setting, compared to previous investments [35]. With additional resources, more support could be provided to the store for implementation, and other factors contributing to the low uptake of the vouchers and reductions on sales of fruit and vegetables could be clarified and addressed. It is likely however that the issues impacting the community at the time which resulted in a high number of forced store closures and amended trading hours influenced voucher uptake and purchases of fruit and vegetables. A strength of HCR was that the voucher incentive was well received by community members and the majority of participants in the evaluation indicated that it helped their family to consume more fruit and vegetables. It was particularly seen as important for mothers with children who needed fruit and vegetables for a healthy start in life.

Another strength of this project was the strong partnerships and relationships formed by the project team with the community, particularly with the local community store as HCR was supported by store managers, staff and at management levels of the store group. Store Managers play an important role in food supply in remote Aboriginal and Torres Strait Islander communities and are therefore essential partners in helping to improve dietary intake [36]. This project illustrates how the store managers can be effectively supported by nutritionists to actively promote the incentive, resulting in increased uptake.

Remote community stores have an important influence on community health through their ability to control the availability and accessibility of both healthy and unhealthy foods [36]. Significant store implementation challenges were observed in this study. This highlighted the difficulties remote retailers face in maintaining normal store operations, in addition to the ability to adequately support health promotion efforts. Investing in assistance for remote retailers to provide healthy foods to communities is critical to the success of any efforts to improve fruit and vegetable purchase and consumption in remote Aboriginal and Torres Strait Islander communities.

5. Conclusions

This mixed methods feasibility study showed high levels of acceptability of the program by community. It also resulted in the identification of several challenges to be considered when implementing a food subsidy strategy or incentive in remote Australia. Investing in remote retailers to overcome the challenges in providing healthy foods is critical to the success of any efforts to improve fruit and vegetable consumption in remote Aboriginal and Torres Strait Islander communities. Additionally, increased investment in a nutrition prevention workforce to implement healthy remote store practices and support retailers to promote nutrition is required.

Feedback from customer interviews suggested that future incentives may be more effective if the reward program was tailored specifically for women with children. A larger scale controlled study targeting women and children may provide greater insight into the use and appropriateness of a fruit and vegetable subsidy in the remote community context.

Consumer food subsidy schemes can help overcome financial barriers and increase affordability of healthy food and drink in remote areas. The high rates of food insecurity in remote Aboriginal and Torres Strait Islander communities are largely a consequence of high rates of unemployment and low incomes compounded by high food costs. Government commitment is needed to reduce the underlying social inequality and to address the affordability of healthy food choices to help close the gap in Aboriginal and Torres Strait Islander health.

Author Contributions: Conceptualization, M.H., C.L., D.L., J.B. and C.B.; Methodology, J.B., C.L., M.H, K.T. and C.B.; Formal Analysis, J.B.; Project administration, C.L.; Supervision, J.B.; Writing-Original Draft Preparation, C.B. and C.L., Writing-Review & Editing, C.B., L.M., C.L., M.H., S.C., J.B., K.C., K.T. and D.L.

Acknowledgments: The authors sincerely thank the store staff and store group, Aboriginal Shire Council members, and community members involved in this study. The authors also thank Susan Jacups and Yvonne Cadet-James who contributed to the development of the paper and Jemma McCutcheon for reviewing the final draft.

References

1. FAO; IFAD; UNICEF; WFP; WHO. The State of Food Security and Nutrition in the World 2018. Building Climate Resilience for Food Security and Nutrition. Available online: http://www.who.int/nutrition/publications/foodsecurity/state-food-security-nutrition-2018-en.pdf?ua=1 (accessed on 20 October 2018).

2. Kuhnlein, H.; Erasmus, B.; Spigelski, D.; Burlingame, B. Indigenous People's Food Systems and Wellbeing: Interventions and Policies for Healthy Communities Food and Agriculture Organization of the United Nations. Available online: http://www.fao.org/docrep/018/i3144e/i3144e.pdf (accessed on 20 October 2018).

3. Australian Bureau of Statistics. Australian Aboriginal and Torres Strait Islander Health Survey: Nutrition Results- Food and Nutrients, 2012-13 Cat No. 4727.0.55.005. Available online: http://www.ausstats.abs.gov.au/ausstats/subscriber.nsf/0/5D4F0DFD2DC65D9ECA257E0D000ED78F/$File/4727.0.55.005%20australian%20aboriginal%20and%20torres%20strait%20islander%20health%20survey,%20nutrition%20results%20%20-%20food%20and%20nutrients%20.pdf (accessed on 20 October 2018).

4. Australian Institute of Health and Welfare. Australia's Health 2018 Cat No. AUS 221. Available online: https://www.aihw.gov.au/getmedia/7c42913d-295f-4bc9-9c24-4e44eff4a04a/aihw-aus-221.pdf.aspx?inline=true (accessed on 20 October 2018).

5. Australian Institute of Health and Welfare. *Australian Burden of Disease Study: Impact and Causes of Illness and Death in Aboriginal and Torres Strait Islander People 2011*; AIHW: Canberra, Australia, 2016.

6. Lee, A.; Ride, K. *Review of Nutrition among Aboriginal and Torres Strait Islander People*; Australian Indigenous HealthInfoNet: Perth, Australia, 2018.

7. Brimblecombe, J.; Maypilama, E.; Colles, S.; Scarlett, M.; Dhurrkay, J.G.; Ritchie, J.; O'Dea, K. Factors Influencing Food Choice in an Australian Aboriginal Community. *Qual. Health Res.* **2014**, 24, 387–400. [CrossRef] [PubMed]

8. Lee, A.J. The Transition of Australian Aboriginal Diet and Nutritional Health. *World Rev. Nutr. Diet.* **1996**, 79, 1–52. [PubMed]

9. Queensland Health. Healthy Food Access Basket. Available online: https://www.health.qld.gov.au/research-reports/reports/public-health/food-nutrition/access (accessed on 15 October 2018).

10. Department of Health. *Northern Territory Market Basket Survey 2016*; Northern Territory Government of Australia: Darwin, Australia, 2017.

11. Pollard, C.; Savage, V.; Landrigan, T.; Hanbury, A.; Kerr, D. *Food Access and Cost Survey 2013 Report*; Department of Health: Perth, Australia, 2015.

12. Australia Bureau of Statistics. 2016 Census QuickStats. Available online: http://quickstats.censusdata.abs.gov.au/census_services/getproduct/census/2016/quickstat/IREG303 (accessed on 1 November 2018).

13. Brimblecombe, J.; O'Dea, K. The role of energy cost in food choices for an Aboriginal population in northern Australia. *Med. J. Aust.* **2009**, 190, 549–551. [PubMed]

14. Drewnowski, A.; Darmon, N. Food choices and diet costs: An economic analysis. *J. Nutr.* **2005**, *135*, 900–904. [CrossRef] [PubMed]

15. World Health Organization. Increasing Fruit and Vegetable Consumption to Reduce the Risk of Noncommunicable Diseases. Available online: https://www.who.int/elena/titles/fruit_vegetables_ncds/en/ (accessed on 1 November 2018).

16. National Health and Medical Research Council. *Australian Dietary Guidelines*; National Health and Medical Research Council: Canberra, Australia, 2013.

17. Deloitte Access Economics. *The Impact of Increasing Vegetable Consumption on Health Expenditure*; Deloitte Access Economics: Canberra, Australia, 2016.

18. Wilson, A. Budget cuts risk halting Australia's progress in preventing chronic disease: Investing in prevention is essential to our nation's long term productivity. *Med. J. Aust.* **2014**, *200*, 558–589. [CrossRef] [PubMed]

19. Thow, A.M.; Jan, S.; Leeder, S.; Swinburn, B. The effect of fiscal policy on diet, obesity and chronic disease: A systematic review. *Bull. World Health Organ.* **2010**, *88*, 609–614. [CrossRef] [PubMed]

20. Thow, A.M.; Downs, S.; Jan, S. A systematic review of the effectiveness of food taxes and subsidies to improve diets: Understanding the recent evidence. *Nutr. Rev.* **2014**, *72*, 551–565. [CrossRef] [PubMed]

21. An, R. Effectiveness of subsidies in promoting healthy food purchases and consumption: A review of field experiments. *Public Health Nutr.* **2013**, *16*, 1215–1228. [CrossRef] [PubMed]

22. Brimblecombe, J.; Ferguson, M.; Chatfield, M.D.; Liberato, S.C.; Gunther, A.; Ball, K.; Moodie, M.; Miles, E.; Magnus, A.; Mhurchu, C.N.; et al. Effect of a price discount and consumer education strategy on food and beverage purchases in remote Indigenous Australia: A stepped-wedge randomised controlled trial. *Lancet Public Health* **2017**, *2*, e82–e95. [CrossRef]

23. Ball, K.; McNaughton, S.A.; Le, H.N.; Gold, L.; Ni Mhurchu, C.; Abbott, G.; Pollard, C.; Crawford, D. Influence of price discounts and skill-building strategies on purchase and consumption of healthy food and beverages: Outcomes of the Supermarket Healthy Eating for Life randomized controlled trial. *Am. J. Clin. Nutr.* **2015**, *101*, 1055–1064. [CrossRef] [PubMed]

24. Black, A.P.; Vally, H.; Morris, P.S.; Daniel, M.; Esterman, A.J.; Smith, F.E.; O'Dea, K. Health outcomes of a subsidised fruit and vegetable program for Aboriginal children in northern New South Wales. *Med. J. Aust.* **2013**, *199*, 46–50. [CrossRef] [PubMed]

25. Thow, A.M.; Downs, S.M.; Mayes, C.; Trevena, H.; Waqanivalu, T.; Cawley, J. Fiscal policy to improve diets and prevent noncommunicable diseases: From recommendations to action. *Bull. World Health Organ.* **2018**, *96*, 201–210. [CrossRef] [PubMed]

26. World Health Organization. *Fiscal Policies for Diet and Prevention on Noncommunicable Diseases Technical Meeting Report, 5–6 May 2015*; World Health Organization: Geneva, Switzerland, 2016.

27. Queensland Government Statistician's Office. Queensland Regional Profiles. Available online: https://statistics.qgso.qld.gov.au/qld-regional-profiles (accessed on 22 October 2018).

28. Steering Committee for the Cape York Food and Nutrition Strategy 2012–2017. *Cape York Food and Nutrition Strategy 2012–2017*; Queensland Health: Brisbane, Australia, 2012.

29. Ferguson, M.; O'Dea, K.; Holden, S.; Miles, E.; Brimblecombe, J. Food and beverage price discounts to improve health in remote Aboriginal communities: Mixed method evaluation of a natural experiment. *Aust. N. Z. J. Public Health* **2017**, *41*, 32–37. [CrossRef] [PubMed]

30. Commonwealth of Australia. National Aboriginal and Torres Strait Islander Health Plan 2013–2023. Available online: http://www.health.gov.au/internet/main/publishing.nsf/content/B92E980680486C3BCA257BF0001BAF01/$File/health-plan.pdf (accessed on 22 October 2018).

31. Australian Bureau of Statistics. Australian Aboriginal and Torres Strait Islander Health Survey: Consumption of Food Groups from the Australian Dietary Guidelines, 2012–13. Available online: http://www.abs.gov.au/AUSSTATS/abs@.nsf/Lookup/4727.0.55.008Main+Features12012-13?OpenDocument (accessed on 29 October 2018).

32. McMahon, E.; Wycherley, T.; O'Dea, K.; Brimblecombe, J. A comparison of dietary estimates from the National Aboriginal and Torres Strait Islander Health Survey to food and beverage purchase data. *Aust. N. Z. J. Public Health* **2017**, *41*, 598–603. [CrossRef] [PubMed]

33. Brimblecombe, J.; Liddle, R.; O'Dea, K. Use of point-of-sale data to assess food and nutrient quality in remote stores. *Public Health Nutr.* **2013**, *16*, 1159–1167. [CrossRef] [PubMed]

34. Brimblecombe, J.; Ferguson, M.; Liberato, S.; O'Dea, K. Characteristics of the community-level diet of Aboriginal people in remote northern Australia. *Med. J. Aust.* **2013**, *198*, 380–384. [CrossRef] [PubMed]

35. Vidgen, H.; Adam, M.; Gallegos, D. Who does nutrition prevention work in Queensland? *Nutr. Diet.* **2015**, *74*, 88–94. [CrossRef] [PubMed]

36. Lee, A.J.; Bonson, A.P.; Powers, J.R. The effect of retail store managers on Aboriginal diet in remote communities. *Aust. N. Z. J. Public Health* **1996**, *20*, 212–214. [CrossRef] [PubMed]

12

Household Food Insecurity Narrows the Sex Gap in Five Adverse Mental Health Outcomes among Canadian Adults

Geneviève Jessiman-Perreault and Lynn McIntyre *

Department of Community Health Sciences, Cumming School of Medicine, University of Calgary, Calgary, AB T2N 1N4, Canada; gjessima@ucalgary.ca
* Correspondence: lmcintyr@ucalgary.ca

Abstract: The sex gap (i.e., the significant difference in an outcome between men and women) in the occurrence of a variety of mental health conditions has been well documented. Household food insecurity has also repeatedly been found to be associated with a variety of poor mental health outcomes. Although both sex and household food insecurity have received attention individually, rarely have they been examined together to explore whether or how these indicators of two social locations interact to impact common mental health outcomes. Using a pooled sample (N = 302,683) of the Canadian Community Health Survey (2005–2012), we test whether sex modifies the relationship between household food insecurity assessed by the Household Food Security Survey Module and five adverse mental health outcomes, controlling for confounding covariates. Although the sex gap was observed among food secure men versus women, males and females reporting any level of food insecurity were equally likely to report adverse mental health outcomes, compared with those reporting food security. Therefore, household food insecurity seems to narrow the sex gap on five adverse mental health outcomes.

Keywords: household food insecurity; mental health; sex; Canadian adults

1. Introduction

The sex gap (i.e., the significant difference in the occurrence of a health outcome between males and females) in mental health conditions has been consistently documented and re-examined [1–3]. The sex gap in mental health outcomes (typically cited as a nearly 2:1 ratio for women versus men reporting depression [4]) has also remained stable across decades. While the exact mechanism underlying drivers of the sex gap in mental health outcomes remains elusive, researchers have begun to examine the sex gap in the context of other important social determinants of health such as age [5], marital status [6], and sexual orientation [7]. This study examines the relationship between sex and five common mental health outcomes in the context of household food insecurity.

1.1. Household Food Insecurity in Canada and Adverse Mental Health Outcomes

Household food insecurity is operationally defined as the lack of access to food because of financial constraints [8] and in Canada, it is measured through national survey responses to the Household Food Security Survey Module (HFSSM) [9,10]. Using this metric, recent national estimates indicate that in 2012, 12.5% of Canadian households experienced some form of food insecurity (4.1% marginal food insecurity, 5.7% moderate food insecurity, and 2.7% severe food insecurity) [8]. Certain subsets of the population—groups most often associated with material deprivation—have a disproportionate risk of reporting household food insecurity; this includes Indigenous Canadians, African Canadians, households that rely on social assistance as their main income source, lone-mother led households, and those who rent rather than own their own home [8].

There is a large and robust body of literature establishing the relationship between household food insecurity and a variety of physical health problems. Adults and children living in food insecure households report poorer physical health; increased physical limitations; and higher prevalence of diabetes mellitus, heart disease, and other chronic conditions [11–13]. Furthermore, those living in food insecure households with pre-existing chronic health problems, such as diabetes, experience increased difficulties managing those conditions [14].

In addition to being associated with poorer physical health, there is a growing body of evidence that household food insecurity is associated with poor mental health and an increased risk of reporting certain mental health conditions, including psychological distress [15], mood and anxiety disorders [12,15], suicidal ideation [15], self-reported fair/poor mental health [16,17], depression [13,17–19], and psychiatric morbidity [20]. Recent research has reported that increasing severity of household food insecurity is associated with a graded increase in the risk of reporting six common mental health outcomes among Canadian adults [21].

Household food insecurity is hypothesized to be associated with poor mental health because of the unique social, physical, and psychological stresses associated with being in a food insecure household [22]. Interestingly, there is evidence that the relationship between household food insecurity and mental health could be bidirectional. Managing a food insecure household is extremely difficult and requires substantial planning [23]; therefore, individuals with pre-existing mental health conditions may be at increased risk of becoming food insecure as a result of the impact of the known symptoms of mental health conditions, such as a lack of energy, fatigue, loss of interest, and impairment of decision making, on the ability of the individual to manage a food insecure household [24,25].

1.2. Household Food Insecurity, Gender/Sex, and Mental Health

Much of the research studying the impact of gender (i.e., the sociocultural expression of biological sex) on household food insecurity and mental health has been conducted on lone mothers. Researchers focusing on this topic have observed that a disproportionate number of food insecure households are led by mothers with a history of depression, psychosis spectrum disorder, or domestic violence [24]. Mothers reporting household food insecurity are also at increased risk of either a major depressive episode or a generalized anxiety disorder at every level of household food insecurity severity (21% for moderate, 30.3% for severe) compared with food secure mothers (16.9%) [19]. Food insecure women may occupy a distinct social position that makes them more susceptible to food management stressors. For example, women have been shown to protect other household members against food insecurity by reducing their food intake to allow other household members to have more food [26,27]. Moreover, women predominantly hold the responsibility for providing and preparing food, which, in the context of food insecurity, may increase levels of stress felt by women [27].

Comparatively little research has been conducted on the mental health of males reporting household food insecurity. The results from in-depth interviews indicate that food insecure men report similar precursors to mental illness as women, such as feelings of powerless, guilt, embarrassment, shame, inequity, and frustration [28]. These emotions, in conjunction with heightened levels of stress associated with food insecurity, could plausibly result in higher levels of mental health conditions. In cross-sectional surveys, men experiencing household food insecurity report a higher prevalence of mood or anxiety disorders compared with food secure men, but those figures are lower than the rates of mood and anxiety disorders observed in food insecure women [12]. Past research on the mental health of males has highlighted that simply being male may not provide equal privilege in mental health, particularly for males who occupy different social locations of disadvantage [29]. We suggest that household food insecurity may be one such social location of disadvantage for males.

This study's research questions are specifically as follows:

1. How is household food insecurity related to the reporting of five adverse mental health outcomes (depressive thoughts in the past month, anxiety disorders, mood disorders, suicidal ideation, and self-reported mental health) in Canadian adult men and women?

2. How is the sex gap in the reporting of five adverse mental health outcomes in Canadian adults changed by concurrent consideration of household food insecurity status, controlling for common socio-demographic covariates?

2. Materials and Methods

2.1. Data Source

The study sample (N = 302,683) was generated by pooling four cycles (Cycle 3.1 [2005], 2007–2008, 2009–2010, and 2011–2012) of the Canadian Community Health Survey (CCHS). The CCHS is a nationally representative series of cross-sectional surveys structured to collect information annually on a variety of issues relating to health including health status, health care utilization, and health determinants [30]. The target population, sampling procedure, and sample sizes are all determined by Statistics Canada. The CCHS is divided by health region and reflects estimates according to health region and province/territories, as well as the Canadian population as a whole. The CCHS collects data from a randomly selected person within a household aged 12 or older residing in a dwelling in the ten provinces and three territories. Individuals living on reserves or Crown land, in institutions, in remote regions, or who are members of the Armed Forces are not included in the survey. The CCHS data sample represents approximately 98% of the Canadian population aged 12 years or older [30]. It is important to note that the survey only captures biological sex, and not gender per se.

The CCHS questions are designed for computer-assisted interviewing with pre-programmed questions, content flow, and allowable responses (ranges or answers). Half of the interviews take place by telephone, while the other half take place in person. Participation in the CCHS is voluntary and responses are kept strictly confidential [30].

Given the difference in sample sizes between the four cycles, the existing survey weights (determined by Statistics Canada) were adjusted depending on their contribution to their total pooled sample sized. Once the individual cycles' sample weights were adjusted, the cycles were combined and the pooled dataset was treated as one sample from a single population with a sample size of N = 515,421 prior to exclusions.

2.2. Exclusion Criteria

The population of interest in this study is working-age Canadian adults, aged 18–64 years, living in the ten provinces. Children aged 12–17 years were excluded from the dataset as mental health concerns differ in youth from adulthood, as do experiences of food insecurity in food insecure households [31]. Respondents aged 65 and older were excluded because seniors have the lowest levels of household food insecurity of the adult demographic in Canada, likely related to receiving seniors' pensions [32]. They also report different mental health problems including more cognitive impairment than working-age adults [33]. In addition, because of challenges of food supply related to isolated geographic areas such as Canada's Northern Territories [34], only respondents from the 10 provinces were included.

Provincial participation in the CCHS is dependent on whether modules of the survey were considered core or optional content in each survey cycle; the measurement of household food insecurity via the Household Food Insecurity Survey Module (HFSSM) was optional in the CCHS 3.1; for that cycle, Newfoundland, Labrador, New Brunswick, Manitoba, and Saskatchewan declined participation [35]. In the 2009–2010 cycle, Prince Edward Island and New Brunswick declined participation in the HFSSM [36]. Pooling four cycles and bootstrapping circumvents problems related to generalizability of the results to the ten provinces, given a substantial sample size was still collected in each of the provinces. Given its importance to the research question, only households who provided a response to the HFSSM were included. After applying exclusions, the total sample size was N = 302,683.

2.3. Measures

2.3.1. Household Food Security Survey Module

Household food insecurity in Canada is measured through the HFSSM. This 18-item questionnaire has been internationally validated and translated into many languages [9]. The HFSSM assesses the food security situation of adults as a group and children as a group within the household over the past 12 months. The HFSSM includes 10 questions measuring household food insecurity in adults and 8 questions measuring household food insecurity in children [30]. Typically, Statistics Canada will compile these to create a derived variable measuring three levels of household food security—food secure, moderate food insecurity, and severe food insecurity. For this study, a four-category household food insecurity variable was used, adding marginal food insecurity, which has demonstrated predictive power in increasing risk of chronic conditions in Canadian adults [12,19,20,37,38]. A description of the creation of the four-level household food insecurity variable is available in Appendix A.

2.3.2. Mental Health Outcome Variables

Five common mental health outcomes collected in the CCHS were included in the analysis: depressive thoughts in the past month, anxiety disorders, mood disorders, mental health status, and suicidal thoughts in the past year. All five outcomes were self-reported, because of the nature of the survey, but respondents were asked to only respond affirmatively to the anxiety and mood disorder questions if they had been so diagnosed by a health professional. These mental health conditions were selected based on their high response rates and their relatively high prevalence rates in Canada. The module including some mental health variables was optional content; as a result, two of the outcomes used in this study (suicidal thoughts, depressive thoughts) were not asked in all provinces. A detailed description of the five mental health outcome variables is presented in Appendix B.

2.3.3. Demographic and Socioeconomic Covariates

Six demographic variables (age, sex, household composition, homeownership, and highest education level in household) were included as covariates and were assessed for effect modification or confounding on the relationship between household food insecurity and adverse mental health outcomes. In addition, variables that measure respondents' race (White, Asian, Indigenous, Other), immigration status (immigrated less than 10 years ago, immigrated 10 or more years ago, Canadian-born), main income source (wages, government assistance, other sources), and inflation-adjusted household income (low income, medium-high income) were also included in the analysis. These covariates were included because of their known association with increased levels of household food insecurity [12,16,17,20,39]. Referent groups were selected based on the lowest prevalence of household food insecurity.

Finally, a cycle variable (2005, 2007/2008, 2009/2010, 2011/2012) was included to determine whether macro-level economic events, such as the 2008–2009 recession in Canada, modified or confounded the relationship between household food insecurity and adverse mental health outcomes.

2.4. Statistical Analysis

Data analysis was conducted at the Prairie Research Data Centre (RDC) using STATA statistical software (version 14, StataCorp, College Station, TX, USA). All estimates were generated with sample weights and 500 bootstrap replicates to approximate the Canadian population, that is, 18–64 year old individuals living in the ten provinces.

Univariate descriptive analyses of all study variables were followed by crude binary logistic regression analyses to assess the proportion of each mental health outcome by level of household food security and by sex, separately, in Canadian adults. Sex-adjusted binary logistic regression models were generated to assess the relationship between household food insecurity and the five mental health outcomes. Finally, interaction terms were created for sex and household food insecurity, and those interactions were included in the sex-adjusted binary logistic regression models to assess for effect modification with each mental health outcome. Reduced (by the removal of non-significant covariates) binary logistic regression analyses were conducted on sex-stratified datasets (one dataset for each sex) to visualize the sex gap for each level of household food insecurity on the odds of reporting five adverse mental health outcomes compared with those who are food secure.

3. Results

Table 1 presents the prevalence and 95% confidence intervals (95% CI) of the study variables. The prevalence of adverse mental health outcomes in this population ranged from 5.3% (5.2%–5.4%) reporting fair/poor mental health to 20.0% (19.6%–20.3%) responding that they had had depressive thoughts in the past month. Approximately 11.8% of the population fulfilled the criteria for some level of household food insecurity (3.7% marginal, 6.7% moderate, and 1.4% severe). Females comprised 50.9% (50.8%–50.9%) of the population.

Table 1. Prevalence (%) and 95% confidence intervals (CI) of study variables (N = 302,683). CCHS—Canadian Community Health Survey.

Variable	Categories	Percent	95% CI
Outcome			
Depressive Thoughts in the Past Month	Yes	20.0	19.6–20.3
Anxiety Disorders	Yes	5.8	5.7–6.0
Mood Disorders	Yes	7.2	7.0–7.3
Suicidal Thoughts in the Past Year	Yes	19.7	18.7–20.7
Mental Health Status	Fair/Poor	5.3	5.2–5.4
Exposure			
Household Food Insecurity Level	Food Secure	88.2	88.0–88.4
	Marginal Food Insecurity	3.7	3.5–3.8
	Moderate Food Insecurity	6.7	6.5–6.9
	Severe Food Insecurity	1.4	1.3–1.5
Covariate	**Categories**	**Mean**	**Standard Deviation**
Age	Continuous (18–64)	42.8	13.5
Covariate	**Categories**	**Percent**	**95% CI**
Sex	Male	49.1	49.1–49.2
	Female	50.9	50.8–50.9
Household Composition	Unattached, living alone	12.5	12.3–12.7
	Single living with others	5.1	5.0–5.3
	Couple, no kids	25.3	25.0–25.5
	Couple with kids <25	45.0	44.7–45.3
	Lone parent, kids <25	6.1	5.9–6.3
	Other/multi-family	6.0	5.9–6.2
Marital Status	Common-law or Married	65.2	64.9–65.4
	Divorced, Widowed, or Separated	9.2	9.0–9.4
	Single	25.7	25.4–25.9
Inflation-Adjusted Income [a]	Low	5.8	5.6–5.9
	Med-High	94.2	94.1–94.4
Income Source	Wages & Salary	88.9	88.7–89.1
	Social Assistance [b]	9.3	9.2–9.5
	Other [c]	2.7	2.6–2.8
Race	White	79.2	78.9–79.6
	Asian	11.7	11.4–11.9
	Indigenous	2.6	2.5–2.7
	Other [d]	6.5	6.3–6.7

Table 1. *Cont.*

Covariate	Categories	Percent	95% CI
Education	Post-Secondary Degree	80.5	80.2–80.7
	Some Post-Secondary	5.4	5.2–5.5
	High School Grad	9.8	9.7–10.0
	Less than High School	4.4	4.2–4.5
Immigration	Immigrated ≥10 years	15.7	15.5–16.0
	Immigrated <10 years	7.5	7.3–7.7
	Canadian Born	76.7	76.4–77.0
Homeownership	Homeowner	73.5	73.1–73.8
	Renter	26.5	26.2–26.9
Cycle of CCHS	3.1	22.2	22.1–22.3
	2007/2008	25.5	25.4–25.6
	2009/2010	25.6	25.6–25.7
	2011/2012	26.6	26.6–26.7

[a] Derived from respondent's total household income before taxes adjusted by Canadian inflation rates for the year the respondent was surveyed [40]. Inflation adjusted income was ranked (low-lower middle, middle, upper middle, and highest) based on the number of people in household and national income thresholds [41,42]. The four-level variable was dichotomized into low and medium-high income. [b] includes the following: benefits from Canada or Quebec pension plan, old age security and guaranteed income supplement, provincial or municipal social assistance or welfare, and child tax benefit. [c] includes the following: retirement pensions, child support, alimony, employment insurance, worker's compensation board, and other. [d] includes those who identify as Black, Latin American, Arab, and Other (multi-racial).

Table 2 presents results from the crude binary logistic regression analysis. The odds ratios were converted to prevalence, and 95% CI are reported for each mental health outcome by level of household food insecurity and by sex, separately. Table 2 also presents the crude sex gap in the reporting of depressive thoughts in the past month, anxiety disorders, mood disorders, suicidal thoughts in the past year, and fair or poor mental health in this population. Table 2 shows that females have a higher prevalence of reporting four out of five mental health outcomes, prior to adjusting for covariates. Males and females have a statistically significant equal prevalence of reporting having had suicidal thoughts in the past year, prior to adjusting for covariates.

Table 2. Results from crude binary logistic regression of household food insecurity and by sex, separately, on five adverse mental health outcomes, presented as prevalence (%) and 95% confidence intervals.

Variable Category	Depressive Thoughts in the Past Month	Anxiety Disorders	Mood Disorders	Suicidal Thoughts in the Past Year	Fair/Poor Mental Health
	Household Food Insecurity Level				
Food Secure	17.5 (17.2, 17.9)	4.8 (4.7, 4.9)	5.8 (5.7, 5.9)	16.8 (15.7, 17.8)	4.0 (3.9, 4.1)
Marginally Food Insecurity	31.1 (28.7, 33.5)	9.9 (9.1, 10.8)	11.4 (10.5, 12.2)	25.6 (21.2, 30.0)	9.2 (8.3, 10.1)
Moderately Food Insecurity	39.8 (37.8,4 1.7)	13.6 (12.8, 14.3)	17.4 (16.6, 18.3)	24.8 (22.0, 27.7)	15.0 (14.2, 15.8)
Severely Food Insecurity	59.3 (55.2, 63.4)	25.4 (23.5, 27.3)	34.2 (32.0, 36.4)	41.0 (36.1, 45.9)	31.1 (28.9, 33.4)
	Sex				
Male	15.1 (14.6, 15.7)	4.1 (4.0, 4.3)	5.0 (4.8, 5.2)	20.9 (19.4, 22.4)	4.8 (4.6, 5.0)
Female	24.7 (24.1, 25.2)	7.5 (7.3, 7.7)	9.3 (9.1, 9.5)	18.8 (17.5, 20.1)	5.8 (5.6, 6.0)

Table 3 presents the sex-adjusted odds of reporting five adverse mental health outcomes for each level of household, compared with those reporting household food security. All five adverse mental health outcomes show increasing odds of reporting adverse mental health outcomes with increasingly severe household food insecurity adjusted for sex, compared with those who are food secure. No interaction, that is, no effect modification, was observed between household food insecurity and sex for any of the five adverse mental health outcomes. Table 3 does, however, show that the sex gap for four of the five mental health conditions persists when controlling for household food insecurity. In sum, household food insecurity at any level is associated with increased odds of reporting five mental health outcomes, compared with those reporting food security, and the sex gap remains when household food insecurity is held constant for all mental health conditions, except suicidal thoughts in the past year.

Table 3. Sex-adjusted binary logistic regression models of household food insecurity and five adverse mental health outcomes, including food insecurity and sex interactions.

Variable Category	Model 1: Depressive Thoughts in the Past Month	Model 2: Anxiety Disorders	Model 3: Mood Disorders	Model 4: Suicidal Thoughts in the Past Year	Model 5: Fair/Poor Mental Health
	Odds Ratio (95% Confidence Interval)				
	Household Food Insecurity Level (food secure = ref)				
Marginal Food Insecurity	2.3 ** (2.0, 2.8)	2.2 ** (1.9, 2.7)	2.3 ** (1.9, 2.7)	1.8 * (1.3, 2.6)	2.4 ** (2.1, 2.9)
Moderate Food Insecurity	3.2 ** (2.8, 3.7)	2.8 ** (2.5, 3.2)	3.2 ** (2.9, 3.6)	1.8 ** (1.4, 2.4)	4.3 ** (3.8, 4.8)
Severe Food Insecurity	8.2 ** (6.3, 10.6)	6.3 ** (5.4, 7.3)	8.4 ** (7.2, 9.7)	3.0 ** (2.2, 4.1)	11.0 ** (9.2, 13.1)
	Sex (male = ref)				
Female	1.9 ** (1.8, 2.0)	1.8 ** (1.7, 1.9)	1.9 ** (1.8, 2.0)	0.9 * (0.7, 1.0)	1.2 ** (1.1, 1.2)
Marginal * Female	0.8 (0.7, 1.0)	0.9 (0.8, 1.2)	0.9 (0.7, 1.0)	0.9 (0.6, 1.5)	1.0 (0.8, 1.2)
Moderate * Female	0.9 (0.7, 1.1)	1.1 (0.9, 1.3)	1.0 (0.9, 1.2)	0.9 (0.6, 1.2)	1.0 (0.8, 1.1)
Severe * Female	0.7 (0.5, 1.0)	1.2 (0.9, 1.4)	1.0 (0.9, 1.3)	1.3 (0.9, 2.0)	1.0 (0.8, 1.2)

$* p < 0.05, ** p < 0.001.$

Figures 1–5 visualize the results from the reduced binary logistic regression analysis stratified by sex. These figures show, separately for males and females, the adjusted odds ratio of respondents experiencing each level of household food insecurity in turn reporting five mental health outcomes, compared with those reporting that they are food secure. The results, adjusted for significant covariates, show that males and females with any level of household food insecurity have no statistically significant difference in the odds ratio for each mental health outcome, compared to those reporting household food security.

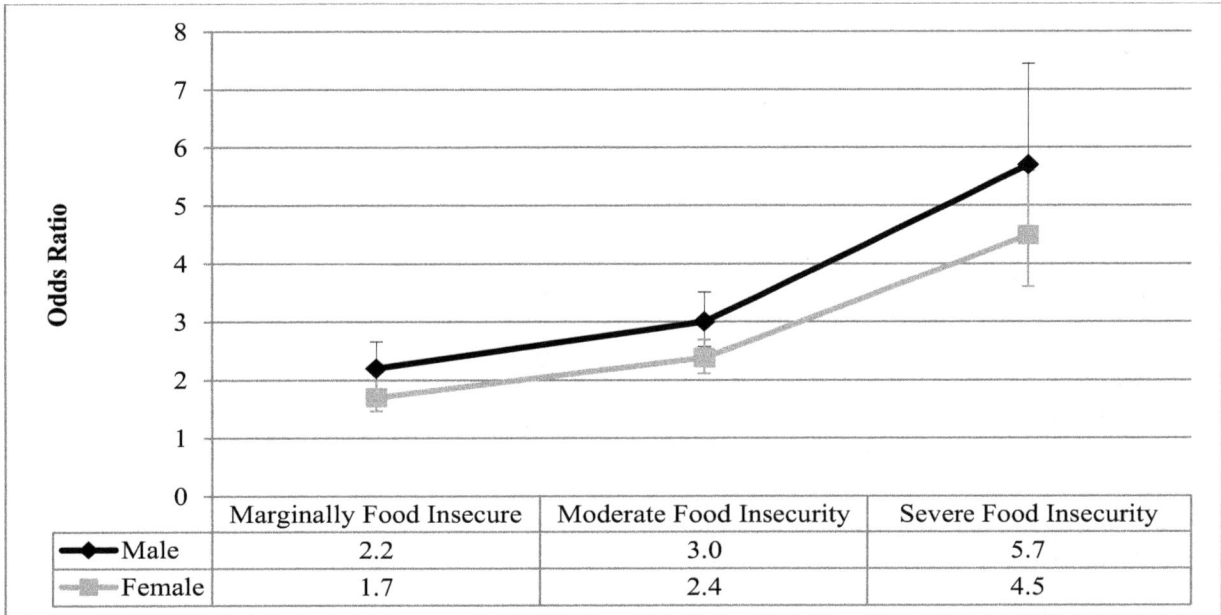

	Marginally Food Insecure	Moderate Food Insecurity	Severe Food Insecurity
Male	2.2	3.0	5.7
Female	1.7	2.4	4.5

Figure 1. Odds ratio of reporting depressive thoughts in the past month for each level of household food insecurity stratified by sex, compared with food secure; results from reduced binary logistic regression.

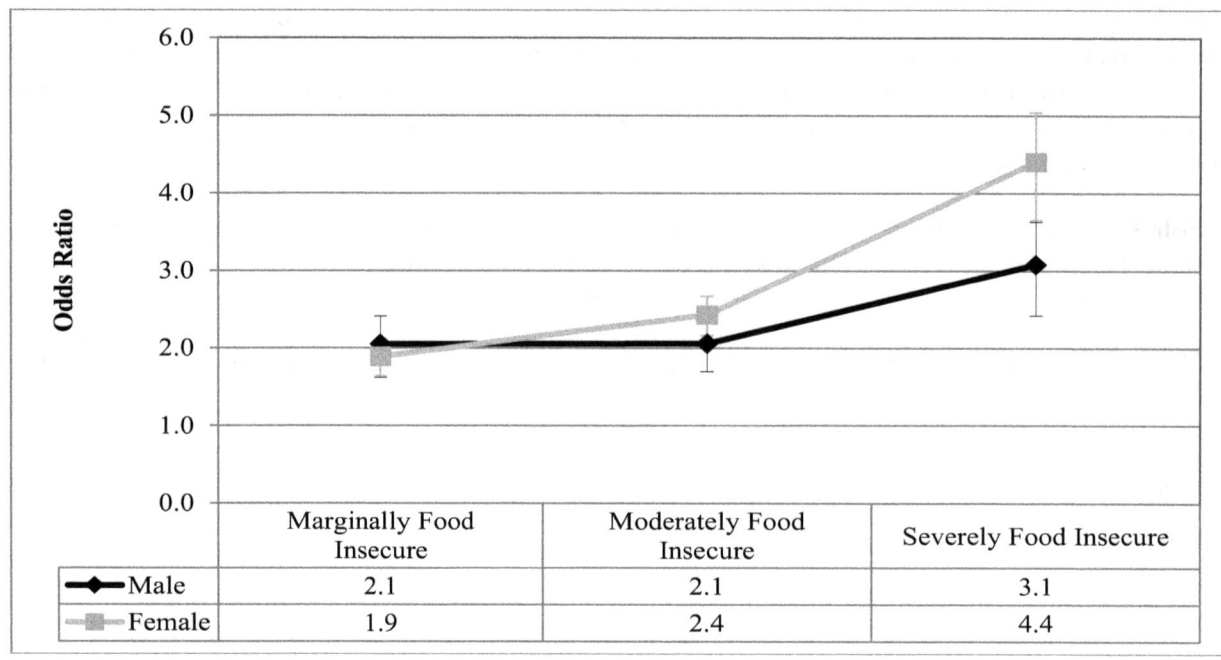

Figure 2. Odds ratio of reporting anxiety disorders for each level of household food insecurity stratified by sex, compared with food secure; results from reduced binary logistic regression.

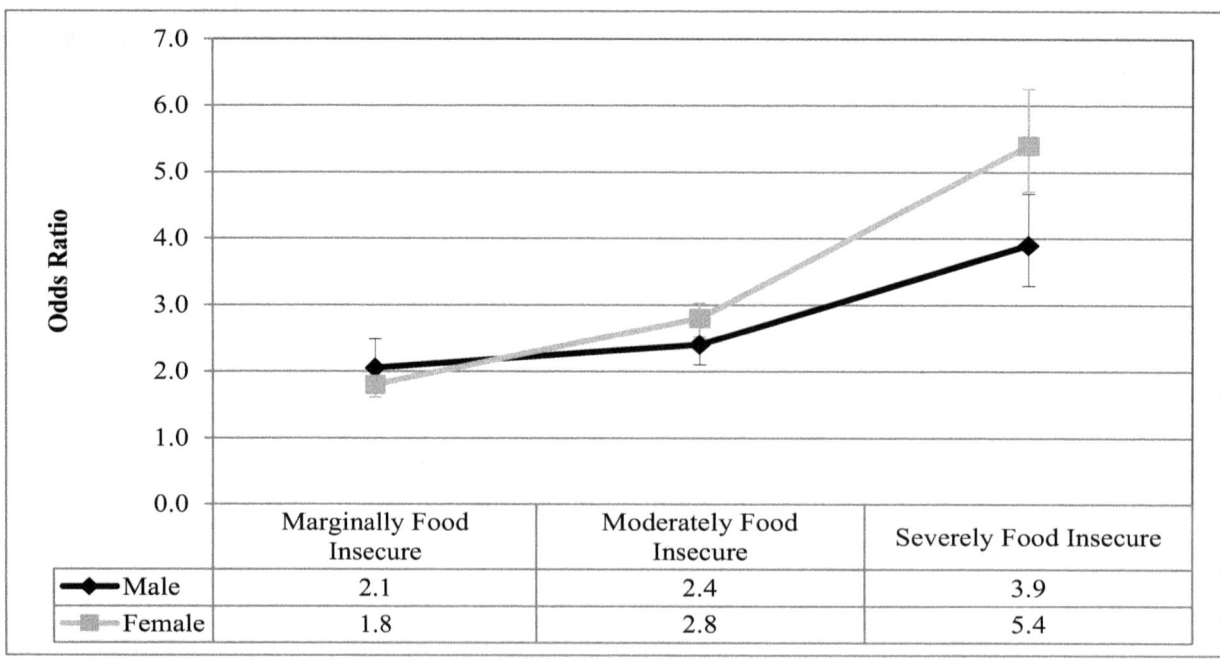

Figure 3. Odds ratio of reporting mood disorders for each level of household food insecurity stratified by sex, compared with food secure; results from reduced binary logistic regression.

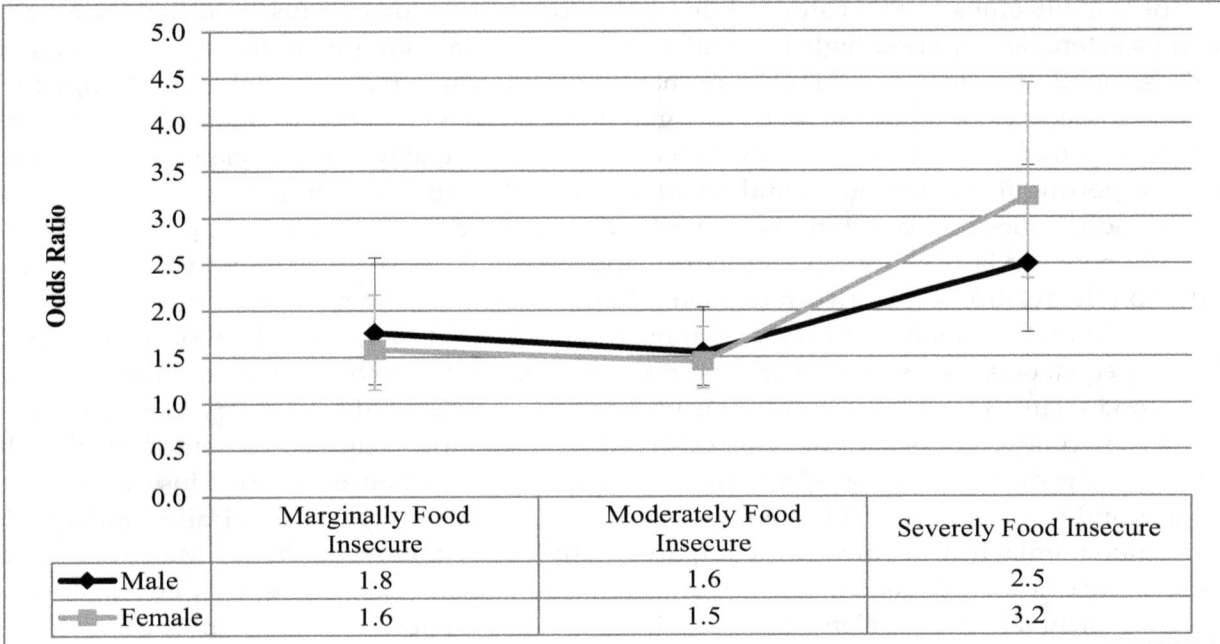

Figure 4. Odds ratio of reporting suicidal thoughts in the past month for each level of household food insecurity stratified by sex, compared with food secure; results from reduced binary logistic regression.

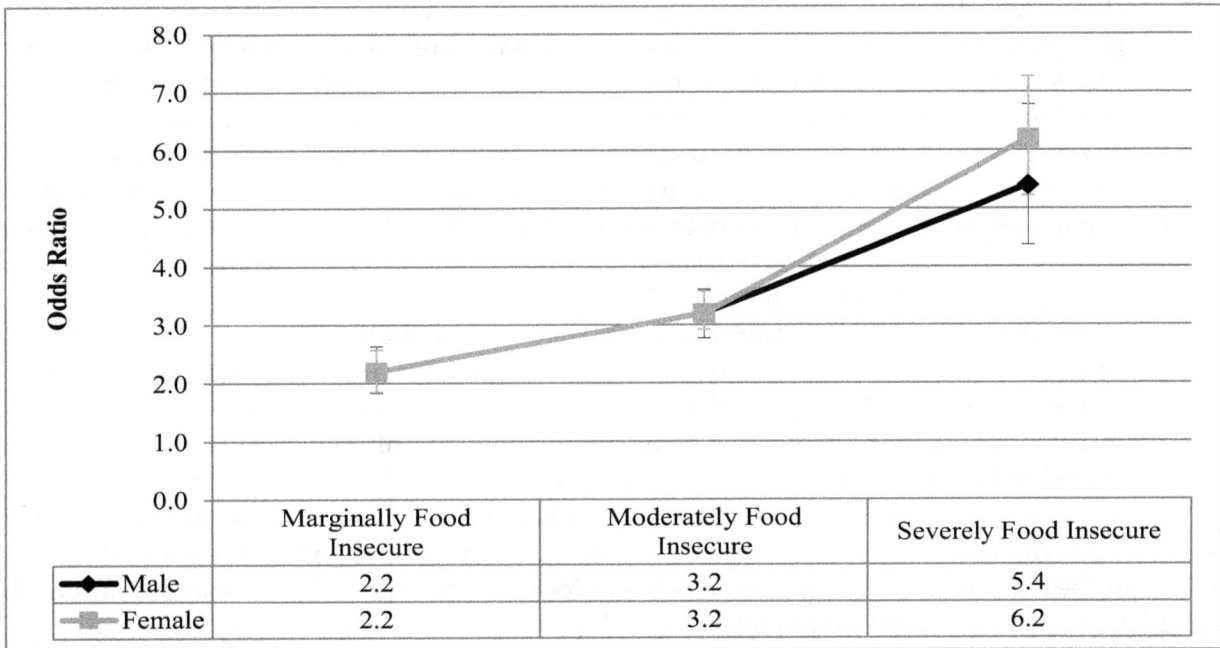

Figure 5. Odds ratio of reporting fair/poor mental health status for each level of household food insecurity stratified by sex, compared with food secure; results from reduced binary logistic regression.

4. Discussion

In recent years, mental health researchers have recognized that separate social locations such as sex and race must be considered together, but in much of the scholarship focusing on mental health conditions, these locations are often treated as independent variables [43]. This type of analysis results in a lack of observability of within-group differences among individuals in different social categories.

From a review of the literature, sex and household food insecurity are two important variables related to the reporting of adverse mental health outcomes. Empirically, this study examined how sex and household food insecurity interact and how that statistical interaction impacts the reporting of mental health outcomes. We first showed that, prior to the inclusion of household food insecurity in the analysis, females reported higher prevalence of depressive thoughts in the past month, anxiety disorders, mood disorders, and fair or poor mental health, compared with males (Table 2), which is aligned with decades of reporting on the sex gap in common mental health outcomes [1–3]. Table 3 shows that even after controlling for sex, household food insecurity was associated with high odds ratios of reporting five common mental health outcomes compared with food secure respondents, and these odds ratios increase with the severity of household food insecurity. Upon analyzing the interaction between household food insecurity and sex (Table 3), sex was found to not be an effect modifier on the relationship between household food insecurity and all five adverse mental health outcomes. Therefore, males and females reporting each level of household food insecurity had statistically equal odds ratios of reporting these adverse mental health outcomes, compared with those who are food secure. In order to confirm this finding, sex-stratified reduced binary logistic regression analyses were conducted for each mental health outcome, and the results are presented graphically in Figures 1–5. The overlapping confidence intervals at each level of household food insecurity indicate that males and females, at each level of household food insecurity, report statistically similar odds of five common mental health outcomes, compared with food secure respondents. Males and females who experience household food insecurity (a chronically stressful experience) may be equally at risk of reporting mental health problems due to their disadvantaged position. It appears that working age adult males' lower rates of reporting or succumbing to mental health outcomes [44,45] are reduced to non-significance once household food insecurity is considered.

This is a novel finding and indicates that the often-reported sex gap in mental health may be true among those who are food secure (who represent most Canadian adults), but among a distinctly disadvantaged population (food insecure), males and females appear to experience a similar mental health burden. Another study focused on the interactions between household food insecurity and sex and its relationship with mental health outcomes, in a high-income country. Carter and associates [46] examined the association between a binary food insecurity measure and psychological distress in New Zealand for males and females separately. The authors found that the sex gap was substantially reduced in the stratified model, but that food insecure females had slightly higher odds of psychological distress than males (using a p-value of <0.1), compared with those who are food secure [46]. The present study advances this work by examining this relationship using a more precise four-level household food insecurity measure that was generated using an internationally adopted and validated tool (i.e., HFSSM). In addition, the present study examines five common adverse mental health outcomes.

Much of the research on the impact of gender on household food insecurity and mental health has been conducted with a study population comprised of females only [16,17,19]. Our results indicate that the relationship between household food insecurity and five adverse mental health outcomes is equally strong in males. Therefore, the chronic stresses associated with household food insecurity [22] could be narrowing the commonly observed sex gap in mental health. This study's findings could indicate that the experience of males and females in food insecure households may be similar. Both groups likely experience substantial psychological, physical, and social stresses (e.g., guilt, shame, powerlessness, and inequality) [22,28] as a result of not having enough money to feed themselves or their families.

Our findings suggest that males and females in a food insecure household experience a similar mental health burden as a result of sharing a more similar social location compared with food secure members of their own sex. The sex gap in mental health outcomes that is often reported for the general population is largely comprised of food secure respondents and appears to have masked the food insecure sub-group's experience of mental health problems, if this important variable is not considered.

4.1. Limitations

The CCHS does not survey some groups that are particularly vulnerable to household food insecurity and mental health problems, specifically First Nations people living on-reserve, homeless populations, and those living in remote regions [47,48]. Researchers estimate that there could be as many as 470,000 additional food insecure people living in Canada that are not included in Statistics Canada's estimate [49]. We cannot assume that the social location of household food insecurity for men and women in these circumstances is the same as the CCHS sample.

While it would be preferable to speak only in terms of gender, the CCHS only delineates by sex and, therefore, sex is used as a variable of interest in this study. Given the self-reported nature of the CCHS, there is potential for measurement error in the mental health outcomes, particularly as a result of social desirability bias—this would result in an underestimation of mental health burden.

The CCHS uses two methods of data collection—computer assisted telephone interviewing (CATI) and computer-assisted person interviewing (CAPI). While there is some evidence in the literature of statistically equal prevalence of self-reported mental health status using CATI and CAPI [50], face-to-face interviewing yields slightly higher reporting of household food insecurity than CATI [51]. This may result in an underestimation of household food insecurity for those responding using CATI.

Finally, type 1 error (the probability of rejecting a null hypothesis that is in fact true [52]) is a threat with a large sample size. In order to circumvent this problem, a bootstrapping method was employed, which effectively narrowed the confidence intervals to increase the difficulty of rejecting the null hypothesis.

4.2. Strengths

This study employs a large and robust dataset, with enough power to examine a four-level household food insecurity variable, using the internationally validated HFSSM. This study uses a nationally representative survey that results in generalizable findings to 98% of the Canadian population aged 18–64 living in the ten provinces. The use of a four-level household food insecurity variable is rare in the literature, despite the predictive power of the marginal group [12,19,37,38].

Finally, this study is novel in that it is one of only two studies to examine the interaction between sex, household food insecurity, and mental health outcomes in high-income countries [46], and the first to examine this phenomenon in Canada, with a four-level food insecurity variable.

5. Conclusions

Although the sex gap in mental health outcomes has been observed and re-examined for decades, few studies have considered whether these important social determinants, sex and food insecurity, have a multiplicative effect on the odds of reporting of mental health problems.

This study showed that the well-documented sex gap in mental health outcomes was reduced to non-significance when household food insecurity was reported. Therefore, household food insecurity appears to act as a chronically stressful condition that overwhelms the capacity of males to either withstand reporting mental health conditions or actually succumb to them. This study suggests that household food insecurity is a social location with public health implications. The high odds of reporting adverse mental health outcomes seen among males experiencing household food insecurity, compared with food secure males, suggest that there is a distinct mental health burden among males experiencing household food insecurity, and that this previously overlooked group is deserving of further study.

Finally, household food insecurity is a modifiable stressor within the complex interplay of sex and mental health. Given the lack of a sex gap in mental health among those with household food insecurity, addressing food insecurity with progressive policy change could result in mental health gains for women, as well as men who share this vulnerability.

Author Contributions: Conceptualization, G.J.P. and L.M.; methodology, G.J.P. and L.M.; formal analysis, G.J.P.; investigation, G.J.P. and L.M.; writing—original draft preparation, G.J.P. and L.M.; writing—review and editing, G.J.P. and L.M.; visualization, G.J.P.; supervision, L.M.; funding acquisition, G.J.P. and L.M.

Acknowledgments: The authors thank and acknowledge the assistance of the staff at the Prairie Regional Data Centre for their advice and guidance.

Appendix A

Table A1. Description of Household Food Insecurity Variable Derived from Household Food Security Survey Module.

Level of Household Food Insecurity	Description of Level	Number of Affirmative Responses
Food Secure	No financial constraints on the ability to fill household's food need.	0 to adult or child food situation questions
Marginally Food Insecure	Worry about running out of food due to financial constraints.	1 food situation question
Moderately Food Insecure	Reductions in quality and/or quantity of food due to financial constraints.	2–5 adult food situation questions or 2–4 child food situation questions
Severely Food Insecurity	Reductions in food intake, missing meals and at its most extreme going a full day without food.	6+ adult food situation questions or 5+ child food situation questions

* adapted from [8].

Appendix B

Table A2. Description of Outcome Variables Included in Study.

Name of Variable	Level of Measurement	Survey Question	Description
Depressive Thoughts in the Past Month	Binary (Yes, No)	"During the past month, about how often did you feel sad or depressed?"	Those who responded all of the time, most of the time, some of the time were coded into the "yes" group. All other respondents were coded into the "no" group.
Major Depressive Episodes in the Past Year	Binary (Yes, No)	The Composite International Diagnostic Interview Short Form (CIDI-SF) measures Major Depressive Episodes (MDE). This subset of questions assesses the depressive symptoms of respondents who felt depressed or lost interest in things for 2 weeks or more in the last 12 months. Respondents are screened into the CIDI-SF based on affirmative responses to the following 2 screening questions, if a respondent answers affirmatively to the screening questions, their depression level is measured based on 7 additional questions.	The classification of depression is based on an affirmative response to the original screening question and 5 out of 9 of the depression questions. This corresponds to a 90% predictive probability of caseness, which closely aligns with the DSM-5 diagnostic guidelines for MDE in adults [53]. This probability expresses the chance that the respondent would have been diagnosed as having experienced a Major Depressive Episode in the past 12 months had they completed the CIDI Long-Form [30].
Anxiety Disorder	Binary (Yes, No)	"Do you have an anxiety disorder such as phobia, obsessive-compulsive disorder or a panic disorder?"	Respondents are reminded that the question is only referring to those conditions diagnosed by a health professional.
Mood Disorder	Binary (Yes, No)	"Do you have a mood disorder such as depression, bipolar disorder, mania or dysthymia?"	Respondents are reminded that the question only refers to those conditions diagnosed by a health professional.
Suicidal Thoughts in the Past Month	Binary (Yes, No)	"Have you ever seriously considered committing suicide or taking your own life? Has this happened in the past 12 months?"	This variable was recoded into a dichotomous variable. In addition, those who answered "not applicable: were coded into the "no" group, given they answered negatively to this question in an earlier prompt.
Self-Reported Mental Health Status	Binary (Fair/Poor, Good/Very Good/Excellent)	"In general, would you say your mental health is: excellent, very good, good, fair, or poor?"	This variable was recoded into a dichotomous variable. "Fair/poor" or "Good/very good/excellent". This variable has been validated and is a reliable measure of general mental health [54].

References

1. ESEMeD/MHEDEA 2000 Investigators; Alonso, J.; Angermeyer, M.C.; Bernert, S.; Bruffaerts, R.; Brugha, T.S.; Bryson, H.; de Girolamo, G.; de Graaf, R.; Demyttenaere, K.; et al. Prevalence of mental disorders in Europe: Results from the European Study of the Epidemiology of Mental Disorders (ESEMeD) project. *Acta Psychiatr. Scand.* **2004**, *109*, 21–27. [CrossRef] [PubMed]

2. Blazer, D.G.; Kessler, R.C.; McGonagle, K.A. The prevalence and distribution of major depression in a national community sample: The National Comorbidity Survey. *Am. J. Psychiatry* **1994**, *151*, 979–986. [CrossRef] [PubMed]

3. Kessler, R.C.; Berglund, P.; Demler, O.; Jin, R.; Koretz, D.; Merikangas, K.R.; Rush, A.J.; Walters, E.E.; Wang, P.S. The epidemiology of major depressive disorder. *JAMA* **2003**, *289*, 3095. [CrossRef] [PubMed]

4. Kessler, R.C. Epidemiology of women and depression. *J. Affect. Disord.* **2003**, *74*, 5–13. [CrossRef]

5. Patten, S.B.; Williams, J.V.A.; Lavorato, D.H.; Wang, J.L.; Bulloch, A.G.M.; Sajobi, T. The association between major depression prevalence and sex becomes weaker with age. *Soc. Psychiatry Psychiatr. Epidemiol.* **2016**, *51*, 203–210. [CrossRef] [PubMed]

6. Simon, R.W. Revisiting the relationship among gender, marital status, and mental health. *Am. J. Sociol.* **2002**, *107*, 1065–1096. [CrossRef] [PubMed]

7. Scott, R.L.; Lasiuk, G.; Norris, C. The relationship between sexual orientation and depression in a national population sample. *J. Clin. Nurs.* **2016**, *25*, 3522–3532. [CrossRef]

8. Tarasuk, V.; Mitchell, A.; Dachner, N. *Household Food Insecurity in Canada, 2012*; PROOF: Toronto, ON, Canada, 2014; Available online: http://proof.utoronto.ca/resources/proof-annual-reports/ (accessed on 1 September 2018).

9. Bickel, G.; Nord, M.; Price, C.; Hamilton, W.; Cook, J. *Guide to Measuring Household Food Security*; United States Department of Agriculture Food and Nutrition Services: Alexandria, VA, USA, 2000.

10. Health Canada. Canadian Community Health Survey. Cycle 2.2, Nutrition (2004)—Income-Related Household Food Security in Canada. 2007. Available online: https://www.canada.ca/content/dam/hc-sc/migration/hc-sc/fn-an/alt_formats/hpfb-dgpsa/pdf/surveill/income_food_sec-sec_alim-eng.pdf (accessed on 1 September 2018).

11. Gucciardi, E.; Vogt, J.A.; DeMelo, M.; Stewart, D.E. Exploration of the relationship between household food insecurity and diabetes in Canada. *Diabetes Care* **2009**, *32*, 2218–2224. [CrossRef]

12. Tarasuk, V.; Mitchell, A.; McLaren, L.; McIntyre, L. Chronic physical and mental health conditions among adults may increase vulnerability to household food insecurity. *J. Nutr.* **2013**, *143*, 1785–1793. [CrossRef]

13. Vozoris, N.T.; Tarasuk, V.S. Household food insufficiency is associated with poorer health. *J. Nutr.* **2003**, *133*, 120–126. [CrossRef]

14. Galesloot, S.; McIntyre, L.; Fenton, T.; Tyminski, S. Food insecurity in Canadian adults receiving diabetes care. *Can. J. Pract. Res.* **2012**, *73*, 261–266. [CrossRef] [PubMed]

15. Davison, K.; Kaplan, B. Food insecurity in adults with mood disorders: Prevalence estimates and associations with nutritional and psychological health. *Ann. Gen. Psychiatry* **2015**, *14*, 21. [CrossRef]

16. Heflin, C.M.; Siefert, K.; Williams, D.R. Food insufficiency and women's mental health: Findings from a 3-year panel of welfare recipients. *Soc. Sci. Med.* **2005**, *61*, 1971–1982. [CrossRef] [PubMed]

17. Siefert, K.; Heflin, C.M.; Corcoran, M.E.; Williams, D.R. Food insufficiency and physical and mental health in a longitudinal survey of welfare recipients. *J. Health Soc. Behav.* **2004**, *22*, 171–186. [CrossRef] [PubMed]

18. Leung, C.W.; Epel, E.S.; Willett, W.C.; Rimm, E.B.; Laraia, B.A. Household food insecurity is positively associated with depression among low-income Supplemental Nutrition Assistance Program participants and income-eligible nonparticipants. *J. Nutr.* **2015**, *145*, 622–627. [CrossRef] [PubMed]

19. Whitaker, R.C.; Phillips, S.M.; Orzol, S.M. Food insecurity and the risks of depression and anxiety in mothers and behavior problems in their preschool-aged children. *Pediatrics* **2006**, *118*, 859–868. [CrossRef] [PubMed]

20. Muldoon, K.A.; Duff, P.K.; Fielden, S.; Anema, A. Food insufficiency is associated with psychiatric morbidity in a nationally representative study of mental illness among food insecure Canadians. *Soc. Psychiatry Psychiatr. Epidemiol.* **2013**, *48*, 795–803. [CrossRef]

21. Jessiman-Perreault, G.; McIntyre, L. The household food insecurity gradient and potential reductions in adverse population mental health outcomes in Canadian adults. *SSM Popul. Health* **2017**, *3*, 464–472. [CrossRef]

22. Hadley, C.; Crooks, D.L. Coping and the biosocial consequences of food insecurity in the 21st century. *Am. J. Phys. Anthropol.* **2012**, *149*, 72–94. [CrossRef]

23. Runnels, V.E.; Kristjansson, E.; Calhoun, M. An investigation of adults' everyday experiences and effects of food insecurity in an urban area in Canada. *Can. J. Community Ment. Health* **2011**, *30*, 157–172. [CrossRef]

24. Melchior, M.; Caspi, A.; Howard, L.M.; Ambler, A.P.; Bolton, H.; Mountain, N.; Moffitt, T.E. Mental health context of food insecurity: A representative cohort of families with young children. *Pediatrics* **2009**, *124*, 564–572. [CrossRef] [PubMed]

25. Wehler, C.; Weinreb, L.F.; Huntington, N.; Scott, R.; Hosmer, D.; Fletcher, K.; Goldberg, R.; Gundersen, C. Risk and protective factors for adult and child hunger among low-income housed and homeless female-headed families. *Am. J. Public Health* **2004**, *94*, 109–115. [CrossRef]

26. McIntyre, L.; Officer, S.; Robinson, L.M. Feeling poor: The felt experience of low-income lone mothers. *Affilia* **2003**, *18*, 316–331. [CrossRef]

27. Olson, C. Food insecurity in women: A recipe for unhealthy trade-offs. *Top. Clin. Nutr.* **2005**, *20*, 321–328. [CrossRef]

28. Hamelin, A.-M.; Beaudry, M.; Habicht, J.-P. Characterization of household food insecurity in Quebec: Food and feelings. *Soc. Sci. Med.* **2002**, *54*, 119–132. [CrossRef]

29. Griffith, D.M. An intersectional approach to men's health. *J. Mens Health* **2012**, *9*, 106–112. [CrossRef]

30. Statistics Canada. *User Guide, Public-Use 2007–2008: Microdata File, Canadian Community Health Survey*; Statistics Canada: Ottawa, ON, Canada, 2008.

31. Fram, M.S.; Frongillo, E.A.; Jones, S.J.; Williams, R.C.; Burke, M.P.; DeLoach, K.P.; Blake, C.E. Children are aware of food insecurity and take responsibility for managing food resources. *J. Nutr.* **2011**, *141*, 1114–1119. [CrossRef] [PubMed]

32. Emery, J.C.H.; Fleisch, V.C.; McIntyre, L. Legislated changes to federal pension income in Canada will adversely affect low income seniors' health. *Prev. Med.* **2013**, *57*, 963–966. [CrossRef]

33. Blazer, D.; Burchett, B.; Service, C.; George, L.K. The association of age and depression among the elderly: An epidemiologic exploration. *J. Gerontol.* **1991**, *46*, 210–215. [CrossRef]

34. Inuit Circumpolar Council. Food Security Across the Arctic. 2012. Available online: http://www.inuitcircumpolar.com/uploads/3/0/5/4/30542564/icc_food_security_across_the_arctic_may_2012.pdf (accessed on 1 September 2018).

35. Statistics Canada. *User Guide, Public-Use 2005: Microdata File, Canadian Community Health Survey*; Statistics Canada: Ottawa, ON, Canada, 2006.

36. Statistics Canada. *User Guide, Public-Use 2009–2010: Microdata File, Canadian Community Health Survey*; Statistics Canada: Ottawa, ON, Canada, 2011.

37. Cook, J.T.; Frank, D.A.; Berkowitz, C.; Black, M.M.; Casey, P.H.; Cutts, D.B.; Meyers, A.F.; Zaldivar, N.; Skalicky, A.; Levenson, S.; et al. Community and international nutrition food insecurity is associated with adverse health outcomes among human infants and toddlers. *J. Nutr.* **2004**, *134*, 1432–1438. [CrossRef]

38. Davison, K.M.; Marshall-Fabien, G.L.; Tecson, A. Association of moderate and severe food insecurity with suicidal ideation in adults: National survey data from three Canadian provinces. *Soc. Psychiatry Psychiatr. Epidemiol.* **2015**, *50*, 963–972. [CrossRef] [PubMed]

39. McIntyre, L.; Wu, X.; Fleisch, V.C.; Emery, H.J.C. Homeowner versus non-homeowner differences in household food insecurity in Canada. *J. Hous. Built Environ.* **2015**, *14*, 349–366. [CrossRef]

40. Statistics Canada. *The Consumer Price Index*; Statistics Canada: Ottawa, ON, Canada, 2016.

41. Canadian Institute for Health Information. *Trends in Income-Related Health Inequalities in Canada: Methodology Notes*; Canadian Institute for Health Information: Ottawa, ON, Canada, 2015.

42. Peel Public Health. *Health in Peel: Determinants and Disparities*; Peel Public Health: Mississauga, ON, Canada, 2011.

43. Van Mens-Verhulst, J.; Radtke, L. Intersectionality and Mental Health: A Case Study. 2008. Available online: https://static1.squarespace.com/static/56fd7e0bf699bb7d0d3ff82d/t/593ab6522e69cf01a44b14d4/1497019986918/INTERSECTIONALITY+AND+MENTAL+HEALTH2.pdf (accessed on 1 September 2018).

44. Galdas, P.M.; Cheater, F.; Marshall, P. Men and health help-seeking behaviour: Literature review. *J. Adv. Nurs.* **2005**, *49*, 616–623. [CrossRef] [PubMed]

45. Kartalova-O'Doherty, Y.; Doherty, T.D. Recovering from recurrent mental health problems: Giving up and fighting to get better. *Int. J. Ment. Health Nurs.* **2010**, *19*, 3–15. [CrossRef] [PubMed]

46. Carter, K.N.; Kruse, K.; Blakely, T.; Collings, S. The association of food security with psychological distress in New Zealand and any gender differences. *Soc. Sci. Med.* **2011**, *72*, 1463–1471. [CrossRef]

47. Loopstra, R.; Tarasuk, V. Food bank usage is a poor indicator of food insecurity: Insights from Canada. *Soc. Policy Soc.* **2015**, *14*, 443–455. [CrossRef]

48. Parpouchi, M.; Moniruzzaman, A.; Russolillo, A.; Somers, J.M. Food insecurity among homeless adults with mental illness. *PLoS ONE* **2016**, *11*, e0159334. [CrossRef]

49. Skinner, K.; Hanning, R.M.; Tsuji, L.J. Prevalence and severity of household food insecurity of First Nations people living in an on-reserve, sub-Artic community within the Mushkegowuk Territory. *Public Health Nutr.* **2014**, *17*, 31–39. [CrossRef]

50. St-Pierre, M.; Béland, Y. Mode effects in the Canadian Community Health Survey: A Comparison of CAPI and CATI. In *Proceedings of the American Statistical Association Meeting, Survey Research Methods*; American Statistical Association: Toronto, ON, Canada, 2004.

51. Kirkpatrick, S.I.; Tarasuk, V. Food insecurity and participation in community food programs among low-income Toronto families. *Can. J. Public Health* **2009**, *100*, 135–139.

52. Oleckno, W.A. *Epidemiology: Concepts and Methods*; Waveland Press: Long Grove, IL, USA, 2008.

53. American Psychiatric Association. *Diagnostic and Statistical Manual of Mental Disorders (DSM-5®)*; American Psychiatric Pub: Arlington, VA, USA, 2013.

54. Mawani, F.N.; Gilmour, H. Validation of self-rated mental health. *Health Rep.* **2010**, *21*, 61–75.

13

Using Cross-Sectional Data to Identify and Quantify the Relative Importance of Factors Associated with and Leading to Food Insecurity

Alison Daly [1,*], **Christina M. Pollard** [1], **Deborah A. Kerr** [1], **Colin W. Binns** [1], **Martin Caraher** [2] and **Michael Phillips** [3]

[1] Faculty of Health Science, School of Public Health, Curtin University, GPO Box U1987, Perth 6845, Western Australia, Australia; C.Pollard@curtin.edu.au (C.M.P.); D.Kerr@curtin.edu.au (D.A.K.); C.Binns@curtin.edu.au (C.W.B.)
[2] Centre for Food Policy, City University of London, Northampton Square, London EC1V 0HB, UK; m.caraher@city.ac.uk
[3] Harry Perkins Institute for Medical Research, University of Western Australia, Perth 6009, Western Australia, Australia; michael.phillips@perkins.uwa.edu.au
* Correspondence: alison.daly@curtin.edu.au

Abstract: Australian governments routinely monitor population household food insecurity (FI) using a single measure—'running out of food at least once in the previous year'. To better inform public health planning, a synthesis of the determinants and how they influence and modify each other in relation to FI was conducted. The analysis used data from the Health & Wellbeing Surveillance System cross-sectional dataset. Weighted means and multivariable weighted logistic regression described and modelled factors involved in FI. The analysis showed the direction and strength of the factors and a path diagram was constructed to illustrate these. The results showed that perceived income, independent of actual income was a strong mediator on the path to FI as were obesity, smoking and other indicators of health status. Eating out three or more times a week and eating no vegetables more strongly followed FI than preceded it. The analysis identified a range of factors and demonstrated the complex and interactive nature of them. Further analysis using propensity score weighted methods to control for covariates identified hypothetical causal links for investigation. These results can be used as a proof of concept to assist public health planning.

Keywords: food insecurity; monitoring; surveillance; determinants; path diagram

1. Introduction

Food security exists "when all people, at all times, have physical, social and economic access to sufficient safe and nutritious food that meets their dietary needs and food preferences for an active and healthy life" [1]. Conversely, food insecurity (FI) is the "limited or uncertain availability of nutritionally adequate and safe foods or the limited or uncertain ability to acquire acceptable food in socially acceptable ways" [2], and is increasing in developed countries [3]. FI is adversely related to diet quality [4–10] and has been associated with the double burden of malnutrition, including undernourishment and obesity [11–13] and additionally it has been associated with poor mental health and socioeconomic disadvantages [14–20].

The complexity and impact of FI has been acknowledged and there is an growing amount of attention being directed to its determinants and how they influence and modify each other, calling for a systemic food system response [21]. FI is a problem of social and economic disadvantage, of which 'running out of food' due to insufficient money is only one component [22]. The complex nature of decisions about food is constrained by both physical access and choice [23], underpinned by the Food and Agricultural Organization's four pillars of availability: Access, utilization, stability and sustainability [24–26]. There is growing consensus regarding the need to focus on and better integrate social and structural factors when developing policies and interventions to improve public health in high income countries [27,28]. Evidence that is accessible to policy makers in the increasingly interrelated and complicated health policy area requires new approaches to research types and analyses [29].

The prevalence of FI in Australia, based on a 2001 review of the literature, showed that the rates were higher among the following groups: Families living with low or unstable incomes, those in remote areas, Aboriginal and Torres Strait Islander people, the unemployed, those living in rental households, single parents, those who were never married, separated or divorced, young adults and the elderly, asylum seekers and migrants, and people with disabilities [30]. FI directly impacts short and long-term health status, contributing to poor physical and psychological health outcomes and Australian health care costs [30]. The paradoxical relationship between FI and obesity has also been demonstrated, also significantly contributing to increasing health care costs [31–34].

Governments are increasingly encouraged to monitor FI, its determinants, mitigating actions, and their effectiveness [35]. Some countries, including Australia, do measure and report the prevalence of FI, including its severity and/or its determinants [36–39], but not routinely. While FI measures are continuously being evaluated and validated to come up with more accurate estimates of FI, the evaluation of the measures generally only contain limited references to determinants [5,40–42]. The severity of FI's effects, as well as its determinants and associated factors are important information used to inform public health planning. Currently there is little recognition among health or social services policy makers regarding the extent of the problem among some population sub-groups, nor the impact of sociodemographic determinants.

This study uses a cross-sectional self-reported dataset (the Western Australian Department of Health's *Health & Wellbeing Surveillance System* 2009–2013, *(HWSS))* to construct a path diagram of variables leading to 'running out of food' at least once in the previous year because of insufficient money. The analysis evaluates the relative importance of variables associated with FI. Specifically, the study aims to: Conduct an analysis to evaluate the relative importance of a range of associated variables with FI; use the results of the analysis to construct a path diagram to FI; propose hypothetical causal paths to and from FI; and suggest how future research and policy can be developed more effectively.

2. Materials and Methods

2.1. Sample and Measures

The HWSS cross-sectional computer-assisted telephone interview survey has measured health and wellbeing indicators (including risk factors) since 2002. Stratified samples by area were drawn from the statewide telephone book *Electronic White Pages* with geocoded addresses. The average participation rate was 90.2%. The 2009 to 2013 dataset, with a total of 21,710 adults aged 18–64 years was analysed. Data were pooled and weighted for probability of selection using iterative proportional fitting with marginal totals for the distribution of Western Australia (WA) residents in 2011 by age, sex and geographic area. The Department of Health in Western Australia datasets are not publicly available. The HWSS was granted ethics approval from the Western Australia Department of Human Research Ethics Committee (HREC 2011/65).

The sociodemographic variables used in this study were: Age, gender, highest level of education attained, living arrangements, area of residence, annual household income (AUD$), perceived discretional income, country of birth employment status and the geographic area based index that reflects socioeconomic advantage and disadvantage (SEIFA) [43]. Self-reported body weight and height, using a correction for over-reported height and under-reported weight [44], was used to estimate the Body Mass Index (BMI) of each respondent. Health-related variables included the self-assessment of: General health, comparison of health with a year prior, psychological distress (using the Kessler 10 index) [45], health risk factors and whether or not the respondent had these variables diagnosed by a doctor. The indicators of self-reported dietary behaviour included daily fruit, vegetable, and low-fat milk intake, as well as weekly take-away food consumption.

2.2. Analysis

The strategy adopted for this analysis was to develop a path diagram to describe a hypothetical model for the network of associations that describe running out of food and its consequences. This method has been used previously [46]. Usually this approach would use a structural equation model (SEM) but the outcome (running out of food or not) was dichotomous, meaning that SEM could not be used. Logistic regression analyses were conducted with a reference group of respondents who did not run out of food. The variables listed in Table 1 were statistically significant at $p \leq 0.1$ and were entered into weighted multivariable logistic regression analyses. While some variables were collected as continuous (e.g., age, K10, fruit, vegetables and physical activity estimates) values, we grouped them based upon accepted guidelines for Australian adults where possible. This was done to avoid assumptions of linearity. Both two way and three way interaction terms between the variables were tested on the final multivariable regression models. Bootstrapping (100 repetitions) produced final model estimates with robust measures used to estimate standard errors for the regression analyses. Results at $p < 0.05$ were considered to be statistically significant and kept in the model. Goodness of fit was assessed using the Hosmer–Lemeshow test. Diagnostic post-estimation tests, including tests for multicollinearity were conducted. The regression results were used to conduct a path diagram where the Bayesian Information Criteria (BIC) [47] was used to determine whether or not an association preceded or came after 'running out of food'. The ordering with the lowest BIC was used to determine the direction of the association. A difference in BIC of 10 or more (considered a very strong indicator) was the minimum value when deciding upon direction of effect. This corresponded to a p value of <0.0004 [48]. The multivariable model was modified to incorporate this information and the path diagram was constructed to reflect the results of the final model. Propensity scores were used to control for potential confounding from the covariates in iterative propensity score weighted logistic regression analyses for four variables. The four variables tested were income, discretional income, eating fast food three or more times a week and eating no vegetables. These four independent variables were operationally defined as variables in the path leading to the outcome of either 'running out of food' or not [49]. Each of these variables were tested for hypothetical causality. All analysis was conducted using Stata 13.1 [50].

3. Results

A total of 709 respondents reported 'running out of food' at least once in the previous twelve months and couldn't afford more (unweighted prevalence = 3.3%; weighted prevalence = 4.0%). The prevalence of variables associated with running out of food at $p < 0.1$ are shown in Table 1. The table presents both the unweighted and weighted prevalences with 95% confidence limits and p values for 'running out of food'. A total of 17,682 correspondents had information for all the variables on Table 1 and this was the sample used to run the multivariable weighted logistic regressions.

Table 2 presents the primary multivariable weighted logistic regression that was used as a basis to create the path analysis. The odds ratios for interaction terms that are presented in the path are estimates based on the results of the regression which either attenuates the effect or enhances the effect. This model showed good fit with the data ($x^2 = 11.02$, $p = 0.27$) and was used as the basis of the path diagram.

Table 1. The unweighted and weighted prevalences of 'running out of food' by sample characteristics, HWSS 2009–2013 (n = 21,705 [a]).

Demographic Variables	Unwght %	Wght %	95% CI	p
18–24	7.8	8.0	[6.5, 9.9]	
25–34	5.1	4.9	[3.8, 6.2]	
35–44	3.6	3.2	[2.6, 4.0]	
45–54	2.8	2.4	[1.9, 2.9]	
55–64	2.0	1.6	[1.3, 2.0]	<0.0001
Tertiary education	1.4	1.9	[1.3, 2.6]	
Less than tertiary education	3.8	4.7	[4.1, 5.3]	<0.0001
Employed	2.2	2.9	[2.5, 3.4]	
Unemployed	11.4	12.6	[9.0, 17.7]	
Home duties	4.3	5.2	[4.0, 6.7]	
Retired	2.3	2.0	[1.3, 3.0]	
Student	7.5	7.1	[4.8, 10.3]	
Unable to work	17.3	17.6	[13.2, 23.0]	<0.0001
Annual household income: over AUD $40,000	1.7	2.4	[2.0, 2.9]	
Annual household income: AUD $20,001–$40,000	7.0	9.6	[7.6, 12.2]	
Annual household income: up to AUD $20,000	15.0	17.8	[14.2, 22.2]	<0.0001
Spend left over money or save some per pay	1.1	1.7	[1.4, 2.0]	
Just enough money to get by per pay	10.6	12.5	[10.7, 14.5]	
Not enough money to get by per pay	17.5	19.0	[15.1, 23.6]	<0.0001
Not aboriginal	3.1	3.8	[3.4, 4.2]	
Aboriginal	12.5	15.0	[9.8, 22.1]	<0.0001
Adults living with others	2.8	3.7	[3.3, 4.2]	
Adults living alone	6.0	6.4	[5.2, 7.8]	<0.0001
Born outside Australia	2.8	2.9	[2.3, 3.7]	
Born in Australia	3.5	4.4	[3.9, 5.0]	0.002
Rents or pays mortgage	4.1	4.6	[4.3, 5.0]	
No mortgage or Government subsidized housing	2.5	3.1	[2.7, 3.4]	0.0003
SEIFA [b] Quintile 5 (least disadvantaged area)	2.4	2.9	[2.3, 3.6]	
SEIFA Quintiles 3,4 (less disadvantaged areas)	3.4	4.5	[3.9, 5.3]	
SEIFA Quintiles 1,2 (most disadvantages areas)	4.0	5.2	[4.2, 6.4]	<0.0001
Has a health care card	10.3	11.3	[9.7, 13.2]	<0.0001
Doesn't have private health insurance	7.0	8.3	[7.2, 9.6]	<0.0001
Has asthma	5.7	6.3	[4.7, 8.4]	0.0011
Some cardiovascular condition	5.8	7.4	[4.9, 11.0]	0.0022
Has cancer	4.5	7.0	[4.3, 11.3]	0.0167
Current mental health (depression/anxiety/other)	9.1	9.7	[8.3, 11.4]	<0.0001
Health rated as fair/poor	8.8	8.9	[7.2, 11.0]	<0.0001
Always or often feel a lack of control over health	12.8	13.9	[11.0, 17.3]	<0.0001
Health rated worse than 12 months ago	7.3	9.4	[7.6, 11.6]	<0.0001
High/very high Kessler 10 score	14.1	14.8	[12.4, 17.6]	<0.0001
BMI 30 or more (in obese range)	4.3	5.2	[4.4, 6.1]	<0.0012
Currently smoking	7.1	8.5	[7.0, 10.3]	<0.0001
Does no leisure time physical activity	4.4	5.5	[4.0, 7.5]	0.0447
Spends four or more hours sitting in leisure time	6.4	7.6	[5.8, 9.8]	<0.0001
Eats 'fast food' [c] three or more times a week	9.1	11.9	[8.3, 17.0]	<0.0001
Uses full fat milk	4.6	5.7	[4.9, 6.7]	<0.0001
Doesn't eat any fruit	6.3	6.4	[4.5, 9.1]	
Eats less than two serves of fruit daily	3.4	4.2	[3.6, 4.9]	
Eats two or more serves of fruit daily	2.7	3.3	[2.8, 4.0]	0.0030
Doesn't eat any vegetables	15.0	14.9	[6.5, 30.4]	
Eats less than five serves daily	3.3	4.0	[3.6, 4.5]	
Eats five or more serves daily	2.3	2.6	[1.7, 3.9]	<0.0012

[a] Sample with no missing values for each sociodemographic variable: Age (n = 21,705); education (n = 21,659); employment status (21,556); income (n = 17,964); perceived spending power (n = 20,959); aboriginal or not (n = 21,694); born in Australia or not (n = 21,704); living arrangements (n = 21,687); own or mortgage/rent (n = 21,705) SEIFA (n = 21,705); [b] SEIFA is an index of relative social disadvantage by area of residence [43] usually presented as quintiles which have been grouped into three levels of social disadvantage for this study; [c] Fast food is operationally defined as take away food such as burgers, pizza, chicken or chips from places like McDonalds, Hungry Jacks, Pizza Hut or Red Rooster.

Table 2. Weighted multivariable logistic regression for associations with running out of food including interaction terms, HWSS 2009–2013 (n = 17,638 [a]) [b].

Main Effects	Odd Ratio (95% CI)	p
35 over	Ref	
18–34 years	5.29 (3.65, 7.65)	0.000
Has tertiary education	Ref	
Does not have tertiary education	1.87 (1.38, 2.54)	0.000
Not Aboriginal	Ref	
Aboriginal	2.07 (1.34, 3.2)	0.001
Household income over $40,000	Ref	
Household income $20,000 to $40,000	1.65 (1.29, 2.1)	0.000
Household income under $20,000	5.28 (3.91, 7.13)	0.000
Can save a bit of money	Ref	
Just enough money to get by	1.08 (0.69, 1.71)	0.730
Not enough money to get by	3.11 (2.17, 4.46)	0.000
Has private health insurance	Ref	
Has no private health insurance	1.80 (1.46, 2.22)	0.000
Does not have doctor diagnosed mental health problem	Ref	
Has a doctor diagnosed mental health problem	2.56 (1.96, 3.35)	0.000
Low or moderate Kessler 10 score	Ref	
High or very high Kessler 10 score	1.65 (1.31, 2.06)	0.000
Health same or better than same time previous year	Ref	
Health worse or much worse than same time previous year	1.70 (1.37, 2.09)	0.000
Does not smoke	Ref	
Smokes	1.58 (1.29, 1.93)	0.000
Is not in Body Mass Index obese range	Ref	
Is in Body Mass Index obese range	1.44 (1.18, 1.76)	0.000
Eats some vegetables daily	Ref	
Eats no vegetables daily	2.40 (1.34, 4.3)	0.003
Eats fast foods less than three times a week	Ref	
Eats fast foods three or more times a week	1.83 (1.11, 3.01)	0.018
Interaction terms		
Has just enough money to get by [#] age 18–24 years	0.56 (0.35, 0.91)	0.019
Has a mental health problem [#] age 18–24 years	0.52 (0.31, 0.86)	0.010
Housing whether or not owned or rented [#] Not enough or just enough money to get by	3.35 (2.41, 4.65)	0.000
Household income under $20,000 [#] Not enough or just enough money to get by	3.05 (1.94, 4.80)	0.000

[a] Logistic reduced the estimation sample as it ran with post stratification adjustment (accounting for new weighted estimation sample); [b] This is the basic model used to determine the direction of effect. Two further models were then produced: One for associations preceding running out of food and one for associations following running out of food. The odd ratios in the path diagram were taken from these two models; [#] Denotes interaction terms between variables: Odds ratios less than 1 attenuate the effect and odds ratios greater than 1 enhance the effect.

The path to 'running out of food' and the associations between variables are shown in Figure 1. The path diagram shows both the main effects and the interaction terms that directly or indirectly influence the primary outcome of 'running out of food'. The models showed a good fit with the data, both for the variables that are associated with 'running out of food' ($\chi^2 = 12.75$; $p = 0.17$) and the possible consequences of 'running out of food' (fast food consumption $\chi^2 = 5.48$; $p = 0.71$; not eating vegetables $\chi^2 = 8.82$; $p = 0.31$).

In Figure 1, the red box represents the outcome measure, demonstrating food insecurity, i.e., 'running out of food' at least once in the previous twelve months. The blue boxes represent sociodemographics that are not able to be changed or are not easily changed. The yellow boxes represent associations which modify other variables on the path to food insecurity as well as being directly associated with food insecurity. The grey boxes represent the hypothesised consequences of food insecurity as informed by the BIC analysis.

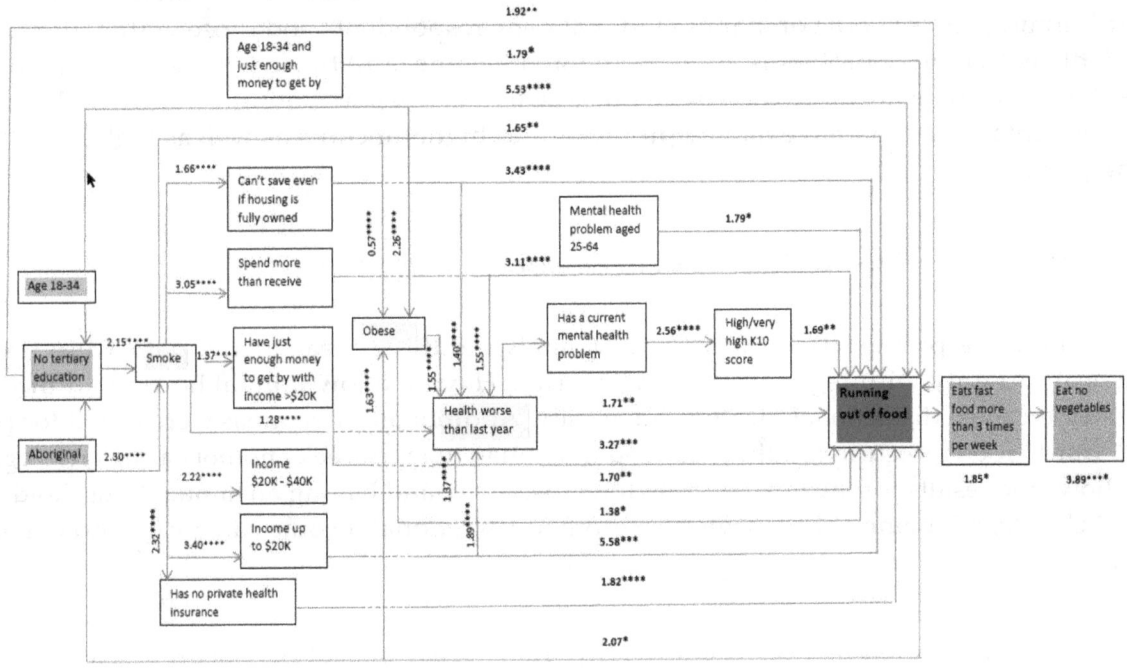

R2 = 0.29 Wald chi2(16) = 643.93 Prob > chi2 = 0.0000

Figure 1. Estimate of probability of eating fast food more than twice a week and eating no vegetables by 'running out of food', adjusted using propensity scores: Showing probable outcomes of 'running out of food', HWSS 2009–2013. * $p < 0.05$; ** $p < 0.01$; *** $p < 0.001$; **** $p < 0.0001$.

3.1. Direct Associations with Food Insecurity

Of the variables regarded as fixed, only three were directly associated with food insecurity: Age group (18–34 years compared to 35–64 years, odds ratio (OR) = 5.53, $p < 0.0001$), prior education level (no tertiary education compared with tertiary education, OR = 1.92, $p < 0.01$) and Aboriginality (of Aboriginal or Torres Strait Islander origin compared with not, OR = 2.07, $p < 0.05$). With the exception of two variables (which are dependent on 'running out of food') all other variables predicted FI. The two variables that were dependent on 'running out of food' were frequent fast food consumption, which subsequently predicted eating no vegetables.

3.2. Effect Modifiers in the Food Insecurity Path

Three variables acted as powerful effect modifiers in the path, shown in the yellow boxes: Smoking, obesity and the perception of worsening health over time (direct association). The size of the effects is shown on the chart as odds rations. To illustrate: Smoking, which is influenced by Aboriginality (OR = 2.30, $p < 0.0001$) and education (OR = 2.15, $p < 0.0001$), has a main effect on 'running out of food' (OR = 1.65, $p < 0.01$) and also acts as an effect modifier for perceived spending power and income (OR = 1.65, $p < 0.01$), income (AUD\$20–40K OR = 2.22, $p < 0.0001$; up to AUD\$20K OR = 3.40, $p < 0.0001$), private health insurance (OR = 1.65, $p < 0.01$) and worsening health status (OR = 1.65, $p < 0.01$).

Obesity influenced by smoking, where aboriginality and younger age has a main effect (OR = 1.38, $p < 0.05$) acts as an effect modifier for worsening health (OR = 1.55 $p < 0.0001$). Worsening health is influenced by smoking, obesity, low income, discretional income, and money problems, which are defined here as any income perceived to be less than needed. It has a main effect (OR = 1.71, $p < 0.01$) and acts as an effect modifier on mental health (OR = 1.71, $p < 0.01$).

Independent associations between younger age and spending power, low income and spending power, money problems, and mental health problems for older respondents are all directly associated with 'running out of food'. Other direct effects include not having private health insurance, having a low income, discretional income and mental health. Mental health also has an indirect effect mediated by high psychological distress, with the score measured by the K10 scale.

Respondents who are younger or who have very low incomes are more than five times as likely to report 'running out of food' compared with older age respondents and those with higher incomes. Respondents with money problems, low discretional income, and those with both low income and low discretional income are more than three times as likely to report 'running out of food' compared with respondents who don't have money problems and higher income as well as higher discretional spending power.

3.3. Adjustment for Covariates and Indicators of Hypothetical Causality

Using iterative propensity score weighted analyses, three areas of the path were tested for hypothetical causality with regard to food insecurity: Having a low annual household income, an inadequate perceived discretional income and obesity. Additionally, two areas were tested for possible causality due to food insecurity: Eating fast food more than twice a week and not eating any vegetables. Table 3 shows the results for the link between food insecurity and having an annual household income of up to AUD$20,000, being able to save versus other discretional income categories and being obese versus not.

Table 3. Estimate of probability of food insecurity ('running out of food' and not being able to afford more) by income, discretional income and obesity, adjusted using propensity scores: Showing probable antecedent factors of 'running out of food', HWSS 2009–2013.

Outcome: 'Running out of Food' at Least Once in the Previous Twelve Months	Coef.	95%	CI	Robust Std. Err	Z	p
Annual household income						
Average effect when income <$20,000	0.038	0.013	0.063	0.013	3.02	0.003
Probability if income is >$20,000	0.028	0.025	0.03	0.001	19.33	<0.001
Discretional income						
Difference between spend left over vs. able to save	0.023	0.014	0.033	0.005	4.85	<0.001
Difference between just enough vs. able to save	0.056	0.046	0.067	0.005	10.48	<0.001
Difference between not enough vs. able to save	0.066	0.048	0.083	0.009	7.38	<0.001
Average probability of outcome for those able to save	0.012	0.009	0.014	0.001	9.05	<0.001
Obesity						
Difference in probability when obese	0.008	0.003	0.013	0.003	3.15	0.002
Average probability of outcome if not obese	0.029	0.026	0.032	0.002	17.88	<0.001

vs = versus.

The first line of Table 3 shows the difference in the probability of 'running out of food' for the population with low income compared with those with a higher income. The second line of the table shows the probability for a reference higher income group 'running out of food'. The overall probability of 'running out of food' for the low income group is the sum of the two coefficients (e.g., 0.038 + 0.028 = 0.066). The next lines of Table 3 show the difference between the population and the reference category(ies) with which they are being compared for the independent variables: Perceived discretional income and obesity. The Supplementary Table S1 shows the full model for incomes above and below $20,000.

Table 4 shows the difference between the population and the reference category(ies) with which they are being compared for eating fast food three or more times a week and not eating vegetables. Eating fast food three or more times a week precedes eating no vegetables (as assessed using BIC in the path analysis).

Table 4. Estimate of probability of eating fast food more than twice a week and eating no vegetables by 'running out of food', adjusted using propensity scores: Showing probable outcomes of 'running out of food', HWSS 2009-2013.

Outcome:	Coef.	95%	CI	Robust Std. Err	Z	p
Eats fast food more than three times a week						
Difference in probability of 'running out of food' vs. not	−0.007	−0.013	−0.0002	0.003	−2.03	0.042
Average probability of outcome when didn't run out	0.019	<0.001	0.017	0.001	17.83	<0.001
Eats no vegetables						
Difference in probability of fast food >2 times weekly	0.029	0.007	0.051	0.011	2.61	0.009
Average probability of FI when fast food <3 times weekly	0.006	0.005	0.007	0.001	10.32	<0.001

4. Discussion

This analysis using a population-based survey resulted in the description of a plausible and quantified pathway to food insecurity, as well as measurement of its dietary impacts. The findings support the hypothesis that food insecurity, measured by whether or not a household ran out of food in the last year, appears to more strongly precede the poor diet indicators of eating fast food three or more times a week and eating no vegetables. While this hypothesis has been proposed previously [51], this proof-of-concept study is the first to quantify both the relative importance of the factors within the feedback loop to food insecurity and the complex nature of the factors leading to it.

The odds of 'running out of food' were higher for younger adults, those without tertiary education and Aboriginal people (odds ratios of 5.53, 2.15 and 2.3 respectively). These findings are consistent with the findings of the Australian national dietary survey which found that the prevalence of food insecurity was higher in Aboriginal populations compared to non-Indigenous Australians (22% compared to 3.7%) [52]. A UK study of 10,452 adults found that different socioeconomic indicators predicted dietary intake, for example, economic access to food, educational attainment and age were related to fruit and vegetable intake and diet costs [53]. The study also showed that dietary costs were not equally important in the causal pathway between socioeconomic position, suggesting that health and diet may be a factor when allocating funding for food [53].

The risk of running out of money for food has been associated with one-off financial stressors such as medical or other expenses due to unexpected events [54] and the price of food has been shown to contribute to food stress among low income families [55]. This current research highlights many other interrelated and potentially changeable factors. Saving ability, at any income level, appears to protect against food insecurity. Financial over-commitment is particularly relevant during times of economic downturn, as has occurred in Western Australia over recent years. The financial stress of housing costs may contribute to food insecurity as people can no longer afford their mortgage or rent, leading to money for food, a discretionary expense, potentially being sacrificed and instead put towards covering housing costs.

Attitudes toward income inequality and how poor people manage their money and cope in stressful situations are underpinned by cultural beliefs, related to blame, plight and privilege [56]. Although most Canadians were willing to accept differences in income related health inequalities such as food insecurity, they were less willing to attribute health inequalities to differences in personal health practices and coping skills [56]. The current study found increased odds of smoking, eating fast food and obesity associated with running out of money to buy food, independent of income level. Similar associations with food insecurity, perceived financial difficulty, smoking, lower fruit and vegetable intake and higher discretionary food intake were found in a representative sample of French households [57].

There are significant associations with not having private health insurance and feeling a lack of control over one's own health, both of which have adjusted odds ratios of 1.9. There is also an increased likelihood of food insecurity associated with social, mental and physical disadvantage as noted in other studies [58]. The number of factors on the path support the notion of deprivation amplification [59]. The results also show that quantification of the degree and direction of effects associated with food insecurity is possible. This quantification lends support to the concept that there may be causality between some of the variables on the path.

According to the theory underlying propensity score methodology as developed by Rosenbaum and Rubin [60], adjustment for propensity scoring removes the influence of confounding by multiple covariates and provides plausible evidence for causation for cross-sectional studies, even though one cannot ascribe any statistical significance to the findings [61]. The results from this current study suggest evidence of a hypothetical causal relationship within the path for the variables presented. The direction of effect is the relative strength of the association, so for example, while obesity may follow FI, it more strongly precedes it. The same applies to eating no vegetables and fast food consumption, which also precede but more strongly follow FI as shown in the path diagram. This is one possible path to FI which provides opportunities to investigate the mechanisms underlying its effects and the mediation illustrated in the path diagram. Other paths to FI can further investigate latent effects such as dietary eating patterns [10]. Unhealthy eating patterns are associated with similar sociodemographics found in the FI pathway of this study [62].

There is value for policy decision makers in quantifying both the relative importance of a range of associations with food insecurity and constructing a path to food insecurity. The path diagram uses a population dataset with enough statistical power to allow for a subsequent investigation of possible causal links, highlighting the need to address the determinants of food insecurity as well as considering the consequences. The complex nature of the path also adds weight to the need for inter-sectoral collaborations to address the various determinants of food security. The results from the path diagram support the need for a system level policy to address this [63,64]. For example, obesity, which in the path diagram more strongly precedes FI has been shown also to follow it [62,65], suggesting the need for a policy that addresses both obesity as well as FI in tandem rather than as a separate policy for each.

The strength of this analysis is that the population survey and large sample size enabled the complex analysis to establish a proof-of-concept study to be undertaken. As with all survey data, there are limitations associated with this research, including some level of non-response and the self-reported nature of the data. The use of sample design weights incorporated in iterative proportional fitting (IFP), also known as 'raking', allowed for adjustment of over and under representation of age, gender and area of residence within the sample. This weighting was also incorporated into the multivariable regression models. The one question measure of food insecurity, based on 'running out of food' and not being able to afford more, does not measure the extent and experience of food insecurity, nor did the self-reported brief diet questions measure actual dietary intake. However, that was not the purpose of this investigation, which was to explore the complex mix of influences leading to FI. A further limitation was the omission of questions relating to attitudinal and lifestyle behaviours which would have allowed for the creation of a model that included these modifiable attributes.

5. Conclusions

The findings support evidence that decisions about food insecurity are complex and interactive, with a variety of factors contributing to the issue. While the single measure of FI cannot be considered adequate to fully estimate the prevalence of FI, the proof-of-concept using this single measure showed expected associations and quantified the effects of 'running out of food' over a range of determinants, such as income and physical and mental wellbeing. The path diagram presented suggests that a wider approach to bringing about change in access and use of food needs to be considered. The findings highlight the need to focus policy effort on mitigating the social determinants of food insecurity and the potential complexity of the pathways to food insecurity. This requires a system approach to policy development for FI and we could encourage policy makers and researchers to use this methodology to explore and quantify the complex relationships leading to food insecurity.

Author Contributions: A.D. was involved in the conception and design of the HWSS; A.D. and C.P. were involved in the conception and design of the NMSS; A.D. and M.P. conceived the approach and analyzed the data; A.D. wrote the first draft of the paper; A.D., C.P., D.K., M.C., C.B., M.P. reviewed and agreed with final drafts of the paper.

Acknowledgments: The Department of Health, Western Australia owns, conducts and funds the Health and Wellbeing Surveillance System (HWSS). The authors are grateful for the ongoing monitoring of nutrition relating attitudes and behaviours and encourage ongoing execution of the survey. Healthway, the Western Australian Health Promotion Foundation, funded the *Food Law, Policy and Communications to Improve Public Health Project (Grant 19986)* to assist the translation of research into practice. The funder had no role in study design, data collection and analysis, decision to publish, or preparation of the manuscript. All sources of funding of the study should be disclosed. A.D. undertook this work as part of her Doctor of Philosophy and received a Healthway Health Promotion Research Scholarship (23342) part of which is being used to support publication.

References

1. Food and Agriculture Organization. *Rome Declaration on World Food Security and World Food Summit Plan of Action: World Food Summit 13–17 November*; FAO: Rome, Italy, 1996.
2. Anderson, S.A. Core indicators of nutritional state for difficult-to-sample populations. *J. Nutr.* **1990**, *120*, 1555–1600. [CrossRef] [PubMed]
3. Riches, G. *Food Bank Nations: Poverty, Corporate Charity and the Right to Food*; Routledge: New York, NJ, USA, 2018.
4. Hanson, K.L.; Connor, L.M. Food insecurity and dietary quality in us adults and children: A systematic review. *Am. J. Clin. Nutr.* **2014**, *100*, 684–692. [CrossRef] [PubMed]
5. Jones, A.D.; Ngure, F.M.; Pelto, G.; Young, S.L. What are we assessing when we measure food security? A compendium and review of current metrics. *Adv. Nutr.* **2013**, *4*, 481–505. [CrossRef] [PubMed]
6. Robaina, K.A.; Martin, K.S. Food insecurity, poor diet quality, and obesity among food pantry participants in hartford, ct. *J. Nutr. Educ. Behav.* **2013**, *45*, 159–164. [CrossRef] [PubMed]
7. Dowler, E. Symposium on 'intervention policies for deprived households' policy initiatives to address low-income households' nutritional needs in the uk. *Proc. Nutr. Soc.* **2008**, *67*, 289–300. [CrossRef] [PubMed]
8. Mook, K.; Laraia, B.A.; Oddo, V.M.; Jones-Smith, J.C. Food security status and barriers to fruit and vegetable consumption in two economically deprived communities of oakland, california, 2013–2014. *Prev. Chronic Dis.* **2016**, *13*, E21. [CrossRef] [PubMed]
9. Tingay, R.S.; Tan, C.J.; Tan, N.C.; Tang, S.; Teoh, P.F.; Wong, R.; Gulliford, M.C. Food insecurity and low income in an english inner city. *J. Public Health Med.* **2003**, *25*, 156–159. [CrossRef] [PubMed]
10. Thornton, L.E.; Pearce, J.R.; Ball, K. Sociodemographic factors associated with healthy eating and food security in socio-economically disadvantaged groups in the uk and victoria, australia. *Public Health Nutr.* **2013**, *17*, 20–30. [CrossRef] [PubMed]
11. Metallinos-Katsaras, E.; Must, A.; Gorman, K. A longitudinal study of food insecurity on obesity in preschool children. *J. Acad. Nutr. Diet.* **2012**, *112*, 1949–1958. [CrossRef] [PubMed]
12. Larson, N.I.; Story, M.T. Food insecurity and weight status among u.S. Children and families: A review of the literature. *Am. J. Prev. Med.* **2011**, *40*, 166–173. [CrossRef] [PubMed]
13. Crawford, P.B.; Webb, K.L. Unraveling the paradox of concurrent food insecurity and obesity. *Am. J. Prev. Med.* **2011**, *40*, 274–275. [CrossRef] [PubMed]
14. Hernandez, D.C.; Marshall, A.; Mineo, C. Maternal depression mediates the association between intimate partner violence and food insecurity. *J. Womens Health* **2014**, *23*, 29–37. [CrossRef] [PubMed]
15. Young, S.L.; Plenty, A.H.; Luwedde, F.A.; Natamba, B.K.; Natureeba, P.; Achan, J.; Mwesigwa, J.; Ruel, T.D.; Ades, V.; Osterbauer, B.; et al. Household food insecurity, maternal nutritional status, and infant feeding practices among hiv-infected ugandan women receiving combination antiretroviral therapy. *Matern. Child Health J.* **2014**, *18*, 2044–2053. [CrossRef] [PubMed]

16. Whitaker, R.C.; Phillips, S.M.; Orzol, S.M. Food insecurity and the risks of depression and anxiety in mothers and behavior problems in their preschool-aged children. *Pediatrics* **2006**, *118*, E859–E868. [CrossRef] [PubMed]

17. Melchior, M.; Chastang, J.F.; Falissard, B.; Galera, C.; Tremblay, R.E.; Cote, S.M.; Boivin, M. Food insecurity and children's mental health: A prospective birth cohort study. *PLoS ONE* **2012**, *7*, e52615. [CrossRef] [PubMed]

18. Muldoon, K.A.; Duff, P.K.; Fielden, S.; Anema, A. Food insufficiency is associated with psychiatric morbidity in a nationally representative study of mental illness among food insecure canadians. *Soc. Psychiatry Psychiatr. Epidemiol.* **2013**, *48*, 795–803. [CrossRef] [PubMed]

19. Pobutsky, A.M.; Baker, K.K.; Reyes-Salvail, F. Investigating measures of social context on 2 population-based health surveys, hawaii, 2010–2012. *Prev. Chron. Dis.* **2015**, *12*, E221.

20. Friel, S. Climate change, food insecurity and chronic diseases: Sustainable and healthy policy opportunities for australia. *N. S. W. Public Health Bull.* **2010**, *21*, 129–133. [CrossRef] [PubMed]

21. Ashe, L.M.; Sonnino, R. At the crossroads: New paradigms of food security, public health nutrition and school food. *Public Health Nutr.* **2013**, *16*, 1020–1027. [CrossRef] [PubMed]

22. Tarasuk, V. Implications of a Basic Income Guarantee for Household Food Insecurity. Northern Policy Institute, 2017. Available online: https://proof.utoronto.ca/wp-content/uploads/2017/06/Paper-Tarasuk-BIG-EN-17.06.13-1712.pdf (accessed on 22 November 2018).

23. Lang, T.; Barling, D.; Caraher, M. Food, social policy and the environment: Towards a new model. *Soc. Policy Adm.* **2001**, *35*, 538–558. [CrossRef]

24. Food and Agriculture Organisation. *Declaration of the World Summit on Food Security 16–18 November*; Food and Agriculture Organisation: Rome, Italiy, 2009.

25. Carletto, C.; Zezza, A.; Banerjee, R. Towards better measurement of household food security: Harmonizing indicators and the role of household surveys. *Glob. Food Secur.* **2013**, *2*, 30–40. [CrossRef]

26. Ecker, O.; Breisinger, C. The Food Security System: A New Conceptual Framework. International Food Policy Research Institute, 2012. Available online: http://ebrary.ifpri.org/cdm/ref/collection/p15738coll2/id/126837 (accessed on 22 November 2018).

27. Rideout, K.; Seed, B.; Ostry, A. Putting food on the public health table: Making food security relevant to regional health authorities. *Can. J. Public Health* **2006**, *97*, 233–236. [PubMed]

28. Bastian, A.; Coveney, J. Local evidenced-based policy options to improve food security in south australia: The use of local knowledge in policy development. *Public Health Nutr.* **2012**, *15*, 1497–1502. [CrossRef] [PubMed]

29. Bell, E. *Research for Health Policy*; Oxford University Press: Oxford, UK, 2009.

30. Caraher, M.; Coveney, J. Public health nutrition and food policy. *Public Health Nutr.* **2004**, *7*, 591–598. [CrossRef] [PubMed]

31. Booth, S.; Smith, A. Food security and poverty in australia-challenges for dietitians. *Aust. J. Nutr. Diet.* **2001**, *58*, 150–156.

32. Tarasuk, V. Health implications of food insecurity. *Soc. Déterm. Health Can. Perspect.* **2004**, 187–200.

33. Dinour, L.M.; Bergen, D.; Yeh, M.-C. The food insecurity–obesity paradox: A review of the literature and the role food stamps may play. *J. Am. Diet. Assoc.* **2007**, *107*, 1952–1961. [CrossRef] [PubMed]

34. Franklin, B.; Jones, A.; Love, D.; Puckett, S.; Macklin, J.; White-Means, S. Exploring mediators of food insecurity and obesity: A review of recent literature. *J. Commun. Health* **2012**, *37*, 253–264. [CrossRef] [PubMed]

35. HLPE, Nutrition and Food Systems. *A Report by the High Level Panel of Experts on Food Security and Nutrition of the Committee on World Food Security*; HLPE: Rome, Italy, 2017.

36. Foley, W.; Ward, P.; Carter, P.; Coveney, J.; Tsourtos, G.; Taylor, A. An ecological analysis of factors associated with food insecurity in south australia, 2002–2007. *Public Health Nutr.* **2010**, *13*, 215–221. [CrossRef] [PubMed]

37. Quine, S.; Morrell, S. Food insecurity in community-dwelling older australians. *Public Health Nutr.* **2006**, *9*, 219–224. [CrossRef] [PubMed]

38. Russell, J.; Flood, V.; Yeatman, H.; Mitchell, P. Prevalence and risk factors of food insecurity among a cohort of older australians. *J. Nutr. Health Aging* **2014**, *18*, 3–8. [CrossRef] [PubMed]

39. Kleve, S.; Davidson, Z.; Gearon, E.; Booth, S.; Palermo, C. Are low-to-middle-income households

experiencing food insecurity in victoria, australia? An examination of the victorian population health survey, 2006–2009. *Aust. J. Prim. Health* **2017**, *23*, 249–256. [CrossRef] [PubMed]

40. Marques, E.S.; Reichenheim, M.E.; de Moraes, C.L.; Antunes, M.M.L.; Salles-Costa, R. Household food insecurity: A systematic review of the measuring instruments used in epidemiological studies. *Public Health Nutr.* **2015**, *18*, 877–892. [CrossRef] [PubMed]

41. McKechnie, R.; Turrell, G.; Giskes, K.; Gallegos, D. Single-item measure of food insecurity used in the national health survey may underestimate prevalence in australia. *Aust. N. Z. J. Public Health* **2018**, *42*, 389–395. [CrossRef] [PubMed]

42. Butcher, L.M.; O'Sullivan, T.A.; Ryan, M.M.; Lo, J.; Devine, A. Utilising a multi-item questionnaire to assess household food security in australia. *Health Promot. J. Aust.* **2018**. [CrossRef] [PubMed]

43. Australian Bureau of Statistics. *Socio-Economic Indexes for Areas (Seifa) 2011*; Australian Bureau of Statistics: Canberra, Australia, 2013.

44. Hayes, A.J.; Kortt, M.A.; Clarke, P.M.; Brandrup, J.D. Estimating equations to correct self-reported height and weight: Implications for prevalence of overweight and obesity in australia. *Aust. N. Z. J. Public Health* **2008**, *32*, 542–545. [CrossRef] [PubMed]

45. Andrews, G.; Slade, T. Interpreting scores on the kessler psychological distress scale (k10). *Aust. N. Z. J. Public Health* **2001**, *25*, 494–497. [CrossRef] [PubMed]

46. Gill, T.K.; Price, K.; Dal Grande, E.; Daly, A.; Taylor, A.W. Feeling angry about current health status: Using a population survey to determine the association with demographic, health and social factors. *BMC Public Health* **2016**, *16*, 588. [CrossRef] [PubMed]

47. Burnham, K.P.; Anderson, D.R. Multimodel inference-understanding aic and bic in model selection. *Sociol. Methods Res.* **2004**, *33*, 261–304. [CrossRef]

48. Raftery, A.E. Bayesian model selection in social research. *Sociol. Methodol.* **1995**, *25*, 111–163. [CrossRef]

49. Little, R.J.; Rubin, D.B. Causal effects in clinical and epidemiological studies via potential outcomes: Concepts and analytical approaches. *Annu. Rev. Public Health* **2000**, *21*, 121–145. [CrossRef] [PubMed]

50. StataCorp. *Stata Statistical Software: Release 13*; StataCorp LP: College Station, TX, USA, 2013.

51. Ramsey, R.; Giskes, K.; Turrell, G.; Gallegos, D. Food insecurity among adults residing in disadvantaged urban areas: Potential health and dietary consequences. *Public Health Nutr.* **2012**, *15*, 227–237. [CrossRef] [PubMed]

52. Australian Bureau of Statistics. *4727.0.55.005-Australian Aboriginal and Torres Strait Islander Health Survey: Nutrition Results-Food and Nutrients, 2012-13*; Australian Bureau of Statistics: Canberra, Australia, 2015.

53. Mackenbach, J.D.; Brage, S.; Forouhi, N.G.; Griffin, S.J.; Wareham, N.J.; Monsivais, P. Does the importance of dietary costs for fruit and vegetable intake vary by socioeconomic position? *Br. J. Nutr.* **2015**, *114*, 1464–1470. [CrossRef] [PubMed]

54. King, S.; Moffitt, A.; Bellamy, J.; Carter, S.; McDowell, C.; Mollenhauer, J. When there not enough to eat: A national study of food insecurity among emergency relief clients. *State Family Report* **2012**, *2*, 137–161. [CrossRef]

55. Landrigan, T.J.; Kerr, D.A.; Dhaliwal, S.S.; Savage, V.; Pollard, C.M. Removing the australian tax exemption on healthy food adds food stress to families vulnerable to poor nutrition. *Aust. N. Z. J. Public Health* **2017**, *41*, 591–597. [CrossRef] [PubMed]

56. Lofters, A.; Slater, M.; Kirst, M.; Shankardass, K.; Quinonez, C. How do people attribute income-related inequalities in health? A cross-sectional study in ontario, canada. *PLoS ONE* **2014**, *9*, e85286. [CrossRef] [PubMed]

57. Bocquier, A.; Vieux, F.; Lioret, S.; Dubuisson, C.; Caillavet, F.; Darmon, N. Socio-economic characteristics, living conditions and diet quality are associated with food insecurity in france. *Public Health Nutr.* **2015**, *18*, 2952–2961. [CrossRef] [PubMed]

58. Stuff, J.E.; Casey, P.H.; Szeto, K.L.; Gossett, J.M.; Robbins, J.M.; Simpson, P.M.; Connell, C.; Bogle, M.L. Household food insecurity is associated with adult health status. *J. Nutr.* **2004**, *134*, 2330–2335. [CrossRef] [PubMed]

59. Macintyre, S. Deprivation amplification revisited; or, is it always true that poorer places have poorer access to resources for healthy diets and physical activity? *Int. J. Behav. Nutr. Phys. Activ.* **2007**, *4*, 32. [CrossRef]

60. Rosenbaum, P.R.; Rubin, D.B. The central role of the propensity score in observational studies for causal effects. *Biometrika* **1983**, *70*, 41–55. [CrossRef]

61.   Habicht, J.P.; Victora, C.G.; Vaughan, J.P. Evaluation designs for adequacy, plausibility and probability of public health programme performance and impact. *Int. J. Epidemiol.* **1999**, *28*, 10–18. [CrossRef] [PubMed]

62.   Daly, A.; Pollard, C.M.; Kerr, D.A.; Binns, C.W.; Phillips, M. Using short dietary questions to develop indicators of dietary behaviour for use in surveys exploring attitudinal and/or behavioural aspects of dietary choices. *Nutrients* **2015**, *7*, 6330–6345. [CrossRef] [PubMed]

63.   Caraher, M.; Furey, S. *The Economics of Emergency Food Aid Provision: A Financial, Social and Cultural Perspective*; Palgrave Macmillan: Basingstoke, UK, 2018.

64.   Steiner, J.F.; Stenmark, S.H.; Sterrett, A.T.; Paolino, A.R.; Stiefel, M.; Gozansky, W.S.; Zeng, C. Food insecurity in older adults in an integrated health care system. *J. Am. Geriat. Soc.* **2018**, *66*, 1017–1024. [CrossRef] [PubMed]

65.   Kaiser, M.L.; Cafer, A. Understanding high incidence of severe obesity and very low food security in food pantry clients: Implications for social work. *Soc. Work Public Health* **2018**, *33*, 125–139. [CrossRef] [PubMed]

14

What can Secondary Data Tell us about Household Food Insecurity in a High-Income Country Context?

Ourega-Zoé Ejebu [1], Stephen Whybrow [2], Lynda Mckenzie [1], Elizabeth Dowler [3],
Ada L Garcia [4], Anne Ludbrook [1], Karen Louise Barton [5], Wendy Louise Wrieden [6]
and Flora Douglas [2,*]

1   Health Economics Research Unit, University of Aberdeen, Aberdeen AB25 2ZD, UK;
    oejebu@abdn.ac.uk (O.E.); l.mckenzie@abdn.ac.uk (L.M.); a.ludbrook@abdn.ac.uk (A.L.)
2   Rowett Institute, University of Aberdeen, Aberdeen AB25 2ZD, UK; stephen.whybrow@abdn.ac.uk
3   Department of Sociology, University of Warwick, Coventry CV4 7AL, UK; Elizabeth.Dowler@warwick.ac.uk
4   Human Nutrition, University of Glasgow, Glasgow G31 2ER, UK; Ada.Garcia@glasgow.ac.uk
5   Division of Food and Drink, Abertay University, Dundee DD1 1HG, UK; K.Barton@abertay.ac.uk
6   Human Nutrition Research Centre and Institute of Health & Society, Newcastle University,
    Newcastle upon Tyne NE2 4HH, UK; Wendy.Wrieden@newcastle.ac.uk
*   Correspondence: f.douglas3@rgu.ac.uk

Abstract: In the absence of routinely collected household food insecurity data, this study investigated what could be determined about the nature and prevalence of household food insecurity in Scotland from secondary data. Secondary analysis of the Living Costs and Food Survey (2007–2012) was conducted to calculate weekly food expenditure and its ratio to equivalised income for households below average income (HBAI) and above average income (non-HBAI). Diet Quality Index (DQI) scores were calculated for this survey and the Scottish Health Survey (SHeS, 2008 and 2012). Secondary data provided a partial picture of food insecurity prevalence in Scotland, and a limited picture of differences in diet quality. In 2012, HBAI spent significantly less in absolute terms per week on food and non-alcoholic drinks (£53.85) compared to non-HBAI (£86.73), but proportionately more of their income (29% and 15% respectively). Poorer households were less likely to achieve recommended fruit and vegetable intakes than were more affluent households. The mean DQI score (SHeS data) of HBAI fell between 2008 and 2012, and was significantly lower than the mean score for non-HBAI in 2012. Secondary data are insufficient to generate the robust and comprehensive picture needed to monitor the incidence and prevalence of food insecurity in Scotland.

Keywords: food insecurity; food poverty; prevalence; household; food surveys; secondary data; Scotland

1. Introduction

Household food insecurity (HFI) is a common problem for low-income households in high-income countries [1–4]. HFI exists when a household experiences the inability "to acquire or consume an adequate quality or sufficient quantity of food in socially acceptable ways, or the uncertainty that one will be able to do so" [5]. It has been empirically established to manifest itself involuntarily across four dimensions: (i) quantity and (ii) quality of food; (iii) psychological impacts; and (iv) socially unacceptable food and ways of obtaining food [6–8]. In high-income countries, food insecurity is more commonly characterised by chronic compromises in dietary quality and anxiety associated with accessing food. In contrast, low and middle income countries most generally experience acute and chronic episodes of food deprivation, hunger, and starvation [8]. Critically, for health and social care policy makers in high-income countries, the experience of food insecurity featuring poor diet quality leads to negative health outcomes i.e., cancer, stroke, cardiovascular disease, diabetes and obesity, and depression [8–15]. Much of the epidemiological evidence highlighting these associations has been generated in the North American context where routine capture of HFI data has taken place for some decades [16]. Nationally representative food security monitoring was established in the U.S. in 1995 with the highest recorded HFI prevalence observed during the global recession of 2008–2009 (14.5% of the population) [17]. While there has been an observed decline in those figures, they remain in the region of 12% of the population (15 million households) [18]. Canadian HFI prevalence runs roughly in line with the U.S. at 11–12% of the population found to have been food insecure since food security monitoring was established there in 1994 [19]. HFI prevalence is also higher in specific population subgroups including households with children, single-parent households and indigenous, black and Hispanic households [18,20], a pattern also observed in Australia and New Zealand [21,22]. It is also widely argued that HFI is an outcome of income insufficiency in relation to necessary household expenditures [20,22–26] and the decisions of policy makers [27]. In the late-2000s, HFI had re-emerged as a subject of public health, social policy, civic and political concern in Scotland and the rest of the UK. This is attributed to an increase in the numbers of people turning to emergency food supply centres (so-called food banks) for help with feeding themselves and their families [28–32]. Food bank use data became a de facto measure of food insecurity across the UK, largely through the high profile reporting of the Trussell Trust, which is one of the best known charitable organizations providing emergency food aid in the UK [33]. Yet the ability of emergency food supply centres to address HFI, or provide an insight into the nature and scale of food insecurity at the local and national level is problematic [6,17,18,34]. In similar international contexts, where it is possible to make comparisons with routinely collected food insecurity data, food bank use data tend to significantly underestimate the prevalence of food insecurity [35,36]. This presents challenges for policy makers tasked with the development, implementation, and evaluation of policy measures aimed at addressing the problem [37]. It is particularly problematic for governments and policy makers given that food banks, as a de facto public policy response to the problem, are unable to meet local demand for food assistance for a variety of inherent resource constraints, unless food is rationed by restricting access for those who want and are able to access them [34,38,39].

It was in this context, and in the absence of any purposively collected and experiential household food insecurity population survey data, that research was undertaken in Scotland, in 2014, to explore the nature and prevalence of HFI. This paper reports on the study component that screened and analysed relevant existing secondary data, with the specific aim of finding out what could be determined about the nature and prevalence of HFI in Scotland, as defined above [5]. The study was also guided by a particular focus on the years preceding the UK economic recession (2008 to 2009) [40] and the period of rapid increase in food prices (2007 to 2012) [41]. Additionally, the analysis included a comparison of the diets of households at risk of food insecurity compared to those at less risk. The paper discusses what analysis of existing data sources is able to reveal (or not) about two of the four defined dimensions of the experience of food insecurity in the Scottish context, i.e., dietary quantity and quality, and reflects on the absence of data on psychological and social experiences, and the implications of this research for future policy making in this area.

2. Materials and Methods

The secondary data analysis proceeded in three stages.

2.1. First stage—Scoping and Data Source Selection

The first stage involved a scoping, consultation and decision making process to identify suitable Scottish data sources to explore food insecurity patterns covering the 2008 UK recession. It was at this stage also that consideration and agreement was reached about the 'at risk' household income threshold that would be used during the analysis, to take account of the lack of a UK food insecurity measure [37].

The threshold level agreed for identifying those at risk of food poverty was equivalised net household income of less than 60% of the median value [42,43], which is the commonly used measure of poverty in the UK. Household income is equivalised to take account of household size and composition (including numbers of adults and children, and their ages [44]). Households below the threshold are referred to as households below average income (HBAI). Households with income above this threshold are referred as non-HBAI. Income was measured before housing costs were deducted [43].

Using the aforementioned HFI definition [5], datasets were identified where relevant variables for analysing HFI trends and prevalence in Scotland were available. Six potentially suitable datasets were identified, with four being rejected. These were, (i) the General Lifestyle Survey [45] (excluded due to difficulties gaining timely data access); (ii) the European Union Statistics on Income and Living Conditions [46] (Scotland is not identified as a separate UK region); the Family Resources Survey [47] (insufficient information on food purchase data); and Kantar Worldpanel [48] (which includes very few low income households and insufficient information to calculate equivalised income). The two remaining datasets, the Living Costs and Food Survey (LCFS) [49] and the Scottish Health Survey (SHeS) [50], were used for this analysis.

The LCFS is an annual stratified random sample survey conducted by the Office for National Statistics. It includes approximately 500 households in Scotland. The survey collects information on household spending patterns from diaries of daily expenditure recorded over a 2-week period. LCFS data from 2007 and 2012 were used for the present study. Variables include weekly household expenditure on food and non-alcoholic drinks brought home, eaten away from home (e.g., at a restaurant or hotel) and take-away items. Weekly food expenditures were adjusted to 2013 prices using the food and non-alcoholic drinks Consumer Price Index (CPI). Food expenditure-to-income ratios were calculated by dividing weekly household food expenditure by weekly equivalised household income using the McClement equivalence scale [44]. Household income was adjusted for inflation using the overall 2013 CPI.

From 2008, the SHeS was conducted annually. It contains information on the prevalence of different health conditions and health-related behaviours, including dietary intake collected on alternate years. Data are collected at an individual (both adults and children) and a household level. It includes around 6500 individual observations in 2008 and 4800 in 2012. Information on usual daily food eating patterns (type of food and frequency of consumption) are provided. SHeS also collects data on annual household income and converts this value to equivalised income using the McClement equivalence scale.

Both datasets were weighted using available sampling weights, which adjust for non-response and to match the population distribution [49,51].

2.2. Second Stage—Prevalence Estimation and Sub Group Analysis

Using both LCFS and SHeS, the second stage involved estimating the numbers of households at risk of being in food poverty, and investigating how prevalence had changed over time, and comparing these changes with data from the Family Resources Survey. Information on household income and prevalence of HBAI from the Family Resources Survey [47] was included to place the Scottish data in the context of data for the whole of the UK. The FRS (Family Resources Survey) is the most comprehensive survey of household financial circumstances using a large sample of UK households, and is the government source for poverty level analyses.

Using LCFS, this stage also included analysis of food expenditure (£) and food-to-income shares (%) between lower and higher income households. Mean weekly expenditure on food and non-alcoholic drinks, and their corresponding values in terms of percentage by food group based on the Eatwell Plate [52] were also calculated. Two-tailed independent t-tests were used to compare mean food expenditure (overall and by food group) and food-to-income shares between HBAI and non-HBAI, and to compare percentage DQI score (see below) between HBAI and non-HBAI and over time.

2.3. Third Stage—Dietary Quality Assessment and Analysis

The third stage involved assessing differences in overall diet quality between those considered at risk, and those not at risk, of being in food poverty. Dietary recommendations are based on the amounts of foods consumed, whereas food and drink are recorded in the LCFS "as purchased". These were adjusted to "as consumed" values per person by accounting for food waste, and food preparation and cooking weight changes [53–55]. Nutrient intakes were calculated using the LCFS food composition database [56].

Within the SHeS, an Eating Habits Module (EHM) assesses consumption of a simple list of foods that are relevant to the Scottish Dietary Goals [57]. The EHM focuses on frequency of consumption of specific foods and was not designed to quantify amounts of foods or nutrients consumed, or meal patterns. It is not possible to assess nutrient intake, household food practices, meal patterns or experiences of the stability of the household food supply from the EHM. The EHM consists of two sections, the first being a series of questions on the consumption of food and drink items to gather information on general eating habits using a food frequency questionnaire methodology. The second assesses fruit and vegetable intake by a 24 h recall method using "everyday" food portion terms (such as tablespoons, cereal bowls and slices). Information on the number and type of fruit and vegetables eaten by respondents the day prior to the interview was used to compare the percentage of individuals in HBAI and non-HBAI reaching the 5-a-day goal for portions of fruit and vegetables.

A more comprehensive measure of diet quality, using the Diet Quality Index (DQI) devised by Barton and colleagues [58,59], was also used to calculate scores for SHeS and LCFS. Diet quality indexes are frequently used to summarise how well an individual's diet compares to a collection of dietary recommendations, based on foods and nutrients considered to be important to health [60]. For example, adherence to the Dietary Guidelines for Americans can be assessed using the Healthy Eating Index, which has been shown to be a valid and reliable index of diet quality [61].

Diet Quality Index scores were calculated for the LCFS (2007 and 2012) and SHeS (2008 and 2012). For the LCFS data, DQI scores were calculated for a combination of foods (fruit and vegetables, fish, and red meat) and nutrients (percentage energy from fat and saturated fat, sugar and complex carbohydrates, and fibre) [58]. For the SHeS data, DQI scores were calculated from seven food components: oil-rich fish; red meat and processed meat; starchy foods; fibre in foods; sugary foods; fatty foods; and fruit and vegetables. The difference in food items used to calculate the DQI is because of the variations in dietary information available from the LCFS and SHeS. Absolute values for the DQI from the two surveys are therefore not directly comparable and have been expressed in the results as a percentage of the maximum possible score for each survey. Higher scores indicate greater adherence to dietary guidelines.

The proportions of food groups contributing to each diet were estimated using the Eatwell Plate recommendations. In the UK, the Eatwell Plate [52] (now updated and renamed the Eatwell Guide) was developed for representing nutrient intake information in a picture format to make dietary recommendations easier for consumers to understand. The Eatwell Plate is a pie-chart diagram consisting of five food group segments, the recommended proportions of which are based on the dietary reference values for the population. The five groups being: 1. bread, rice, potatoes, pasta and other starchy foods (starchy, which should make up around 33% of the diet), 2. fruit and vegetables (F&V, 33%), 3. milk and dairy foods (dairy, 15%), 4. meat, fish, eggs, beans and other non-dairy sources of protein (protein, 12%) and 5. foods and drinks that are high in fat or sugar, or both (HFHS, 8%).

Statistical analyses were carried out using STATA Version 13 (StataCorp LP, College Station, Texas, TX, USA) and SPSS Version 22 (SPSS/IBM Corp, Armonk, New York, NY, USA).

3. Results

3.1. Households at Risk of Food Insecurity—Prevalence Estimates

Table 1 shows the number and proportion of HBAI estimated in the LCFS, SHeS, and from the FRS.

Table 1. Prevalence of households below 60% median income in Living Costs and Food Survey (LCFS), Scottish Health Survey (SHeS) and the Family Resources Survey (FRS), along with mean weekly expenditure and measures of diet quality.

Year of Survey	LCFS		SHeS			FRS	
	2007	2012	2008	2012		2007/8	2012/13
Scottish observations (households)	501	483	3567	2697		NA	NA
Monthly equivalised median household income (£)	£2079	£2039	£1842	£1954		£1699	£1907
Poverty threshold * (£)	£1247	£1223	£1105	£1172		£1019	£1144
Percentage of HBAI (Number)	23.4% (117)	18.9% (92)	26.3% (940)	23.4% (632)		17%	16%
Percentage of non-HBAI (Number)	76.7% (384)	81.1% (391)	73.6% (2627)	76.6% (2065)		NA	NA
Weekly expenditure on food and drinks (£)—HBAI $$	£54.08 [48.30–59.86]	£53.85 [45.11–62.6]	NA	NA		NA	NA
Weekly expenditure on food and drinks (£)—non-HBAI $$	£102.14 [95.41–108.87]	£86.73 [81.43–92.02]	NA	NA		NA	NA
p-values of mean food expenditure between HBAI and non-HBAI	$p < 0.001$	$p < 0.001$					
Weekly expenditure on food and drinks (% income)—HBAI $$	30.7% [22.36–39.04]	29.4% [23.19–35.53]	NA	NA		NA	NA
Weekly expenditure on food and drinks (% income)—Non-HBAI $$	14.1% [13.14–15.06]	15.5% [14.38–16.59]	NA	NA		NA	NA
p-values of food-to-income ratios between HBAI and non-HBAI	$p < 0.001$	$p < 0.001$					
DQI score (%)—HBAI	35.1% [31.9–38.3]	36.2% [31.8–40.5]	50.4%	48.5%		NA	NA
DQI score (%)—non-HBAI	36.5% [34.7–38.4]	34.7% [33.0–36.5]	51.6%	51.6%		NA	NA
p-values of DQI scores between HBAI and non-HBAI	$p = 0.327$	$p = 0.506$					

* 60% of monthly equivalised median household income (£). $$ weekly food includes grocery shopping, non-alcoholic drinks, food eaten away from home (e.g., at a restaurant or hotel) and take-away food. Confidence interval into [brackets]. HBAI: households below average income.

Prevalence estimates from the LCFS and SHeS are similar. In contrast, the results using LCFS data are weighted to adjust for non-response and to match population distributions, and give higher levels than those in the FRS. However, all estimates show an apparent decline in the prevalence of HBAI between 2007 and 2012.

Table 1 also shows the mean weekly expenditure on food (including food eaten away from home and take away food) and non-alcoholic drinks using LCFS. Results are displayed for HBAI and non-HBAI for 2007 and 2012, respectively. HBAI spent less actual money per week on food than non-HBAI (Table 1) ($p < 0.001$ in both years), but the proportion (%) of equivalised household income spent on food was approximately twice the proportion spent by non-HBAI ($p < 0.001$ in both years). There is a slight decrease in both food expenditure and the share of food expenditure to income from 2007 to 2012 for HBAI. However, there is a bigger drop in food expenditure by non-HBAI combined with an increasing share of income being spent on food. This suggests that non-HBAI had more discretion to reduce food spending in the face of declining real incomes during the period of recession.

3.2. Dietary Analysis and Assessment

Table 2 reports the (mean) weekly expenditure of HBAI and non-HBAI, by Eatwell Plate food group, as well as the corresponding percentage share of income (%). In contrast to the results in Table 1, any other food expenditure (e.g., food eaten away from home and take-away food) are excluded from this calculation.

For each food group, while HBAI spend significantly less of their weekly income in pounds (£), they spend proportionately (%) more in comparison to non-HBAI ($p < 0.001$ for each food group in both years). There is no statistically difference of expenditure between HBAI and non-HBAI for Non-alcoholic drinks in year 2012 and 'Other' food (for both years).

Non-HBAI households spend more on both 'healthy' food (fruit and vegetables) and 'unhealthy food' (foods high in fat and sugar (HFHS)), suggesting that poor dietary choices are not necessarily determined solely by spending power. Meat and other sources of proteins, and HFHS represent the largest share of food expenditure in both HBAI and non-HBAI alike. Noticeably, fruit and vegetables constitute the third largest food expenditure in both household types.

Figure 1 shows the percentage of SHeS individuals from HBAI and non-HBAI by number of portions of fruits and vegetables consumed on the day prior to the interview. In both years, there is a marked difference in the proportion of individuals reaching the 5-a-day target between those in HBAI and non-HBAI (14% and 32%, $p < 0.001$ in 2008 and 12% and 21%, $p < 0.001$ in 2012). Respondents in HBAI were more likely to report consuming no, or only one portion of, fruit or vegetables the previous day compared to their non-HBAI counterparts.

The proportion of individuals in HBAI who reported eating no fruit and vegetables the day prior to the interview was higher in 2012 (18%) than in 2008 (11%). Nevertheless, 14% of individuals from HBAI reported eating five or more portions of fruits and vegetables in 2008; this proportion fell to 11% by 2012. However, there was little change in the proportion of individuals from non-HBAI eating five or more portions of fruits and vegetables over time (22% and 21% respectively).

Examination of the DQI scores calculated from the LCFS revealed no significant differences between HBAI and non-HBAI households for percentage DQI score (35.1% and 36.5%, $p = 0.327$ in 2007, and 36.2% and 34.7%, $p = 0.506$ for 2012) (Table 1). Examination of the DQI score based on the SHeS data showed the overall mean percentage DQI scores were similar in 2008 for HBAI and non HBAI (50.4% and 51.6% respectively, $p = 0.196$). However, by 2012, the overall percentage DQI score was significantly lower for HBAI than non-HBAI (48.5% and 51.6% respectively, $p = 0.001$).

Table 2. Mean weekly expenditure * (£ and % of income) of HBAI (households below average income.) and non-HBAI, by food group.

Food type	2007 HBAI	2007 non-HBAI	p-values 2007	2012 HBAI	2012 non-HBAI	p-values 2012
Starchy food	£5.91 [5.16–6.67]; 2.49% [1.80–3.17]	£8.06 [7.45–8.66]; 0.87% [0.79–0.94]	$p < 0.001$; $p < 0.001$	£5.28 [4.24–6.31]; 3.01% [2.06–3.95]	£6.93 [6.42–7.43]; 1.25% [1.13–1.37]	$p = 0.005$; $p < 0.001$
Fruits and vegetables	£6.85 [5.73–7.97]; 2.54% [2.00–3.09]	£12.83 [11.82–13.85]; 1.31% [1.20–1.41]	$p < 0.001$; $p < 0.001$	£7.22 [5.59–8.86]; 3.70% [2.81–4.59]	£10.83 [9.98–11.69]; 1.86% [1.69–2.03]	$p < 0.001$; $p < 0.001$
Milk and dairy	£5.16 [4.47–5.85]; 2.09% [1.64–2.53]	£7.75 [7.02–8.46]; 0.83% [0.75–0.90]	$p < 0.001$; $p < 0.001$	£5.10 [4.26–5.94]; 2.71% [2.13–3.28]	£6.28 [5.84–6.73]; 1.09% [1.01–1.1]	$p = 0.015$; $p < 0.001$
Meat and protein	£12.22 [10.53–13.92]; 4.20% [3.53–4.87]	£19.87 [18.35–21.38]; 2.09% [1.92–2.25]	$p < 0.001$; $p < 0.001$	£12.08 [9.67–14.48]; 6.52% [4.82–8.23]	£18.2 [16.70–19.71]; 3.15% [2.86–3.44]	$p < 0.001$; $p < 0.001$
HFHS	£10.72 [9.26–12.19]; 4.71% [3.07–6.36]	£19.39 [17.69–21.10]; 2.07% [1.88–2.27]	$p < 0.001$; $p = 0.0018$	£11.78 [9.80–13.76]; 5.95% [4.91–6.99]	£17.12 [15.81–18.44]; 3.05% [2.75–3.35]	$p < 0.001$; $p < 0.001$
Non-alcoholic drinks	£1.07 [0.84–1.30]; 0.37% [0.28–0.45]	£1.72 [1.46–1.98]; 0.18% [0.15–0.21]	$p < 0.001$; $p < 0.001$	£1.11 [0.78–1.44]; 0.71% [0.25–1.17]	£1.46 [1.22–1.71]; 0.25% [0.21–0.30]	$p = 0.095$; $p = 0.053$
Other food	£0.08 [0.01–0.14]; 0.03% [0.004–0.05]	£0.13 [0.003–0.23]; 0.02% [0.00–0.03]	$p = 0.3756$; $p = 0.4632$	£0.05 [0.01–0.09]; 0.02% [0.006–0.04]	£0.14 [0.08–0.20]; 0.03% [0.02–0.04]	$p = 0.014$; $p = 0.856$
Total *	£42.01 [37.40–46.65]; 16.42% [13.26–19.60]	£69.73 [65.06–74.41]; 7.37% [6.82–7.90]	$p < 0.001$; $p < 0.001$	£42.62 [35.77–49.47]; 22.62% [18.05–27.18]	£60.96 [57.24–64.70]; 10.68% [9.99–11.37]	$p < 0.001$; $p < 0.001$
Observations	117	384		92	391	

* Excludes spending on food eaten away from home and takeaway food. Confidence interval into [brackets]. p-values represent the statistical differences between HBAI and non-HBAI for (i) mean weekly expenditure and (ii) food-to-income ratios respectively. Source: computed by the authors based on LCFS 2007 and 2012. Weighted and adjusted for inflation.

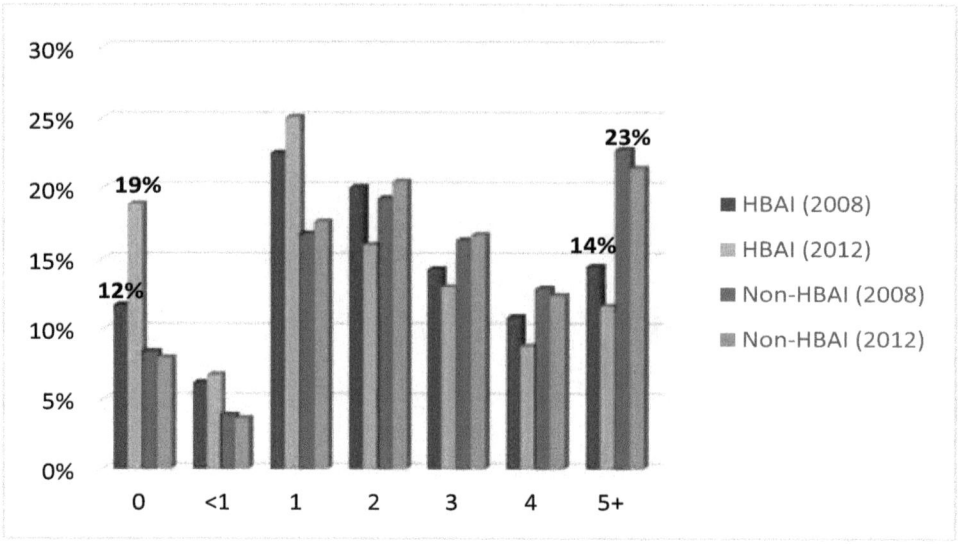

Figure 1. Percentage of individuals from HBAI (households below average income.) and non-HBAI by fruit and vegetables consumption (number of portions on the day prior to the interview). Source: computed by the authors based on SHeS (2008 and 2012)—weighted data.

4. Discussion

This study aimed to establish what could be determined about the nature and prevalence of household food insecurity in Scotland from secondary data. The scoping study established that it was possible to gain only a partial picture of HFI in the Scottish context, allowing a focus on quantity and quality of diets. Therefore, the subsequent analyses centered on an exploration of food expenditure-to-income shares and levels of food expenditure, and a dietary quality analysis of foods purchased and reported as consumed. The analysis focused on HBAI and non-HBAI households, over the period following the recent economic recession. Consequently, this discussion proceeds in two parts, focusing firstly on the findings of the 'partial picture' data able to be accessed and analysed, and secondly, reflecting on the policy and practice implications arising from the lack of routine capture of psychosocial domain data of the experience of household food insecurity in the population.

4.1. Household Expenditure and Food and Nutrition Security

This analysis revealed that low income households in Scotland have continued to allocate a greater income share (%) to food over the period following the recession, with food expenditure a particularly prominent component of all household expenditure, compared to wealthier households. This is consistent with the expenditure patterns reported for the whole of the UK [62]. Findings from the current study suggest that the HBAI group had less margin to reduce food expenditure than their wealthier counterparts. For, at the same time that there was a reduction in food spending for this group, the income share devoted to it increased, as it did for non-HBAI. These findings also align with the current position, as more recent UK figures suggest that increases in food prices have continued to exacerbate the situation of low-income households due to the larger income share they devote to food expenditure, compared with higher income households [63]. Given the relative stasis of, and in many cases decline in, household incomes in low income households in the UK [64], the net effect on those lower income households is that they probably have less available income to spend on other essential household items.

Indeed, although there appear to be few differences in the diets of HBAI and non-HBAI when the frequencies of consumption of all key food groups were compared using the DQI, in both the LCFS and SHeS data, the consistent exception is in fruit and vegetable consumption. Fruit and vegetable consumption is commonly used as proxy indicator of diet quality. Lower income households have lower expenditure on fruit and vegetables than do higher income households (LCFS); and their self-reported consumption was lower compared with non-HBAI (SHeS). These results from the SHeS partially support previous research indicating that the quality of dietary intake is poor across all income groups in Scotland, but tends to be worse in the poorer households [65], and that these effects have worsened over time. Overall, the indicators of HFI and the subsequent analysis used in this study are innovative and could be adapted in other studies to bridge the gap in the literature.

As this research was designed to examine the usefulness of existing relevant data sources in enabling the characterization of HFI in Scotland, it is important to note that the SHeS is designed to estimate frequency of consumption rather than provide estimates of the amounts of foods consumed. This makes interpretation of dietary quality difficult, since the Scottish Dietary Targets are based on amounts of food groups consumed. It is conceivable that those on the lowest incomes have already made all possible adjustments to expenditure and cannot further reduce spending, as argued above [62]. This finding might also be explained by the relatively short shelf life of fresh fruit and vegetables, which often makes such items relatively unattractive to purchase compared to other less perishable items for those whose room for financial manoeuver is more limited.

Consequently, when considering and interpreting these findings, it is important to note that virtually no attention had been paid to people's lived experience of food insecurity in Scotland until very recently. No study has focused on the experience of food (in)security in the context of other necessary household expenditures [66], that might explain these patterns of difference in diet quality and, for example, expenditure on fruit and vegetables. Why these patterns persist, despite longstanding educational campaigns exhorting the benefits of healthy eating, has also not been investigated. Where empirical research (in high income country contexts) has been conducted to investigate the direct perspectives and motivations of different socioeconomic households regarding "healthy" food provisioning and meal preparation (as opposed to drawing inferences from dietary pattern data), low income/food insecure households are no less likely than their wealthy counterparts to express a desire to consume healthy food [67]. Indeed, there is some evidence to suggest that very low-income households possess significant food knowledge and skills, and employ multiple strategies with the aim of feeding the family nutritious foods [68–72]. The evidence presented above regarding income shares devoted to food in Scotland in recent years suggests that the capacity for very low income households to be able to take action according to their aspirations and preferences could be constrained; which is consistent with the views of health, social care and third sector practitioners supporting economically and social vulnerable groups in Scotland [73].

The analysis also revealed an apparent decrease in the proportion of households whose household income fell below 60% of the median income value between 2007 and 2012, which some may construe to mean a subsequent decline in the numbers of households affected by food insecurity. The poverty threshold used in this study was based on the median income of each sample survey, and not the UK or Scottish median income; this might partially explain disparities in the percentage of HBAI within the FRS. In addition, since the "HBAI at risk marker" is based on a single threshold each year, any change in the overall nature of the distribution of equivalised household income between survey years could affect the position of the median relative to the mean equivalised income. This could influence the proportion of households above and below the poverty threshold level. Median income was likely to be falling in real terms due to the recession. Existing Scottish Government surveys and reports provide a more thorough and complete view of the prevalence of poverty per se [74,75].

In addition, the food poverty threshold used in this study (<60% of the median equivalised household income) masks the experiences of households with considerably lower incomes, which are also likely to be underrepresented in the datasets used in this analysis. Individuals whose household income is below 50% or 40% of the UK median income are considered as living in severe or extreme poverty, respectively [74]. Moreover, those just above or below this threshold may be quite similar, and experience similar financial difficulties from increased household costs.

Furthermore, households living on remote Scottish islands are not included in the LCFS, for data collection cost reasons. This is an important omission, given that incomes are known to be lower in rural areas, and that those living in remote and rural areas in Scotland need to spend "10–40% more on everyday requirements than elsewhere in the UK" [76]. In the LCFS, sampling variability was also affected by a higher non-response rate of households whose head had no post-school qualification or was in a manual social class group [56]. In the SHeS, deprived areas were over-sampled however [56]. In both LCFS and SHeS, weights were used to reduce the effect of non-response bias so that the sample distribution matches the population distribution in terms of region, age group and sex [49,77].

However, international evidence derived from jurisdictions where food insecurity is routinely monitored shows that while household income is an important determinant, it does not fully explain the circumstances of all those who are food insecure. Housing costs (i.e., mortgage, rent, fuel and insurances), and other necessary household expenditures (such as travel and debt) have been shown to significantly contribute to the observed prevalence of food insecurity [78,79].

4.2. Study Implications

While the current analysis revealed some important and worrying patterns of population dietary deterioration in HBAI households at the same time as they are apportioning more and more of their income to food expenditure in Scotland, it also revealed some crucial gaps in the available data. For example, it was not possible to show which groups of people were most at risk from food insecurity. As highlighted previously, in other high income jurisdictions it has been possible to identify specific household types that are more at risk of severe and enduring HFI, and with it, the theoretical possibility of targeted policy interventions [18,20]. The need for this data has been brought into sharp relief in recent times in the UK as a recently published report by the UN Rapporteur for Extreme Poverty and Human Rights expressed great concern for the working poor, female-headed households, children and those living with disabilities, pensioners, asylum seekers and refugees and those living in rural poverty as most at risk of extreme poverty in the UK at the present time [80].

An analysis of children living in households at risk of HFI was not possible either. Such analysis would be very informative considering the latest finding of a UNICEF report [81]. It revealed that in 2014, 19.7% children aged 0–17 were living in HBAI in the UK. Whilst this stands below the average of developed countries (21.0%), it is an indication of the extent to which HFI affects vulnerable groups.

Another important gap revealed was the lack of data that could provide a picture of the people and groups who were affected by uncertainty/anxiety associated with being able to afford to feed oneself or the family. Nor was it possible to determine the duration and frequency of these types of experiences at the household level. Based on U.S. observational studies [6], markers of food deprivation are regarded as more sensitive than income-based measures alone, in capturing not only the material aspects of deprivation (largely caused by income poverty), but also its combined biological and psychosocial effects on health and well-being. A number of international studies have also concluded that the experience of HFI is likely to be impacting human health as much through 'non-nutritional' mechanisms, such as worry, anxiety, feelings of deprivation, and social isolation, as through nutritional routes [6,82–84].

Indirect measures of HFI, such as food availability, purchasing power, consumption patterns and anthropometric measures were deemed to be insufficient for HFI monitoring and the evaluation of interventions intended to address it as far back as the late 1970's [85]. Within other high-income country contexts, where routine HFI monitoring takes place, a now significant body of research has linked HFI with negative physical and psychological health consequences [16,68,86,87]. It is also known to impair chronic condition management [88,89] and is independently associated with increased health care use and costs [90].

Therefore, it has been encouraging to witness the discussion and policy shifts in recent years highlighting the need for routine monitoring of HFI across the UK. However, there is still no agreement about the means and measures by which this should be done, with policy differences emerging within the different nations of the UK regarding these [91,92]. For example, the Scottish Government have recently accepted the main recommendations of the Independent Working Group on Food Poverty in Scotland [93] and have introduced a HFI measure (a derivative of the UN Food Insecurity Experience Scale) [94] into the SHeS. The SHeS operates on a continuous annual reporting basis, and provides sufficient data for each individual health board area in Scotland to understand their population health dynamics over time, and has the potential for data linkage with other population data sets including disease registers [95]. The SHeS is specifically funded to monitor population health outcomes and trends. Therefore, the inclusion of a HFI measure in this survey should make it possible to determine the effectiveness of policy interventions intended to address HFI, as well as understanding the role of HFI in the poor health outcomes of the Scottish population. The benefits of placing this measure here, and with it the potential routine capture the more multi-dimensional HFI experience, are manifold. Firstly, it provides the facility to assess and monitor food insecurity experience for different subgroups (e.g., geographic location, age, ethnicity, household type, occupational status and health status). Secondly, embedded HFI monitoring in such a survey enables data linkage with other population data sets including disease registers, and therefore enables better scrutiny of the impact of food insecurity experience on population health outcomes [95]. Thirdly, the inclusion of a such HFI measure also provides the facility to monitor prevalence and severity (if not chronicity), and with it the potential to develop better understanding of the role different HFI experiences (in terms of nature and severity) has in relation to health outcomes within the Scottish population, something that was beyond the scope of this study. Fourthly, it should also provide a robust means to determine the effectiveness of policy interventions intended to address HFI. Indeed, it is important to stress the benefits of introducing and retaining such a measure compared to the HFI indicator used in Europe, which uses a more unidimensional indicator that is based primarily on the prevalence of the household's inability to afford meat/fish/poultry (or a vegetarian equivalent) every second day [25]. Fifthly as the SHeS survey routinely also captures household income data, it should be possible to monitor and model changes in HFI prevalence in the context of changing national and household economic circumstances and social policy changes, something one-off cross-sectional studies cannot undertake. There have been calls for a similar type of measure to be introduced in England and Wales [96].

In 2003, the UK Food Standards Agency used a piloted questionnaire based on the USDA (United States Department of Agriculture) experience to investigate household food security in a UK-wide survey of diet and nutrition in low-income households [97]. A similar questionnaire was used in the Food Standard Agency's 'Food and You' consumer survey in England in 2016 [98]. However, this seems unlikely to offer the same depth and functionality as the data collected by the SHeS going forward. In addition, none of the measures mentioned above include questions about children's food security status. This is a serious omission given the reported levels of child poverty and so-called 'holiday hunger' in the UK, relating to the important role that is played by provision of free school meals to low income families during term time [99], and the associated poor child health and educational outcomes that have been observed in international contexts where children's HFI status is captured and recorded [100].

It is important also to acknowledge that, while routine food insecurity measurement offers the potential to characterise and monitor HFI prevalence more comprehensively, and provides a means to evaluate policy and programmatic interventions aimed at addressing it, challenges will remain in capturing the experiences of homeless and destitute individuals and families, and representing them in secondary data. Routine HFI monitoring and evaluation endeavors must therefore also include direct qualitative engagement with those highly vulnerable groups and the services and/or agencies responsible for their care and support, to inform and evaluate social, economic and health policy changes intended to address HFI [73]. In addition, whilst periodic episodes of absolute food deprivation are a public health and ethical concern of any country, it is also the case that the less severe experience of food insecurity resulting in chronic dietary quality compromises over time, is likely to be the more prevalent experience in high income countries like Scotland. This is an important distinction to be able to capture as accurately as possible as chronic food insecurity experience is considered to be as damaging to health and well-being over the long term as periodic deprivation experiences [68] and this phenomenon needs more research attention in HFI monitoring work in the UK and elsewhere than it currently receives. Related to this is the need in the UK to develop a better understanding to the impact of food insecurity on chronic or long-term health condition management in the UK [73]. Having a clearer picture of the severity and chronicity of people's HFI experience as well as national and subnational prevalence would assist researchers and policy makers to develop more insight into this overlooked health care issue, and create better informed policy responses to address HFI in the Scotland and elsewhere in the UK.

5. Conclusions

This study provided a partial picture of the prevalence of HFI in Scotland. It revealed that low income households have been consuming a diet that has further deteriorated in nutritional quality over the period following the recession and have been spending a significantly higher proportion of their household incomes compared to wealthier households. Other important dimensions of HFI are unavailable for scrutiny for monitoring and evaluation purposes. Additional or alternative measures to identify at-risk households are required to inform the development and evaluation of policy and programmatic interventions intended to address the problem. Routine and systematic monitoring would not only enable HFI incidence and prevalence to be better characterised, but would enable the relationship between household-level problems of food insecurity and changing social and economic conditions to be monitored and understood. In order to develop, implement and evaluate social and public health policy interventions intended to reduce the numbers of households affected by food insecurity, the routine capture of household food insecurity data suitable for Scottish and UK population health monitoring is urgently needed.

Author Contributions: Conceptualisation, F.D., A.L.G., S.W., L.M., A.L., E.D.; methodology, O.E., S.W., L.M., A.G., A.L., K.L.B., W.L.W., F.D.; validation formal analysis O.E., S.W., L.M., K.L.B., A.L.G.; data curation O.E., S.W., L.M.; writing—original draft preparation O.E.; F.D.; writing—review and editing F.D., O.E., S.W., L.M., K.L.B., A.L., A.L.G., E.D.; supervision A.L., L.M.; project administration F.D.; funding acquisition F.D., L.M., S.W., A.L., E.D.

Acknowledgments: This study was also like to acknowledge Bill Gray NHS Health Scotland and Dionne MacKison formerly of NHS Health Scotland for their professional review and support during the project. The authors would also like to acknowledge the anonymous reviewers of this manuscript, whose observations and suggestions improved this paper.

References

1.   Tarasuk, V.; Dachner, N.; Hamelin, A.M.; Ostry, A.; Williams, P.; Bosckei, E.; Poland, B.; Raine, K. A survey of food bank operations in five Canadian cities. *BMC Public Health* **2014**, *14*, 1234. [CrossRef] [PubMed]

2.   Martin-Fernandez, J.; Grillo, F.; Parizot, I.; Caillavet, F.; Chauvin, P. Prevalence and socioeconomic and geographical inequalities of household food insecurity in the Paris region, France, 2010. *BMC Public Health* **2013**, *13*, 486. [CrossRef] [PubMed]

3.   Pfeiffer, S.; Ritter, T.; Hirseland, A. Hunger and nutritional poverty in Germany: Quantitative and qualitative empirical insights. *Crit. Public Health* **2011**, *21*, 417–428. [CrossRef]

4.   Reeves, A.; Loopstra, R.; Stuckler, D. The growing disconnect between food prices and wages in Europe: Cross-national analysis of food deprivation and welfare regimes in twenty-one EU countries, 2004–2012. *Public Health Nutr.* **2017**, *20*, 1414–1422. [CrossRef] [PubMed]

5. Radimer, K.L.; Olson, C.M.; Campbell, C.C. Development of indicators to assess hunger. *J. Nutr.* **1990**, *120*, 1544–1548. [CrossRef] [PubMed]

6. Habicht, J.-P.; Pelto, G.; Frongillo, E.; Rose, D. Conceptualization and instrumentation of food insecurity. In Proceedings of the Workshop on the Measurement of Food Insecurity and Hunger, Washington, DC, USA, 15 July 2004.

7. Fram, M.S.; Bernal, J.; Frongillo, E.A. *The Measurement of Food Insecurity Among Children: Review of Literature and Concept Note*; Innocenti Working Paper No. 2015-08; UNICEF Office of Research: Florence, Italy, 2015.

8. Tarasuk, V. *Discussion Paper on Household and Individual Food Insecurity*; Health Canada: Ottawa, ON, Canada, 2001; Volume 13.

9. Patil, S.P.; Craven, K.; Kolasa, K.M. Food insecurity: It is more common than you think, recognizing it can improve the care you give. *Nutr. Today* **2017**, *52*, 248–257. [CrossRef]

10. Butcher, L.; Ryan, M.; O'Sullivan, T.; Lo, J.; Devine, A. What drives food insecurity in Western Australia? How the perceptions of people at risk differ to those of stakeholders. *Nutrients* **2018**, *10*, 1059. [CrossRef]

11. Ward, P.R.; Verity, F.; Carter, P.; Tsourtos, G.; Coveney, J.; Wong, K.C. Food stress in Adelaide: The relationship between low income and the affordability of healthy food. *J. Environ. Public Health* **2013**, *2013*, 968078. [CrossRef]

12. Gundersen, C.; Ziliak, J.P. Food Insecurity And Health Outcomes. *Health Aff. (Millwood)* **2015**, *34*, 1830–1839. [CrossRef]

13. Maynard, M.; Andrade, L.; Packull-McCormick, S.; Perlman, C.; Leos-Toro, C.; Kirkpatrick, S. Food Insecurity and Mental Health among Females in High-Income Countries. *Int. J. Environ. Res. Public Health* **2018**, *15*, 1424. [CrossRef] [PubMed]

14. Martin, M.S.; Maddocks, E.; Chen, Y.; Gilman, S.E.; Colman, I. Food insecurity and mental illness: Disproportionate impacts in the context of perceived stress and social isolation. *Public Health* **2016**, *132*, 86–91. [CrossRef] [PubMed]

15. Butland, B.; Jebb, S.; Kopelman, P.; McPherson, K.; Thomas, S.; Mardell, J.; Parry, V. *Foresight, Tackling Obesities: Future Choices*; UK Government Office for Science: London, UK, 2007.

16. Nord, M. What have we learned from two decades of research on household food security? *Public Health Nutr.* **2014**, *17*, 2–4. [CrossRef]

17. Riches, G.; Silvasti, T. Hunger in the rich world: Food aid and right to food perspectives. In *First World Hunger Revisited*; Springer: Berlin, Germany, 2014; pp. 1–14.

18. Coleman-Jensen, A.; Rabbitt, M.; Gregory, C.; Singh, A. *Household Food Security in the United States in 2015*; ERR-215; U.S. Department of Agriculture, Economic Research Service: Washington, DC, USA, September 2016.

19. Riches, G.; Tarasuk, V. Canada: Thirty years of food charity and public policy neglect. In *First World Hunger Revisited*; Springer: Berlin, Germany, 2014; pp. 42–56.

20. Tarasuk, V.; Mitchell, A.; Dachner, N. *Household Food Insecurity in Canada, 2014: Research to Identify Policy Options to Reduce Food Insecurity*; Research to Identify Policy Options to Reduce Food Insecurity (PROOF): Toronto, ON, Canada, 2016.

21. Rosier, K. *Food Insecurity in Australia: What Is It, Who Experiences It and How Can Child and Family Services Support Families Experiencing It?* Australian Commonwealth Government: Melbourne, Australia, 2011.

22. Carter, K.N.; Lanumata, T.; Kruse, K.; Gorton, D. What are the determinants of food insecurity in New Zealand and does this differ for males and females? *Aust. N. Z. J. Public Health* **2010**, *34*, 602–608. [CrossRef]

23. Riches, G. Food banks and food security: Welfare reform, human rights and social policy. Lessons from Canada? *Soc. Policy Adm.* **2002**, *36*, 648–663. [CrossRef]

24. Loopstra, R.; Reeves, A.; Taylor-Robinson, D.; Barr, B.; McKee, M.; Stuckler, D. Austerity, sanctions, and the rise of food banks in the UK. *BMJ* **2015**, *350*, h1775. [CrossRef] [PubMed]

25. Davis, O.; Geiger, B.B. Did Food Insecurity rise across Europe after the 2008 Crisis? An analysis across welfare regimes. *Soc. Policy Soc.* **2017**, *16*, 343–360. [CrossRef]

26. Dowler, E. Food banks and food justice in 'Austerity Britain'. In *First World Hunger Revisited*; Springer: Berlin, Germany, 2014; pp. 160–175.

27. McIntyre, L.; Patterson, P.B.; Mah, C.L. The application of 'valence' to the idea of household food insecurity in Canada. *Soc. Sci. Med.* **2019**, *220*, 176–183. [CrossRef]

28.   Cooper, N.; Purcell, S.; Jackson, R. Below the Breadline: The Relentless Rise of Food Poverty in Britain. Available online: https://policy-practice.oxfam.org.uk/publications/below-the-breadline-the-relentless-rise-of-food-poverty-in-britain-317730 (accessed on 27 December 2018).

29.   Government, H.U. Hansard Report of House of Commons Food Banks Debate 18th December. 2013. Available online: http://www.publications.parliament.uk/pa/cm201314/cmhansrd/cm131218/debtext/131218-0003.htm (accessed on 20 August 2018).

30.   Ashton, J.R.; Middleton, J.; Lang, T. Open letter to Prime Minister David Cameron on food poverty in the UK. *Lancet* **2014**, *383*, 1631. [CrossRef]

31.   Duggan, E. The Food Poverty Scandal that Shames Britain: Nearly 1m People Rely on Handouts to Eat—And Benefit Reforms May Be to Blame. Available online: https://www.independent.co.uk/news/uk/politics/churches-unite-to-act-on-food-poverty-600-leaders-from-all-denominations-demand-government-u-turn-on-9263035.html (accessed on 27 December 2018).

32.   Sosenko, F.; Livingstone, N.; Fitzpatrick, S. *Overview of Food Aid Provision in Scotland*; Scottish Government: Edinburgh, UK, 2013.

33.   Trust, T. UK Food Bank Use Continues to Rise. 2017. Available online: https://www.trusselltrust.org/2017/04/25/uk-foodbank-use-continues-rise/ (accessed on 6 August 2018).

34.   Bazerghi, C.; McKay, F.H.; Dunn, M. The role of food banks in addressing food insecurity: A systematic review. *J. Community Health* **2016**, *41*, 732–740. [CrossRef]

35.   Loopstra, R.; Tarasuk, V. The relationship between food banks and household food insecurity among low-income Toronto families. *Can. Public Policy* **2012**, *38*, 497–514. [CrossRef]

36.   Loopstra, R.; Tarasuk, V. Food bank usage is a poor indicator of food insecurity: Insights from Canada. *Soc. Policy Soc.* **2015**, *14*, 443–455. [CrossRef]

37.   Food Foundation. *Household Food Insecurity: The Missing Data*; The Food Foundation: London, UK, 2016.

38.   Iafrati, S. "We're not a bottomless pit": Food banks' capacity to sustainably meet increasing demand. *Volunt. Sect. Rev.* **2018**, *9*, 39–53. [CrossRef]

39.   Poppendieck, J. *Sweet Charity?: Emergency Food and the End of Entitlement*; Penguin: London, UK, 1999.

40.   Crossley, T.F.; Low, H.; O'Dea, C. Household consumption through recent recessions. *Fisc. Stud.* **2013**, *34*, 203–229. [CrossRef]

41.   Griffith, R.; O'Connell, M.; Smith, K. *Food Expenditure and Nutritional Quality over the Great Recession*; IFS Briefing Note BN143; Institute of Fiscal Studies: London, UK, 2013.

42.   Adams, N.; Carr, J.; Collins, J. *Households Below average Income: An Analysis of the Income Distribtution, 1994/95 to 2010/11*; Department for Work and Pensions: London, UK, 2012.

43.   McGuinness, F. *Poverty in the UK: Statistics*; House of Commons Library: London, UK, 2018.

44.   McClements, L.D. Equivalence scales for children. *J. Public Econ.* **1977**, *8*, 191–210. [CrossRef]

45.   UK Data Service. General Lifestyle Survey. 2017. Available online: https://discover.ukdataservice.ac.uk/series/?sn=200019 (accessed on 5 April 2017).

46.   Eurostat. European Union Statistics on Income and Living Conditions EU-SILC. 2017. Available online: http://ec.europa.eu/eurostat/web/microdata/european-union-statistics-on-income-and-living-conditions (accessed on 5 April 2017).

47.   Service, U.D. Family Resources Survey. 2017. Available online: https://discover.ukdataservice.ac.uk/series/?sn=200017 (accessed on 5 April 2017).

48.   Kantar. Kantar World Panel. 2017. Available online: https://www.kantarworldpanel.com/global/Consumer-Panels (accessed on 5 April 2017).

49.   Department for Environment, Food and Rural Affairs. Living Costs and Food Survey. 2015. Available online: https://www.ons.gov.uk/file?uri=/peoplepopulationandcommunity/personalandhouseholdfinances/incomeandwealth/methodologies/livingcostsandfoodsurvey/livingcostsfoodtechnicalreport2015.pdf (accessed on 5 November 2017).

50.   Scottish Health Survey. 2015. Available online: http://discover.ukdataservice.ac.uk/series/?sn=2000047 (accessed on 27 December 2018).

51.   Scottish Government. Scottish Household Survey—Survey Details. 2009. Available online: http://www.gov.scot/Topics/Statistics/16002/Methodology (accessed on 27 December 2018).

52. Food Standards Agency. The Eatwell Plate. Available online: https://www.gov.uk/government/publications/the-eatwell-guide (accessed on 25 March 2014).

53. Barton, K.L.; Wrieden, W.L.; Sherriff, A.; Armstrong, J.; Anderson, A.S. Trends in socio-economic inequalities in the Scottish diet: 2001–2009. *Public Health Nutr.* **2015**, *18*, 2970–2980. [CrossRef] [PubMed]

54. Wrieden, W.; Armstrong, J.; Anderson, A.; Sherriff, A.; Barton, K. Choosing the best method to estimate the energy density of a population using food purchase data. *J. Hum. Nutr. Diet.* **2015**, *28*, 126–134. [CrossRef] [PubMed]

55. Wrieden, W.L.; Armstrong, J.; Sherriff, A.; Anderson, A.S.; Barton, K.L. Slow pace of dietary change in Scotland: 2001–2009. *Br. J. Nutr.* **2013**, *109*, 1892–1902. [CrossRef] [PubMed]

56. Office for National Statistics. *Living Costs and Food Survey. User Guide Volume A—Introduction*; Office for National Statistics: Newport, UK, 2013.

57. Scottish Government. *Revised Dietary Goals*; Scottish Government: Edinburgh, UK, 2013.

58. Barton, K.L. An Exploratory Analysis of the Scottish Diet 2001–2009 Using Household Purchase Data. Ph.D. Thesis, Universtiy of Dundee, Dundee, UK, 2014.

59. Armstrong, J.; Sherriff, A.; Wrieden, W.L.; Brogan, Y.; Barton, K.L. *Deriving and Interpreting Dietary Patterns in the Scottish Diet: Further Analysis of the Scottish Health Survey and Expenditure and Food Survey*; Food Standards scotland: Aberdeen, UK, 2009.

60. Waijers, P.M.; Feskens, E.J.; Ocké, M.C. A critical review of predefined diet quality scores. *Bri. J. Nutr.* **2007**, *97*, 219–231. [CrossRef]

61. Guenther, P.M.; Kirkpatrick, S.I.; Reedy, J.; Krebs-Smith, S.M.; Buckman, D.W.; Dodd, K.W.; Casavale, K.O.; Carroll, R.J. The Healthy Eating Index-2010 Is a Valid and Reliable Measure of Diet Quality According to the 2010 Dietary Guidelines for Americans1–3. *J. Nutr.* **2013**, *144*, 399–407. [CrossRef]

62. Department for Environment, Food & Rural Affairs. *Family Food*; Department for Environment, Food & Rural Affairs: London, UK, 2012.

63. Department for Environment, Food & Rural Affairs. *Food Statistics in Your Pocket 2017: Prices and Expenditure*; Department for Environment, Food & Rural Affairs: London, UK, 2018.

64. Thompson, S. *The Low-Pay, No-Pay Cycle*; Joseph Rowntree Foundation: York, UK, 2015.

65. Food Standards Scotland. *The Scottish Diet Needs to Change: Situation Report Update*; Food Standards Scotland: Aberdeen, UK, 2018.

66. Douglas, F.; Ejebu, O.Z.; Garcia, A.; MacKenzie, F.; Whybrow, S.; McKenzie, L.; Ludbrook, A.; Dowler, E. *The Nature and Extent of Food Poverty in Scotland*; NHS Health Scotland: Glasgow, UK, 2015.

67. Nevarez, L.; Tobin, K.; Waltermaurer, E. Food Acquisition in Poughkeepsie, NY: Exploring the Stratification of "Healthy Food" Consciousness in a Food-Insecure City. *Food Cult. Soc.* **2016**, *19*, 19–44. [CrossRef]

68. Tarasuk, V. A critical examination of community-based responses to household food insecurity in Canada. *Health Educ. Behav.* **2001**, *28*, 487–499. [CrossRef] [PubMed]

69. Hamelin, A.-M.; Mercier, C.; Bédard, A. Discrepancies in households and other stakeholders viewpoints on the food security experience: A gap to address. *Health Educ. Res.* **2009**, *25*, 401–412. [CrossRef] [PubMed]

70. Hamelin, A.M.; Mercier, C.; Bédard, A. Needs for food security from the standpoint of Canadian households participating and not participating in community food programmes. *Int. J. Consum. Stud.* **2011**, *35*, 58–68. [CrossRef]

71. Harden, J.; Dickson, A. Low-income mothers' food practices with young children: A qualitative longitudinal study. *Health Educ. J.* **2015**, *74*, 381–391. [CrossRef]

72. Douglas, F.; Sapko, J.; Kiezebrink, K.; Kyle, J. Resourcefulness, desperation, shame, gratitude and powerlessness: Common themes emerging from a study of food bank use in northeast Scotland. *AIMS Public Health* **2015**, *2*, 297–317. [CrossRef] [PubMed]

73. Douglas, F.; MacKenzie, F.; Ejebu, O.-Z.; Whybrow, S.; Garcia, A.L.; McKenzie, L.; Ludbrook, A.; Dowler, E. "A Lot of People Are Struggling Privately. They Don't Know Where to Go or They're Not Sure of What to Do": Frontline Service Provider Perspectives of the Nature of Household Food Insecurity in Scotland. *Int. J. Environ. Res. Public Health* **2018**, *15*, 2738. [CrossRef]

74. Scottish Government. *Severe Poverty in Scotland*; Scottish Government: Edinburgh, UK, 2015.

75. Scottish Government. *Poverty and Income Inequality in Scotland 2009–10*; Scottish Government: Edinburgh, UK, 2015.

76. Hirsch, D.; Bryan, A.; Davis, A.; Smith, N. *A Minimum Income Standard for Remote and Rural Scotland*; Highlands and Islands Enterprise: Inverness, UK, 2013.

77. ScotCen Social Research. *Scottish Health Survey, 2012: User Guide*; Scottish Government: Edinburgh, UK, 2013.

78. Fafard, A.-A.; Tarasuk, V. Shelter Expenditures Increase Vulnerability to Household Food Insecurity. *FASEB J.* **2015**, *29*, 261.6.

79. Sriram, U.; Tarasuk, V. Economic predictors of household food insecurity in Canadian metropolitan areas. *J. Hunger Environ. Nutr.* **2016**, *11*, 1–13. [CrossRef]

80. Alston, P. Statement on Visit to the United Kingdom, by Professor Philip Alston, United Nations Special Rapporteur on Extreme Poverty and Human Rights. 2018. Available online: https://www.ohchr.org/EN/NewsEvents/Pages/DisplayNews.aspx?NewsID=23881&LangID=E (accessed on 14 December 2018).

81. UNICEF. *Building the Future: Children and the Sustainable Development Goals in Rich Countries*; UNICEF: New York, NY, USA, 2017.

82. Kirkpatrick, S.I.; McIntyre, L.; Potestio, M.L. Child hunger and long-term adverse consequences for health. *Arch. Pediatr. Adolesc. Med.* **2010**, *164*, 754–762. [CrossRef]

83. Seligman, H.K.; Laraia, B.A.; Kushel, M.B. Food insecurity is associated with chronic disease among low-income NHANES participants. *J. Nutr.* **2009**, *140*, 304–310. [CrossRef]

84. Gowda, C.; Hadley, C.; Aiello, A.E. The association between food insecurity and inflammation in the US adult population. *Am. J. Public Health* **2012**, *102*, 1579–1586. [CrossRef] [PubMed]

85. Marques, E.S.; Reichenheim, M.E.; de Moraes, C.L.; Antunes, M.M.; Salles-Costa, R. Household food insecurity: A systematic review of the measuring instruments used in epidemiological studies. *Public Health Nutr.* **2015**, *18*, 877–892. [CrossRef]

86. Muldoon, K.A.; Duff, P.K.; Fielden, S.; Anema, A. Food insufficiency is associated with psychiatric morbidity in a nationally representative study of mental illness among food insecure Canadians. *Soc. Psychiatry Psychiatr. Epidemiol.* **2013**, *48*, 795–803. [CrossRef] [PubMed]

87. Fitzpatrick, T.; Rosella, L.C.; Calzavara, A.; Petch, J.; Pinto, A.D.; Manson, H.; Goel, V.; Wodchis, W.P. Looking beyond income and education: Socioeconomic status gradients among future high-cost users of health care. *Am. J. Prev. Med.* **2015**, *49*, 161–171. [CrossRef]

88. Seligman, H.K.; Davis, T.C.; Schillinger, D.; Wolf, M.S. Food insecurity is associated with hypoglycemia and poor diabetes self-management in a low-income sample with diabetes. *J. Health Care Poor Underserved* **2010**, *21*, 1227–1233. [PubMed]

89. Chan, J.; DeMelo, M.; Gingras, J.; Gucciardi, E. Challenges of diabetes self-management in adults affected by food insecurity in a large urban centre of Ontario, Canada. *Int. J. Endocrinol.* **2015**, *2015*, 903468. [CrossRef] [PubMed]

90. Tarasuk, V.; Cheng, J.; de Oliveira, C.; Dachner, N.; Gundersen, C.; Kurdyak, P. Association between household food insecurity and annual health care costs. *Can. Med. Assoc. J.* **2015**, *187*, 429–436. [CrossRef] [PubMed]

91. All-Party Parliamentary Inquiry into Hunger in the United Kingdom. *Feeding Britain: A Strategy for Zero Hunger in England, Wales, Scotland and Northern Ireland*; Children's Society: London, UK, 2014.

92. Scottish Food Comission. *Scottish Food Commission Interim Report*; Scottish Food Comission: Edinburgh, UK, 2016.

93. Scottish Government. *Dignity: Ending Hunger Together in Scotland—The Report of the Independent Working Group on Food Poverty*; Scottish Government: Edinburgh, UK, 2016.

94. Cafiero, C.; Nord, M.; Viviani, S. *Methods for Estimating Comparable Prevalence Rates of Food Insecurity Experienced by Adults throughout the World*; IOP Publishing: Bristol, UK, 2016.

95. Observatory, S.P.H. Scottish Health Survey. 2016. Available online: http://www.scotpho.org.uk/publications/overview-of-key-data-sources/surveys-cross-sectional/scottish-health-survey (accessed on 17 July 2017).

96. Tait, C. *Hungry for Change: The Final Report of the Fabian Commission on Food and Poverty*; Fabian Society: London, UK, 2015.

97. Nelson, M.; Erens, B.; Bates, B.; Church, S.; Boshier, T. *Low Income Diet and Nutrition Survey*; TSO: London, UK, 2007; Volume 3.

98.   Agency, F.S. 'Food and You' Survey Wave 4. 2017. Available online: https://www.food.gov.uk/science/research-reports/ssresearch/foodandyou (accessed on 28 March 2017).

99.   Machin, R.J. Understanding holiday hunger. *J. Poverty Soc. Justice* **2016**, *24*, 311–319. [CrossRef]

100.   Cook, J.T.; Frank, D.A. Food security, poverty, and human development in the United States. *Ann. N. Y. Acad. Sci.* **2008**, *1136*, 193–209. [CrossRef]

Healthy Diets in Rural Victoria—Cheaper than Unhealthy Alternatives, yet Unaffordable

Penelope Love [1,2,*][iD], Jillian Whelan [3][iD], Colin Bell [3][iD], Felicity Grainger [2], Cherie Russell [1,2][iD], Meron Lewis [4] and Amanda Lee [4,5]

[1] Institute for Physical Activity and Nutrition (IPAN), Deakin University, Geelong 3220, Australia; caru@deakin.edu.au
[2] School of Exercise and Nutrition Sciences, Deakin University, Geelong 3220, Australia; fgrainge@deakin.edu.au
[3] School of Medicine, Global Obesity Centre, Deakin University, Geelong 3220, Australia; jill.whelan@deakin.edu.au (J.W.); colin.bell@deakin.edu.au (C.B.)
[4] The Australian Prevention Partnership Centre (TAPPC), Sax Institute, Sydney 2007, Australia; meron.lewis@saxinstitute.org.au (M.L.); amanda.lee@saxinstitute.org.au (A.L.)
[5] School of Public Health, University of Queensland, Herston QLD 4006, Australia
* Correspondence: penny.love@deakin.edu.au

Abstract: Rural communities experience higher rates of obesity and reduced food security compared with urban communities. The perception that healthy foods are expensive contributes to poor dietary choices. Providing an accessible, available, affordable healthy food supply is an equitable way to improve the nutritional quality of the diet for a community, however, local food supply data are rarely available for small rural towns. This study used the Healthy Diets ASAP tool to assess price, price differential and affordability of recommended (healthy) and current diets in a rural Local Government Area (LGA) (pop ≈ 7000; 10 towns) in Victoria, Australia. All retail food outlets were surveyed (*n* = 40). The four most populous towns had supermarkets; remaining towns had one general store each. Seven towns had café/take-away outlets, and all towns had at least one hotel/pub. For all towns the current unhealthy diet was more expensive than the recommended healthy diet, with 59.5% of the current food budget spent on discretionary items. Affordability of the healthy diet accounted for 30–32% of disposable income. This study confirms that while a healthy diet is less expensive than the current unhealthier diet, affordability is a challenge for rural communities. Food security is reduced further with restricted geographical access, a limited healthy food supply, and higher food prices.

Keywords: Healthy Diets ASAP tool; food security; food prices; diet affordability; rural communities; INFORMAS

1. Introduction

'If it's not available or you cannot afford it, then you cannot eat it even if you wanted to!'. [1] (p. 363)

The cost of food and the financial resources to procure it are key economic determinants of food choice [1]. Food security is defined as the physical, social and economic access to a stable and safe food supply, in sufficient quantity and quality to meet dietary needs and food preferences, within an environment that supports a healthy and active lifestyle [2]. In high income countries, like Australia, people identified as being most at risk for food insecurity have typically been those on low incomes, experiencing homelessness, refugees and migrants, and Aboriginal and Torres Strait Islander communities [3]. More recently, however, households on middle incomes, experiencing financial stress, have been identified as food insecure [3]. The national food insecurity prevalence of 4% [4] for Australia is therefore considered an underestimation, with predictions of 10–25% of households in some areas being food insecure [3].

The link between food insecurity and overweight/obesity [5] is of particular concern given the global prevalence of this complex public health problem [6]. In Australia, 25% of children and 63% of adults are overweight/obese [4], with rural Australian communities generally experiencing higher rates of obesity and decreased food security than their urban counterparts [7]. Despite having a higher disease burden, rural communities in Australia are frequently overlooked and under-researched regarding prevention, and therefore less informed about appropriate solutions. Providing an accessible, available and affordable healthy food supply is a well-established [8,9] and equitable way to improve the nutritional quality of food consumed by a community or population [10].

Unhealthy diets, and associated overweight/obesity, are now the major preventable risk factor contributing to the burden of disease [11], yet adherence to the Australian Dietary Guidelines is poor [12]. Unhealthy diets are caused by a range of complex and inter-related determinants including 'obesogenic' food environments, defined as an environment that promotes weight gain and hinders weight loss, affecting food promotion, availability, accessibility and affordability [9]. A key determinant is the perception that healthy diets are expensive and a barrier to the purchase of healthier foods [13]. Increased food prices, poorer quality produce and a limited variety of healthier options are primary contributors to food insecurity for Australian households [14]. The price and affordability of a healthy diet is of particular concern for rural communities where geographic location and low population density pose significant challenges for the food supply chain, resulting in an infrequent supply of healthy food to at risk communities [15], often of poorer quality [16] and less varied in terms of product brand, size and type [17,18]. A lack of infrastructure in these areas with low-density transport networks and high car dependency also make access to food outlets more difficult than in larger towns and cities [15].

Food pricing information in Australia has most commonly been collected using "healthy food basket" (HFB) methodology, using a predefined list of indicator food items representative of the total diet for different reference households [13]. Different HFB methodology exists across Australian States and Territories, with Victoria using the Victorian Healthy Food Basket (VHFB) comprising 44 listed food items. The VHFB approach poses limitations for small rural towns with food stores that often do not meet the inclusion criterion to stock at least 90% of the listed food items [19] as well as not including generic food product brands which are becoming increasingly prominent in Australian food stores [20].

The recent development of the Healthy Diets Australian Standardised Affordability and Price (ASAP) tool, through the global INFORMAS (International Network for Food and Obesity/non-communicable diseases Research, Monitoring and Action Support) network, may overcome these challenges. The Healthy Diets ASAP tool seeks to provide a standardised method to assess and compare the price and affordability of the recommended Australian diet with the current Australian diet [21–23], to enable informed community specific food supply decisions. The Healthy Diets ASAP tool comprises 76 food items [23] indicative of the recommended Australian diet (based on the quantitative modelled Foundation Diets within the Australian Dietary Guidelines) [24] and the current Australian diet (based on reported dietary intakes within the Australian Health Survey 2011–2012) [25]. Food item prices ($n = 43$), adjusted for edible proportion, representative of the recommended Australian diet encompass the five food groups (fruit; vegetables and legumes; grain/cereal foods; meats, poultry, fish and alternatives; milk, yoghurt, cheese and alternatives); and unsaturated oils and spreads. Additional food item prices ($n = 33$) representative of the current Australian diet include discretionary high in saturated fats, sugars, salt and/or alcohol (described as energy dense) and considered not necessary as part of a healthy diet. Discretionary items include cakes, biscuits, pastries, pies; chocolate, confectionary, ice confections; butter, cream, spreads which contain predominantly saturated fats; potato chips, crisps and other fatty or salty snack foods; sugar-sweetened soft drinks and cordials; sports and energy drinks; and alcoholic drinks) [24] (p. 144).

This study assessed and compared the price, price differential (relative price) and affordability of the recommended Australian diet (as defined by the Australian Dietary Guidelines) and the current Australian diet (as described by the Australian Health Survey) for a small rural Local Government Area in Victoria, Australia. Ethical approval for this study was obtained through Deakin University (HEAG-H 80_2016).

2. Materials and Methods

2.1. Study Context and Selection of Study Site

The LGA selected for this study was determined by its rurality, modifiable chronic disease risk factor profile, and limited exposure to State-funded health promotion/obesity prevention initiatives.

The study LGA is predominately a rural area, growing mainly wheat, barley, oilseeds and legumes, and grazing sheep [26]. Geographically classified as remote (population size 5000–10,000), the LGA is described as having moderate accessibility based on minimum road distance from populated localities to nearest service centres [27]. At the time of this study, the LGA had a total population of 6674 residents across 7158 km^2, comprising one main town (≈2300 residents), eight small towns (≈130 to 800 residents) and eight smaller localities (<100 residents) [26]. The LGA is subdivided into three wards (north, central, south) defined by electoral boundaries, influencing the provision of services and creating three distinct community hubs within the LGA. The LGA scores below the regional State average on the Index of Relative Disadvantage, with up to 59% of families in some towns on low incomes; a high proportion of people aged over 65 and people with a disability; and high levels of social isolation [28,29]. Compared with State averages, the LGA experiences a high prevalence of overweight (38.3% vs. Victorian average 31.2%) and obesity (38.3% vs. Victorian average 18.8%); low fruit and vegetable consumption (4.5% vs. Victorian average 5.2%); high sugar sweetened beverage consumption (30.3% vs. Victorian average 15.9%); high take-away meal consumption (80.9% eating takeaway once per week vs. Victorian average 71.2%); and similar levels of food insecurity (4.6%) [30].

2.2. Selection of Data Collection Tool

The Healthy Diets ASAP tool was used to collect food pricing information (Supplementary File S1) [21,23] for the recommended Australian diet, defined by the Australian Dietary Guidelines (ADG) [24], and the current Australian diet, described by the Australian Health Survey (AHS) [25] (Table 1). The current Australian diet is comparable with that reported for the study LGA [30]; namely; low daily fruit consumption (LGA 1.3 serves vs. AHS 1.2 serves vs. ADG 2 serves); low daily vegetable consumption (LGA 2.5 serves vs. AHS 2.7 serves vs. ADG 5 serves).

Table 1. Comparison of the recommended and current Australian diets for males and females (19–50 years) [12].

Food Groupings (Recommended Serves/Day)	Australian Dietary Guidelines—Recommended Dietary Intakes		Australian Health Survey—Current Dietary Intakes	
	Males	Females	Males	Females
Bread and Cereals	6	6	5.2	3.7
Fruit	2	2	1.2	1.1
Vegetables	6	5	2.8	2.7
Dairy	2.5	2.5	1.6	1.3
Meat and alternatives	3	2.5	2.2	1.6
Discretionary items	0	0	6.4	4.2

2.3. Selection of Retail Food Outlets

Thirty-nine retail food outlets (supermarkets, general stores, bakeries, take-away outlets, cafes, hotels/pubs and service stations) were identified across the LGA using the community directory available on the LGA website. Validation of these business listings, using 'ground truthing' (physically viewing and recording of outlets) [31], identified that three outlets had closed and four new outlets had opened. All outlets operating at the time of the study were surveyed ($n = 40$). These outlets were located across ten towns within the LGA.

2.4. Data Collection

Assistance was provided by AL and ML regarding the use of the Healthy Diets ASAP tool protocols [23] and data were collected by four researchers, working in pairs (PL, JW, FG, CR), within one week in June 2017. As per protocol, within each town, all supermarkets and general stores were surveyed first, followed by bakeries, take-away outlets, cafes, hotels/pubs, and service stations. Permission to participate was obtained verbally from each outlet manager immediately prior to data collection, with all outlets agreeing to participate. Data collected included usual price for specified brands and sizes; sale/special promotion price if usual price was unavailable; price of cheapest brand if specified brand was unavailable; price of nearest larger size (or nearest smaller size) if specified size was unavailable; and cheapest usual price for loose fresh produce. Alternate product brand names and sizes were recorded. Unavailable items were cross checked with outlet managers to determine if out of stock or never stocked. Information for out of stock items was provided by outlet managers, and never stocked items were recorded as missing.

2.5. Data Entry

Eleven data sheets were compiled representing the main town with two supermarkets, and the nine smaller towns each with one supermarket or general store. Data entry was done by F.G. and C.R. with all entries cross-checked by PL and JW. As per protocol, missing items within an outlet were allocated the mean price for that item from all other outlets across the LGA.; and price conversions were calculated for alternate product sizes. The Healthy Diets ASAP tool uses the reference household of two parents (one full-time employed; one part-time employed) and two children (boy aged 14 years; girl aged 8 years). Median disposable family income for this reference household was derived from recent census data for the LGA, calculated at $AUD2358/fortnight [26]. Using the Healthy Diets ASAP tool protocol, indicative minimum disposable income for this reference household was calculated based on minimum wage rates, family tax benefits and relevant welfare payments derived from the Australian Government Department of Human Services [32], calculated at $AUD2167.24/fortnight as detailed in Table 2. The LGA scores below the regional State average on the Index of Relative Disadvantage [28] with only 7.3% of households on high incomes [26].

2.6. Data Analysis

Data were analysed to explore price differential and affordability of the recommended diet and current diet for the reference household for the whole LGA; by ward (south, central and north); and each town within the LGA. Mean food prices were used for whole of LGA and by ward analyses. Price differentials were compared using the following metrics: total diet; each of the five food groups (fruit; vegetables/legumes; grains/cereals; meats/nuts/seeds/eggs; and milk/yoghurt/cheese); unsaturated oils/spreads; discretionary items (take-away foods, soft drinks, alcoholic beverages). Data were also entered into SPSS version 25 and Wilcoxon-signed ranks test were used to compare total diet costs between towns, and between the northern, central and southern areas of the LGA. Affordability of the recommended diet and current diet was calculated as a proportion of household income using median and indicative minimum disposable incomes for an average and low income household, respectively.

Table 2. Low income household calculations ($AUD) for reference household of two parents with two children within the Local Government Area (adult male; adult female; boy 14 years; girl 8 years).

Assumptions [a]	Fortnightly Income	
The family is privately renting a 3 bedroom house at $130/week	Paid employment—adult male	$1390.04
The adult male works on a permanent basis at national minimum wage * ($18.29/h) for 38 h/week	Paid employment—adult female	$219.00
The adult female works on a part-time basis at national minimum wage * ($18.29/h) for 6 h/week	Family Tax Benefit A ^	$420.70
Both children attend school and are fully immunised	Family Tax Benefit A supplement	$55.87
None of the family are disabled	Family Tax Benefit B ^^	$108.64
The family have some emergency savings that earn negligible interest	Family Tax Benefit B Supplement	$13.62
The family has negligible tax deductions	Clean Energy Supplement	$9.94
	Rent Assistance **	$132.61
	INCOME TAX PAID #	−$185.66
	TOTAL FORTNIGHTLY INCOME	**$2167.24**

[a] Verification of assumptions: https://profile.id.com.au/; * Minimum Wage: https://www.fairwork.gov.au/how-we-will-help/templates-and-guides/fact-sheets/minimum-workplace-entitlements/minimum-wages. # current-national-minimum-wage; ^ Family Tax A: https://www.humanservices.gov.au/customer/enablers/payment-rates-family-tax-benefit-part; ^^ Family Tax B: https://www.humanservices.gov.au/customer/enablers/payment-rates-family-tax-benefit-part-b; ** Rent Assistance: Full amount of rent assistance paid to couple with 1 or 2 children if rent is >$436.19 per fortnight, minimum rent is $229.8/fortnight. Full amount is $155.26/fortnight. Rent assistance is paid at the rate of 75 cents for every dollar of rent paid in excess of that threshold up to the maximum rate applicable to the person. Rental at $260/fortnight; rent assistance = 155.26 − [260 − 229.80 × 0.75] = $132.61 https://www.humanservices.gov.au/individuals/enablers/how-much-rent-assistance-you-can-get; # Income tax paid: (income tax due + income tax offset + remote area tax offset) => −5147.45 + 372.29 + 0 = $4775.16; Annual income tax due: tax bracket >$37,000 − $87,000 => $3572 plus 32.5c for each $1 over $37,000; Annual income at $41,847.52; Tax paid = 3572 + [(41,847.52 − 37,000.00) × 0.325] = $5147.45; Annual income tax offset: available if taxable income is <$66,667. Maximum tax offset of $445 applies if taxable income is $37,000 or less. This amount is reduced by 1.5 cents for each dollar over $37,000. Annual income at $41847.52; Tax offset = 445 − [(41,847.52 − 37,000.00) × 0.015] = $372.29 https://www.ato.gov.au/individuals/income-and-deductions/offsets-and-rebates/low-income-earners/.

3. Results

Forty retail food outlets were included in the study, located across 10 towns, and categorized as supermarkets ($n = 5$), general stores ($n = 6$), bakeries ($n = 2$), take-away outlets ($n = 6$), cafés ($n = 7$), hotels/pubs ($n = 12$) and service stations ($n = 2$) (Table 3). The majority of outlets ($n = 14$) were in the main town, with a range of 2–5 outlets in the smaller towns. Supermarkets were located in four towns; two in the main town and one each in the three next most populated towns. General stores were located in the six remaining towns. All towns had at least one hotel/pub, and the majority of towns had a café and/or take-away outlet. Three towns, all with populations less than 150, had no cafés or take-away outlets (Figure 1).

Pricing for the recommended and current diets, using the reference household, are presented for the whole LGA, and the southern, central and northern communities of the LGA in Figure 2 and Appendix A. Figure 2 also illustrates the contribution of the cost of component food groups to total diet costs. Data for each town is available in Supplementary File S2.

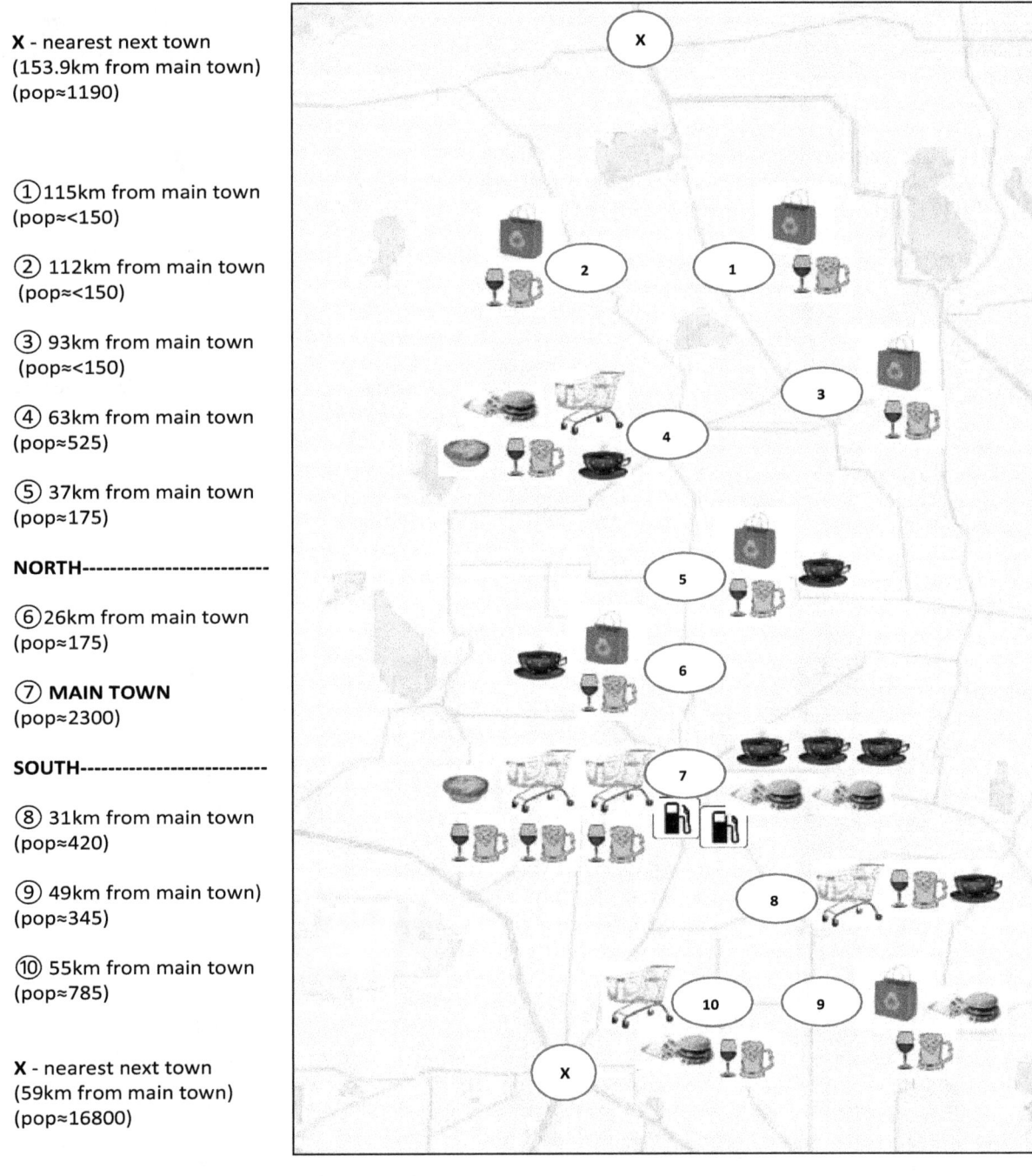

X - nearest next town
(153.9km from main town)
(pop≈1190)

① 115km from main town
(pop≈<150)

② 112km from main town
(pop≈<150)

③ 93km from main town
(pop≈<150)

④ 63km from main town
(pop≈525)

⑤ 37km from main town
(pop≈175)

NORTH------------------------

⑥ 26km from main town
(pop≈175)

⑦ **MAIN TOWN**
(pop≈2300)

SOUTH------------------------

⑧ 31km from main town
(pop≈420)

⑨ 49km from main town)
(pop≈345)

⑩ 55km from main town
(pop≈785)

X - nearest next town
(59km from main town)
(pop≈16800)

LEGEND:
Supermarket   **General Store**   **Service Station**   **Bakery**

Take-away   **Hotel/Pub**   **Café**   **pop = population of town**

(x)   **Nearest town outside LGA boundary**   (#)   **Town in LGA (km from main town in LGA)**

Figure 1. Distribution of food retail outlets across ten towns within the Local Government Area indicating type of outlet and distance (km) of towns from the main town (https://www.google.com/maps).

Table 3. Number and type of retail food outlet surveyed across the Local Government Area (LGA).

Retail Food Outlet by Town		Super-Market [a]	General Store [b]	Bakery	Take-Away	Café	Hotel/Pub	Service Station	Total Outlets by Town
North of LGA	Town 1		1				1		2
	Town 2		1				1		2
	Town 3		1				1		2
	Town 4	1		1	1	1	1		5
	Town 5		1			1	1		3
Centre of LGA	Town 6		1			1	1		3
	Town 7	2		1	3	3	3	2	14
South of LGA	Town 8	1				1	1		3
	Town 9		1		1		1		3
	Town 10	1			1		1		3
Total Outlets by Type		5	6	2	6	7	12	2	40

[a] Supermarket—chain store, selling food products predominantly, open for extended hours on most day; [b] General stores—privately owned, selling food products and other items, open for limited hours.

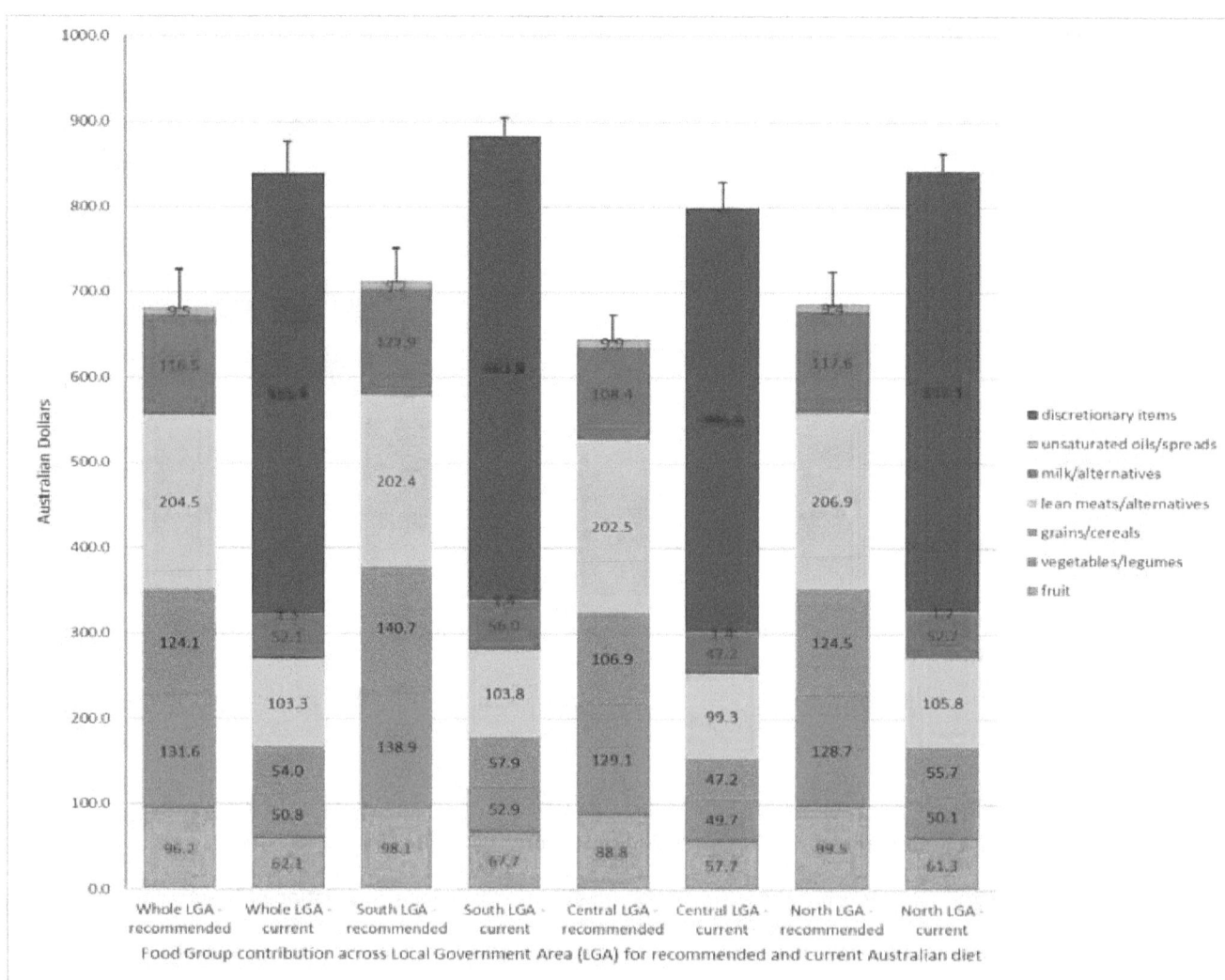

Figure 2. Food group contribution and total diet costs for recommended and current diets for the Local Government Area ($AUDmean ± SD per fortnight).

Across the LGA, the recommended diet was cheaper than the current diet ($AUD702.41 ± 44.80 vs. $AUD866.19 ± 37.54 per fortnight/reference household), costing an average 81.1% of the current diet budget. Within the current diet, expenditure for all five food groups was less than half what would be required to achieve recommended intakes of these foods; namely, fruit and vegetables (13% current vs. 32% required); grains/cereal-based foods (6.2% current vs. 17.7% required); lean meats, poultry, fish, eggs (11.9% current vs. 29.1% required); and milk, cheese, yoghurt (6.0% vs. 16.6%). The majority of the current diet budget was spent on discretionary items (59.5%), particularly take-away foods/beverages (18.1%) and alcoholic beverages (11.2%).

For each of the three LGA wards, the recommended diet was cheaper than the current diet, costing an average 81.3% of the current diet budget for southern and northern wards, and an average of 80.4% for central towns (Supplementary File S2). Food item prices were higher in the southern (8.7%) and northern (5.5%) towns than the central towns in the LGA. Food item prices in the southern towns were highest for four of the five food groups (especially fruits, grains, and milk, cheese and yoghurt); take-away food items were the most expensive (approximately 12–13%); and sugar-sweetened beverages were the cheapest. For towns in the centre of the LGA, take-away food items were the cheapest and sugar-sweetened beverages the most expensive (approximately 19–23%). For both the southern and northern towns, price differences were greatest for grains (approximately 15–19%) and milk, cheese and yoghurt (approximately 10–16%) than the other five food groups.

Across the LGA the cost of the current diet was statistically significantly higher than the recommended diet at $p < 0.05$. There were no significant differences between the three LGA wards.

Affordability of the recommended and current diets was calculated using median and indicative minimum disposable incomes for an average and low income household, respectively (Table 4). Across the LGA, the recommended diet ($AUD702.41 ± 44.80/fortnight/reference household) would expend 30–32% of a median and low income household, respectively; and the current diet ($AUD866.19 ± 37.54/fortnight/reference household) would expend 37–40% of a median and low income household. Affordability of the recommended diet as a proportion of household income was similar for the southern and northern towns, approximately 2% higher than towns in the centre of the LGA.

Availability of food items listed on the Healthy Diets ASAP tool protocol ($n = 76$) varied across the ten towns within the LGA. All items were available within the main town, which had two supermarkets and twelve other food retail outlets. Towns with supermarkets appeared to have fewer missing food items (3–12 missing items) compared to towns with only a general store (18–38 missing items). Most commonly missing food items were low fat yoghurt and low fat cheese (available only in the main town); cooked whole chicken (available in two towns); canned sweetcorn (no added salt) and extra virgin olive oil (both available in three towns); and unsalted peanuts (available in four towns). Yoghurt (full or reduced fat) was unavailable in five towns. Specific product brands and product sizes were unavailable for 36 (47%) and 43 (75%) of the listed food items, respectively, requiring substitution with price of cheapest brand and price of nearest larger (or nearest smaller) size. As per protocol, missing items within an outlet were allocated the mean price for that item from all other outlets across the LGA, thereby minimizing effects to food budget calculations.

Table 4. Affordability (% household income) of the recommended diet and current diet across the Local Government Area (LGA) for the reference household by median and low income ($AUD).

LGA Area and Town	Median Household Income ($2358)		Low Household Income ($2167)	
	Recommended Diet (%)	Current Diet (%)	Recommended Diet (%)	Current Diet (%)
Whole of LGA	30	37	32	40
Town 1	28	36	30	39
Town 2	28	37	31	40
Town 3	32	37	35	41
Town 4	30	32	33	34
Town 5	32	38	34	42
North of the LGA	30	37	33	40
Town 6	27	35	30	38
Town 7	27–30	33–36	30–32	36–40
Centre of the LGA	28	35	31	38
Town 8	31	37	33	40
Town 9	33	39	36	42
Town 10	29	39	32	42
South of the LGA	30	37	32	40

4. Discussion

This study assessed the price, price differential (relative price) and affordability of the recommended and current diets in a small rural LGA in Victoria, Australia. Study findings confirm the paradoxical co-existence of food insecurity, low income and obesity, linked to limited geographical access to a healthy, fresh food supply; limited variety of healthy food options; the ubiquitous availability of highly palatable energy-dense foods, drinks and discretionary items; higher overall food prices; and low incomes reducing affordability of a healthy diet.

Findings suggest that a healthy diet, consistent with national dietary guidelines, is less expensive than the current diet consumed by Australians. For some rural towns, this differential may be as much as 18.9%. The Healthy Diets ASAP tool has only recently been used within Australia, with available studies of the pilot approach limited to urban areas reporting a finding of 16.3% for a low income household [21]. These findings challenge the perception that a healthy diet is more expensive, as described in a systematic review of food pricing studies across 10 countries (excluding Australia) [33] which found little difference between the cost of healthier and unhealthy dietary patterns. As explained by Lewis and Lee [13], studies included in this review did not consider the contribution of alcoholic beverages or most other discretionary items[1] to the cost of the diet nor the application of a goods and sales tax (GST) exemption to certain food items. The inclusion of discretionary items is important in the Australian context, as over a third (35%) of the total daily intake of Australians comprises discretionary items in the form of biscuits, cakes, confectionary, sugar-sweetened beverages and alcoholic beverages [12]. Additionally Australia applies a 10% GST exemption to basic, healthy foods in the five food groups such as fruit, vegetables, bread, fresh meat, eggs and milk [34], increasing the affordability of these food items.

On average the income of Australian families in rural and remote areas is 15–20% lower than in metropolitan areas, which together with higher food prices in these areas, makes it difficult to afford a healthy diet [15]. While purchasing a recommended diet may be less expensive than the current diet, findings from this study highlight that it would account for almost a third of the budget for median (30%) and low (32%) income households in the LGA. These levels of affordability align with those reported by the Healthy Diets ASAP pilot tool, where a recommended diet accounted for 20–29% of a low income household budget in an urban area [21]. Study findings are similar however to research using 'healthy food basket' methodologies which found the recommended diet accounted for between 26–32% of a low income household budget across urban and rural towns of South Australia [17], Victoria [16,35] and Queensland [36]. While there is no accepted benchmark for affordability of a healthy diet [22], relative unaffordability is commonly associated with food costs accounting for 30% or more of the household budget [1,35]. Recently, Ward et al. [17] have proposed that 'food stress' occurs when food costs account for 25% or more of the household income.

Australian studies consistently show significant increases in food pricing as one moves from inner city to suburban to regional and rural areas [16,17,35,36]. "Out-shopping", purchasing food outside of one's local area from a larger centre, is therefore a common practice in rural areas [37] to benefit from lower prices and greater variety. In this study, differences in food prices were observed across the LGA, with prices 8–10% higher in the south. Furthermore, a comparison of the cost of a 'Victorian Healthy Food Basket' for the LGA ($AUD528.41), with neighbouring regional towns ($AUD438.30—town population ≈ 17,000; $AUD453.34—town population ≈ 30,000) reveals that food prices are lower in regional towns outside the LGA boundary [38,39]. In addition to higher food pricing and out-shopping, rural communities often experience low density transport networks, leading to an increased reliance on motor vehicles, with associated time, fuel and vehicle maintenance costs, when purchasing food [15].

This study also found that the majority of the food budget was spent on discretionary items (59.5%), of which take-away foods comprised 18%. The Australian Dietary Guidelines food price indexes report [40] estimates that 58.2% of the 2014 household food budget was spent on discretionary items; and Lee et al. [21] report a similar figure of 58% for households in an urban area. While study findings on discretionary item expenditure are higher than reported by others, they do align with the Victorian Population Health Survey [30], with the LGA having high sugar sweetened beverage consumption (30.3% vs. Victorian average 15.9%), low fruit and vegetable consumption (4.5% vs. Victorian average 5.2%) [30]; and high take-away meal consumption (80.9% eating takeaway once per week vs. Victorian average 71.2%).

While a recommended diet may cost less than the current diet, it would appear that price is not the main driver of food choice for this community. In addition to the cost of foods, LGA residents have reported poor quality, limited variety (especially culturally appropriate foods), and inadequate or unreliable public transport as other reasons limiting their food choices [28]. The abundant supply of 'convenience' outlets (bakeries, take-away outlets, cafes, hotels/pubs, service stations) also appears to meet consumer demand for convenience [32] and taste [14], overcoming the challenges of limited geographic access, busy lifestyles and limited cooking skills, while also contributing to the local economy.

The rising cost of foods [16] combined with a limited number of food retail outlets, stocking a reduced variety of food items, lowers the likelihood of rural communities adhering to a healthier diet [41]. Rural areas with few supermarkets and several 'convenience' outlets have been found to have higher food prices, and limited availability of fresh produce and healthier food choices, particularly skim/low fat milk, whole wheat bread, fruits and vegetables [42]. Of the 40 food retail outlets included in this study, 11 (27.5%) were supermarkets and general stores selling predominantly healthy five food group items; and 29 (72.5%) were 'convenience' outlets selling predominately discretionary and take-away food items. Rural towns in Victoria have consistently been excluded from 'Victorian Healthy Food Basket' studies as they do not meet the inclusion criterion of stocking at least 90% (40 of 44) of listed food items [16,19]. Similarly, this study found that healthier food items were frequently unavailable in smaller general stores compared with supermarkets.

There is potential for supermarkets to increase variety and quality of fresh and healthy food options; provide competitive, lower pricing for healthy foods; and improve geographic access in areas described as 'food deserts' [41]. However, studies in the United States show that while supermarkets improve the perceptions of healthy food access amongst residents, improvements in net availability of healthy foods may be minimal, with residents continuing to shop outside their local area; more food stores stocking a wider variety of all food products; and greater market segmentation with 'convenience' outlets reducing stocks of healthy foods [41]. Positive impacts on food pricing however may be experienced with healthy foods offered at lower prices and discretionary item prices increasing as 'convenience' outlets attempt to compensate for reduced stocks of healthy foods [41]. In Australia, supermarkets are described by Pulker et al. [43] (p. 1) as having *"a powerful position in the Australian food system . . . . . . acting as gate-keepers between food producers and consumers"*, thereby influencing the range and price of food choices available, and shaping consumer preferences and social norms. While Australian supermarkets demonstrate some commitment to nutrition promotion and the prevention of obesity, Sacks et al. [44] argue that more is needed across this sector, especially to address the availability, affordability and promotion of healthy food choices.

In contrast to the establishment of new supermarkets, improvements to existing stores is suggested as a less time consuming and less expensive strategy to improve the variety and relative price of healthy food options in underserved areas with 'food deserts' [41]. In-store activities found to be feasible and acceptable to food retailers in rural communities, with modest levels of effectiveness, appear to focus predominately on health promotional practices, such as the provision of recipes and shopping lists for healthy meals, in-store displays with healthy samples, promotional signage within the store, and point-of-purchase signage for fruits and vegetables [45]. In a recent systematic review of 30 studies across nine countries regarding the effectiveness of food pricing strategies, Gittelsohn et al. [46] found that nearly all studies ($n = 27$) used in-store pricing strategies to promote healthy foods, most commonly fruits and vegetables (usually through price discounts, coupons and vouchers). Few studies ($n = 6$) used pricing strategies to specifically discourage unhealthy foods such as sugar-sweetened beverages and foods high in fat and/or sugar (using a price increase). It was noted that using pricing strategies that target only fruits and vegetables may be difficult for small retail outlets to implement, especially in low income communities, as fresh produce is often hard to source and highly perishable; and therefore any price incentives should cover a broad range of healthy food items [46].

In one of few studies exploring the perspectives of retailers, Kim et al. [47] found that small store owners in a low income community, regardless of their ethnic background, regarded customer preferences and wholesaler availability of food products as critical barriers to the provision of healthy options. The stocking of 'low customer demand' items was perceived to be a high-risk investment resulting in possible sales loss. When queried about pricing strategies, concerns were raised about offering discounts on multiple items given the small range of products the stores usually stocked. Retailers felt that discounts created price fluctuations and customer dissatisfaction when prices returned to normal. They also described the availability and pricing/discounting of items as being highly dependent on what wholesalers can offer [47].

Rural communities in Australia are serviced by long food supply chains which are not flexible to sudden changes or able to keep inventories to a minimum; instead they encourage the delivery of set quotas of items with a long shelf life [15]. Small stores not aligned to major supermarket chains are therefore at a disadvantage in acquiring fresh produce regularly and at competitive prices. Strategies to improve and/or subsidise the freighting of food to remote Australian communities have been suggested for communities who face similar challenges of vast distances, extreme temperatures and variable road conditions [48,49]. For example, 'group freight buying' where a group of stores combines their volumes to fill transport units on a geographically logical freight route that are not at full capacity, resulting in increased service frequency and/or lower freight costs per unit transported [49]. Such strategies will require leadership across all levels of government, and a strong commitment to the development and implementation of a National Nutrition Policy [50] and a National Food Plan that considers health [51].

At a policy level, food pricing options exist in the form of taxation, subsidisation, or a combination of these [22,52]. The taxing of unhealthy foods is considered of benefit for raising revenue as well as an effective strategy to improve dietary behaviours [53]; and subsidising healthy food is considered of benefit in making these foods more affordable and also, though to a smaller effect, appear to improve dietary behaviours [21,52]. For Australia, the exemption of 'healthy' foods from goods and sales tax (GST) is a means of reducing 'food stress' for low income families. Without this safeguard, Lee et al. [21] estimate that the cost of a healthy (recommended) diet would increase by approximately 10%, with the likelihood of a greater proportion of the food budget being spent on discretionary items.

5. Strengths and Limitations

To our knowledge, this is the first study in rural Australia to utilize the Healthy Diets ASAP tool to explore the price, price differential and affordability of the recommended and current diet. This study was also able to survey all supermarkets and general stores given the relative low number of outlets available, thereby providing a true representation for this LGA. While an advantage to data collection, a small sample size of retail outlets poses limitations for statistically analysis.

As a cross sectional study, data collection reflects a single time point, occurring on random days of the week during Winter, and therefore pricing information is indicative of seasonal and wholesaler availability at that time. 'Ground truthing' was used to identify and verify the presence of operational food stores, however food environments are constantly subject to change, and food stores included in this study may have since closed and/or new businesses opened.

No data was collected regarding consumer shopping venue preferences, especially the phenomena of 'out-shopping' which is known to occur anecdotally; nor other means through which food items may be obtained such as the community garden, food swaps, the food pantry or food bank. It was also out of scope for this study to conduct in-depth interviews with food store owners which may have elicited information regarding food pricing strategies.

The Healthy Diets ASAP tool was a practical and time efficient survey to conduct across the LGA. While some product brands/sizes were different to those specified on the protocol, the tool allowed for alternate brands/sizes to be included. The use of average prices for missing/unavailable items may have led to an underestimation of the cost of the diet for these towns as residents would have travelled to purchase this item elsewhere. Information on unavailable items will be used to update the tool for greater utility. The tool has been developed for different reference households, with the default being two adults and two children. It may be necessary to enable a wider application to other reference households to better reflect the demographics of rural, remote communities with higher numbers of elderly couples with no children and single-parent families.

6. Conclusions

This study confirms that while a healthy diet is less expensive than the current unhealthy diet, affordability is a challenge for Australians living in rural Victoria, especially for families on median or low incomes. For these communities, food security is compromised by limited geographical access to food retail outlets, with most outlets, especially in smaller towns, offering a reduced variety of healthy food choices at higher prices.

Implications for research: Research shows that rural, remote communities have poor adherence to recommended dietary guidelines, experience higher rates of overweight/obesity and associated chronic disease, and are disproportionately affected by the influence of their food environment compared with their urban counterparts. There appears to be a gap, however, in research regarding the influence of food environments among rural communities. Continued research in this area is therefore warranted to improve our understanding and identification of important determinants of diet for these Australian communities.

Implications for practice and policy: It would appear that price is not the main driver of food choice for rural, remote Australian communities. A preference for unhealthier foods, that meet the needs of convenience and taste, undermines the establishment of a reliable demand-supply cycle that would be economically viable for small food retailers. The challenge of food distribution across vast distances to provide affordable, quality produce also serves as a barrier within rural communities affecting accessibility and availability of supply. Understanding the associations between these factors will help to shape appropriate interventions needed at the individual, organizational, community and policy level. It is evident that a combination of strategies is required, including public health campaigns and programs targeting the individual to improve food literacy knowledge and skills; interventions in food retail outlets to improve affordability and promotion of healthier foods/drinks; establishing alternative community-led food supply options such as food cooperatives, farmers' markets and community gardens; safeguarding agricultural land use and monitoring the zoning of fast food retail outlets through local, regional and state government planning mechanisms; developing a flexible, responsive food supply chain; and retaining a General Sales Tax (GST) exemption for basic healthy foods.

Author Contributions: P.L. and J.W. conceived and designed the study with input from C.B.; A.L. and M.L. provided expertise on the Healthy Diets ASAP tool methodology; P.L., J.W., F.G. and C.R. undertook data collection and analysis; M.L. cross-checked data analysis; P.L. led the writing of the manuscript with input from all authors. All authors approved the manuscript for submission.

Acknowledgments: The authors thank all retail outlet owners within the study area for their willingness and time to participate in this study.

Appendix

Table A1. Price of recommended and current diets for the Local Government Area (using a reference household of two parents and two children).

Northern LGA = towns 1,2,3,4,5; Central LGA = towns 6,7; Southern LGA = towns 8,9,10	Whole LGA—Recommended Diet	Whole LGA—Current Diet	Southern LGA—Recommended Diet	Southern LGA—Current Diet	Central LGA—Recommended Diet	Central LGA—Current Diet	Northern LGA—Recommended Diet	Northern LGA—Current Diet
TOTAL DIET $mean ±sd	702.41 ± 44.89	866.19 ± 37.54	733.31 ± 39.70	901.38 ± 20.87	661.96 ± 27.66	823.23 ± 29.55	708.14 ± 37.96	870.86 ± 21.02
CORE 5 FOOD GROUP FOODS $mean +sd (%total diet cost)	702.41 ± 44.89 (100.0%)	343.47 ± 26.93 (39.65%)	733.31 ± 39.70 (100%)	360.24 ± 23.33 (39.97%)	661.96 ± 27.66 (100%)	318.79 ± 19.23 (38.72%)	708.14 ± 37.96(100%)	348.20 ± 22.15 (39.98%)
FRUIT $mean ±sd (%total diet cost)	96.20 ± 13.89 (13.70%)	62.06 ± 11.45 (7.16%)	98.14 ± 15.29 (13.38%)	67.73 ± 12.11 (7.51%)	88.77 ± 2.48 (13.41%)	57.65 ± 2.35 (7.00%)	99.49 ± 15.30 (14.05%)	61.31 ± 12.87 (7.04%)
VEGETABLES/LEGUMES $mean ±sd (%total diet cost)	131.61 ± 8.71 (18.74%)	50.77 ± 4.39 (5.86%)	138.87 ± 1.15 (18.94%)	52.90 ± 2.75 (5.87%)	129.14 ± 10.15 (19.51%)	49.74 ± 5.13 (6.04%)	128.74 ± 7.80 (18.18%)	50.10 ± 4.26 (5.75%)
FRUIT & VEG/LEGUMES $mean ±sd (%total diet cost)	227.81 ± 18.81 (32.43%)	112.83 ± 13.00 (13.03%)	237.01 ± 15.77 (32.32%)	120.64 ± 12.67 (13.38%)	217.90 ± 11.33 (32.92%)	107.39 ± 7.33 (13.04%)	228.23 ± 21.02 (32.23%)	111.41 ± 13.66 (12.79%)
GRAINS/CEREALS $mean ±sd (%total diet cost)	124.11 ± 17.69 (17.67%)	53.98 ± 5.13 (6.23%)	140.70 ± 13.93 (19.19%)	57.93 ± 3.86 (6.43%)	106.86 ± 8.71 (16.14%)	47.22 ± 2.06 (5.74%)	124.50 ± 13.52(17.58%)	55.68 ± 2.63 (6.39%)
LEAN MEATS & ALT $mean ±sd (%total diet cost)	204.48 ± 9.05 (29.11%)	103.27 ± 6.56 (11.92%)	202.41 ± 11.03 (27.60%)	103.80 ± 6.06 (11.44%)	202.54 ± 10.10 (30.60%)	99.32 ± 7.22 (12.06%)	206.88 ± 5.94 (29.22%)	105.76 ± 5.08 (12.14%)
MILK & ALT $mean ±sd (%total diet cost)	116.54 ± 6.64 (16.59%)	52.08 ± 4.82 (6.01%)	122.86 ± 3.30 (16.75%)	55.99 ± 4.79 (6.21%)	108.40 ± 5.41 (16.38%)	47.17 ± 2.80 (5.73%)	117.64 ± 2.83 (16.61%)	52.67 ± 2.94 (6.05%)
UNSATURATED OILS/SPREADS $mean +sd (%total diet cost)	9.47 ± 0.86 (1.35%)	1.30 ± 0.19 (1.15%)	9.16 ± 1.25 (1.25%)	1.43 ± 0.19 (0.16%)	9.92 ± 0.22 (1.50%)	1.36 ± 0.07 (0.17%)	9.39 ± 0.69 (1.33%)	1.19 ± 0.17 (0.14%)
WATER $mean +sd (%total diet cost)	20.00 ± 5.90 (2.85%)	20.00 ± 5.90 (2.31%)	21.18 ± 8.31 (2.89%)	21.18 ± 8.31 (2.35%)	16.33 ± 5.55 (2.47%)	16.33 ± 5.55 (1.98%)	21.50 ± 2.32 (3.04%)	21.50 ± 2.32 (2.47%)
ALL DISCRETIONARY FOODS $mean +sd (%total diet cost)		515.42 ± 22.77 (59.50%)		534.77 ± 28.41 (59.33%)		496.63 ± 17.77 (60.33%)		515.08 ± 5.49 (59.15%)
TAKE-AWAY FOODS $mean +sd (%total diet cost)		156.67 ± 15.29 (18.09%)		172.48 ± 19.10 (19.13%)		149.97 ± 3.06 (18.22%)		151.20 ± 9.14 (17.36%)
ARTIFICIALLY SWEETENED BEVERAGES $mean +sd (%total diet cost)		7.31 ± 1.10 (0.84%)		6.37 ± 0.93 (0.71%)		7.81 ± 0.91 (0.95%)		7.58 ± 0.96 (0.87%)
SUGAR SWEETENED BEVERAGES$mean +sd (%total diet cost)		44.03 ± 6.66 (5.08%)		38.37 ± 5.63 (4.26%)		47.05 ± 5.46(5.72%)		45.61 ± 5.79 (5.24%)
ALCOHOLIC BEVERAGES $mean +sd (%total diet cost)		97.33 ± 9.74 (11.24%)		102.63 ± 12.40 (11.39%)		88.45 ± 6.96 (10.74%)		99.47 ± 4.30 (11.42%)

References

1. Burns, C.; Friel, S. It's time to determine the cost of a healthy diet in Australia. *ANZJPH* **2007**, *31*, 363–365. [CrossRef]

2. HLPE. *Food Security and Climate Change*; Committee on World Food Security: Rome, Italy, 2012.

3. McKechnie, R.; Turrell, G.; Giskes, K.; Gallegos, D. Single-item measure of food insecurity used in the national health survey may underestimate prevalence in Australia. *ANZJPH* **2018**, *42*, 389–395. [CrossRef] [PubMed]

4. ABS. *Australian National Health Survey—First Results 2014–2015*; Australian Bureau of Statistics: Canberra, Australia, 2015.

5. Franklin, B.; Jones, A.; Love, D.; Puckett, S.; Macklin, J.; White-Means, S. Exploring mediators of food insecurity and obesity: A review of recent literature. *J. Community Health* **2012**, *37*, 253–264. [CrossRef] [PubMed]

6. Abarca-Gómez, L.; Abdeen, Z.A.; Hamid, Z.A.; Abu-Rmeileh, N.M.; Acosta-Cazares, B.; Acuin, C.; Adams, R.J.; Aekplakorn, W.; Afsana, K.; Aguilar-Salinas, C.A.; et al. Worldwide trends in body-mass index, underweight, overweight, and obesity from 1975 to 2016: A pooled analysis of 2416 population based measurement studies in 128·9 million children, adolescents, and adults. *Lancet* **2017**, *390*, 2627–2642. [CrossRef]

7. AIHW. *Australian Burden of Disease: Impact of Overweight and Obesity as a Risk Factor for Chronic Conditions*; Australian Institute of Health and Welfare: Canberra, Australia, 2017.

8. Glanz, K.; Johnson, L.; Yaroch, A.L.; Phillips, M.; Ayala, G.X.; Davis, E.L. Measures of retail food store environments and sales: Review and implications for healthy eating initiatives. *J. Nutr. Educ. Behav.* **2016**, *48*, 280.e1–288.e1. [CrossRef] [PubMed]

9. Swinburn, B.A.; Sacks, G.; Hall, K.D.; McPherson, K.; Finegood, D.T.; Moodie, M.L.; Gortmaker, S.L. The global obesity pandemic: Shaped by global drivers and local environments. *Lancet* **2011**, *378*, 804–814. [CrossRef]

10. Backholer, K.; Spencer, E.; Gearon, E.; Magliano, D.J.; McNaughton, S.A.; Shaw, J.E.; Peeters, A. The association between socio-economic position and diet quality in Australian adults. *Public Health Nutr.* **2016**, *19*, 477–485. [CrossRef] [PubMed]

11. AIHW. *Australian Burden of Disease Study: Impact and Causes of Illness and Deaths in Australia 2011*; Australian Institute of Health and Welfare: Canberra, Australia, 2016.

12. ABS. *Australian Health Survey—Consumption of Food Groups from the Australian Dietary Guidelines 2011–2012*; Australian Bureau of Statistics: Canberra, Australia, 2016.

13. Lewis, M.; Lee, A. Costing 'healthy' food baskets in Australia—A systematic review of food price and affordability monitoring tools, protocols and methods. *Public Health Nutr.* **2016**, *19*, 2872–2886. [CrossRef] [PubMed]

14. State Government of Victoria. *Victorian Population Health Survey 2012*; Department of Health and Human Services: Melbourne, Australia, 2016.

15. National Rural Health Alliance. *Food Security and Health in Rural and Remote AUSTRALIA*; Rural Industries Research and Development Corporation, Australian Government: Deakin West, ACT, Australia, 2016.

16. Palermo, C.; McCartan, J.; Kleve, S.; Sinha, K.; Shiell, A. A longitudinal study of the cost of food in victoria influenced by geography and nutritional quality. *ANZJPH* **2016**, *40*, 270–273. [CrossRef] [PubMed]

17. Ward, P.R.; Coveney, J.; Verity, F.; Carter, P.; Schilling, M. Cost and affordability of healthy food in rural South Australia. *Rural Remote Health* **2012**, *12*, 1938. [PubMed]

18. Innes-Hughes, C.; Boylan, S.; King, L.; Lobb, E. Measuring the food environment in three rural towns in New South Wales, Australia. *Health Promot. J. Aust.* **2012**, *23*, 129–133. [CrossRef]

19. Palermo, C.E.; Walker, K.Z.; Hill, P.; McDonald, J. The cost of healthy food in rural Victoria. *Rural Remote Health* **2008**, *8*, 1074. [PubMed]

20. Chapman, K.; Innes-Hughes, C.; Goldsbury, D.; Kelly, B.; Bauman, A.; Allman-Farinelli, M. A comparison of the cost of generic and branded food products in Australian supermarkets. *Public Health Nutr.* **2013**, *16*, 894–900. [CrossRef] [PubMed]

21. Lee, A.J.; Kane, S.; Ramsey, R.; Good, E.; Dick, M. Testing the price and affordability of healthy and current (unhealthy) diets and the potential impacts of policy change in Australia. *BMC Public Health* **2016**, *16*, 315. [CrossRef] [PubMed]

22. Lee, A.; Mhurchu, C.N.; Sacks, G.; Swinburn, B.; Snowdon, W.; Vandevijvere, S.; Hawkes, C.; L'Abbe, M.; Rayner, M.; Sanders, D.; et al. Monitoring the price and affordability of foods and diets globally. *Obes. Rev.* **2013**, *14* (Suppl. 1), 82–95. [CrossRef]

23. Lee, A.; Kane, S.; Lewis, M.; Good, E.; Pollard, C.M.; Landrigan, T.J.; Dick, M. Healthy Diets ASAP—Australian Standardised Affordability and Pricing methods protocol. *BMC Nutr. J.* **2018**, *17*, 88. [CrossRef] [PubMed]

24. NHMRC. *Australian Dietary Guidelines*; National Health and Medical Research Council: Canberra, Australia, 2013. Available online: http://www.eatforhealth.gov.au (accessed on 26 August 2018).

25. ABS. *Australian Health Survey—First Results 2011–2012*; Australian Bureau of Statistics: Canberra, Australia, 2012.

26. ABS. Census of Population and Housing—Quickstats, Community Profiles and Datapacks User Guide. Available online: http://quickstats.censusdata.abs.gov.au/census_services/getproduct/census/2016/quickstat/LGA27630 (accessed on 28 August 2017).

27. AIHW. *Rural, Regional and Remote Health: A Guide to Remoteness Classifications*; Australian Institute of Health and Welfare: Canberra, Australia, 2004.

28. Wimmera Primary Care Partnership. *Wimmera Population Health and Wellbeing Profile 2016*; Wimmera Primary Care Partnership: Horsham, Victoria, Australia, 2016.

29. State Government of Victoria. *Change and Disadvantage in the Grampians Region, Vvictoria*; Department of Planning and Community Development: Melbourne, Australia, 2011.

30. State Government of Victoria. *Victorian Population Health Survey 2014: Modifiable Risk Factors Contributing to Chronic Disease in Victoria*; Department of Health and Human Services: Melbourne, Australia, 2016.

31. Caspi, C.E.; Friebur, R. Modified ground-truthing: An accurate and cost-effective food environment validation method for town and rural areas. *IJBNPA* **2016**, *13*, 37. [CrossRef] [PubMed]

32. Australian Government Department of Human Services. Social and Health Payments and Services. Available online: https://www.humanservices.gov.au/ (accessed on 28 August 2017).

33. Rao, M.; Afshin, A.; Singh, G.; Mozaffarian, D. Do healthier foods and diet patterns cost more than less healthy options? A systematic review and meta-analysis. *BMJ Open* **2013**, *3*, e004277. [CrossRef] [PubMed]

34. Australian Taxation Office, A.G. GST-Free Food. Available online: https://www.ato.gov.au/Business/GST/In-detail/Your-industry/Food/GST-and-food/?anchor=GSTfreefood (accessed on 3 July 2018).

35. Rossimel, A.; Han, S.S.; Larsen, K.; Palermo, C. Access and affordability of nutritious food in metropolitan Melbourne. *Nutr. Diet.* **2016**, *73*, 13–18. [CrossRef]

36. Harrison, M.; Lee, A.; Findlay, M.; Nicholls, R.; Leonard, D.; Martin, C. The increasing cost of healthy food. *ANZJPH* **2010**, *34*, 179–186. [CrossRef] [PubMed]

37. Bardenhagen, C.J.; Pinard, C.A.; Pirog, R.; Yaroch, A.L. Characterizing rural food access in remote areas. *J. Community Health* **2017**, *42*, 1008–1019. [CrossRef] [PubMed]

38. State Government of Victoria. *VLGA Food Scan Report: Mildura Rural City Council*; Healthy Together Victoria: Mildura, Australia, 2013.

39. Wimmera Food Security Group. *Victorian Healthy Food Basket Survey—Summer 2016–2017*; Wimmera Primary Care Partnership: Horsham, Victoria, Australia, 2017.

40. ABS. Australian Dietary Guideline Food Price Indexes Series 6401.1. Available online: http://www.abs.gov.au/AUSSTATS/abs@.nsf/Previousproducts/6401.0Feature%20Article1Dec%202015?opendocument&tabname=Summary&prodno=6401.0&issue=Dec%202015&num=&view= (accessed on 12 November 2017).

41. Ghosh-Dastidar, M.; Hunter, G.; Collins, R.L.; Zenk, S.N.; Cummins, S.; Beckman, R.; Nugroho, A.K.; Sloan, J.C.; Wagner, L.; Dubowitz, T. Does opening a supermarket in a food desert change the food environment? *Health Place* **2017**, *46*, 249–256. [CrossRef] [PubMed]

42. Vilaro, M.; Barnett, T. The rural food environment: A survey of food price, availability, and quality in a rural Florida community. *Food Public Health* **2013**, *3*. [CrossRef]

43. Pulker, C.E.; Trapp, G.S.A.; Scott, J.A.; Pollard, C.M. What are the position and power of supermarkets in the Australian food system, and the implications for public health? A systematic scoping review. *Obes. Rev.* **2018**, *19*, 198–218. [CrossRef] [PubMed]

44. Sacks, G.; Robinson, E.; Cameron, A.; INFORMAS. *Inside Our Supermarkets—Assessment of Company Policies and Committments Related to Obesity Prevention and Nutrition*; Deakin University: Melbourne, Australia, 2018.

45. Martinez-Donate, A.P.; Riggall, A.J.; Meinen, A.M.; Malecki, K.; Escaron, A.L.; Hall, B.; Menzies, A.; Garske, G.; Nieto, F.J.; Nitzke, S. Evaluation of a pilot healthy eating intervention in restaurants and food stores of a rural community: A randomized community trial. *BMC Public Health* **2015**, *15*, 136. [CrossRef] [PubMed]

46. Gittelsohn, J.; Trude, A.C.B.; Kim, H. Pricing strategies to encourage availability, purchase, and consumption of healthy foods and beverages: A systematic review. *Prev. Chronic Dis.* **2017**, *14*, E107. [CrossRef] [PubMed]

47. Kim, M.; Budd, N.; Batorsky, B.; Krubiner, C.; Manchikanti, S.; Waldrop, G.; Trude, A.; Gittelsohn, J. Barriers to and facilitators of stocking healthy food options: Viewpoints of Baltimore city small storeowners. *Ecol. Food Nutr.* **2017**, *56*, 17–30. [CrossRef] [PubMed]

48. *Freight Improvement Toolkit*; National Rural Health Alliance: Canberra, ACT, Australia, 2007.

49. Queensland Health. *Vegetable and Fruit Supply to South West Queensland: An Information Paper*; Queensland Government: Brisbane, Australia, 2006.

50. Lee, A.; Baker, P.; Stanton, R.; Friel, S.; O'Dea, K.; Weightman, A. *Scoping Study to Inform the Development of the New National Nutrition Policy*; (rft 028/1213); Released under FOI, March 2016; QUT, Australian Department of Health and Ageing: Queensland, Brisbane, Australia, 2013.

51. *The People's Food Plan*; Australian Food Sovereignty Alliance: Canberra, ACT, Australia, 2013.

52. Kern, D.M.; Auchincloss, A.H.; Stehr, M.F.; Roux, A.V.D.; Moore, L.V.; Kanter, G.P.; Robinson, L.F. Neighborhood prices of healthier and unhealthier foods and associations with diet quality: Evidence from the multi-ethnic study of atherosclerosis. *Int. J. Environ. Res. Public Health* **2017**, *14*, 1394. [CrossRef] [PubMed]

53. Powell, L.M.; Maciejewski, M.L. Taxes and sugar-sweetened beverages. *JAMA* **2018**, *319*, 229–230. [CrossRef] [PubMed]

Charitable Food Systems' Capacity to Address Food Insecurity

Christina M. Pollard [1,*] [iD], Bruce Mackintosh [2] [iD], Cathy Campbell [1], Deborah Kerr [1] [iD], Andrea Begley [1] [iD], Jonine Jancey [1], Martin Caraher [3] [iD], Joel Berg [4] and Sue Booth [5]

[1] Faculty of Health Science, School of Public Health, Curtin University, GPO Box U1987, Perth 6845, Australia; Cathy.Campbell555@gmail.com (C.C.); D.Kerr@curtin.edu.au (D.K.); A.Begley@curtin.edu.au (A.B.); J.Jancey@curtin.edu.au (J.J.)
[2] School of Agriculture and Environment, The University of Western Australia, 35 Stirling Highway, Crawley, Perth 6009, Australia; bruce.mackintosh@uwa.edu.au
[3] Centre for Food Policy, City University of London, Northampton Square, London EC1V 0HB, UK; m.caraher@city.ac.uk
[4] Hunger Free America, 50 Broad Street, Suite 1103, New York 10004, NY, USA; JBerg@hungerfreeamerica.org
[5] College of Medicine & Public Health, Flinders University, GPO Box 2100, Adelaide 5000, Australia; sue.booth@flinders.edu.au
*   Correspondence: C.Pollard@curtin.edu.au

Abstract: Australian efforts to address food insecurity are delivered by a charitable food system (CFS) which fails to meet demand. The scope and nature of the CFS is unknown. This study audits the organisational capacity of the CFS within the 10.9 square kilometres of inner-city Perth, Western Australia. A desktop analysis of services and 12 face-to-face interviews with representatives from CFS organisations was conducted. All CFS organisations were not-for–profit and guided by humanitarian or faith-based values. The CFS comprised three indirect services (IS) sourcing, banking and/or distributing food to 15 direct services (DS) providing food to recipients. DS offered 30 different food services at 34 locations feeding over 5670 people/week via 16 models including mobile and seated meals, food parcels, supermarket vouchers, and food pantries. Volunteer to paid staff ratios were 33:1 (DS) and 19:1 (IS). System-wide, food was mainly donated and most funding was philanthropic. Only three organisations received government funds. No organisation had a nutrition policy. The organisational capacity of the CFS was precarious due to unreliable, insufficient and inappropriate financial, human and food resources and structures. System-wide reforms are needed to ensure adequate and appropriate food relief for Australians experiencing food insecurity.

Keywords: food insecurity; charitable food services; food charity; food system; nutrition; voluntary failure

1. Introduction

The health consequences of socio-economic disadvantage, including homelessness, are increasingly seen in high income countries, including Australia [1–4]. Food insufficiency is closely associated with poor mental and physical health [5–8] and is common among people who are homeless [5,9,10].

Cities attract vulnerable populations experiencing food insecurity as they provide concentrated food and support services. The types of people accessing inner-city charitable food services (CFS) are highly variable and include people who are homeless or domiciled and in financial difficulty due to a range of circumstances, those living in hostel and shelters, backpackers, and women fleeing from domestic violence. The inner-city precinct of Perth, the capital city of Western Australia, covers

10.9 square kilometres with a population of about 32,000 people. The Perth Homeless Registry showed that the number of street-present people increased from 192 to 319 between 2012 and 2016 [11]. Over 80% had been homeless for six months or more and 52% had complex comorbidities of existing medical conditions, mental illness and substance use disorders [11].

Concerns have been raised regarding the ongoing capacity of food relief systems in both Australia and the United States (U.S.) to meet the increasing demand [12,13]. There is also evidence of sub-optimal nutritional quality in the food provided [14,15]. Australia's response to food insecurity is at a critical point given the increasing need, the absence of government-funded food assistance such as in the U.S. [15] and the diminishing welfare safety net [16]. Australian Government welfare policies designed to reduce poverty—for example, the Australian Age Pension [17], Family Tax Benefit and the Child Care Subsidy [18] and Newstart Allowance [19]—provide assistance to low income earners and may assist in improving food security; however, the evidence for the increasing demand for food relief suggests they are inadequate.

Food charity, the delivery of donated, unsaleable, or waste food by the voluntary (non-profit) sector, is the dominant response to food insecurity in Australia [12]. This charitable food system (CFS), originally designed to provide immediate short-term food relief, is struggling as food insecurity and the demand for food assistance is chronic and increasing [12,20]. In 2015, there were 3000 to 4000 food relief services nationally [12]. The demand for food relief services increased in 2016, up 8% from 2015 [21].

Although short-term need is assumed in Australia [22], there is evidence of long-term reliance on the CFS [23,24]. The Australian response to food insecurity has been described as ad hoc with numerous small voluntary organisations providing food assistance [25]. Internationally, researchers have questioned whether the expansion and reliance on food charity and food banking is the appropriate response to food insecurity in developed countries, based on users' negative experiences of shame and being stigmatised and poor quality or limited food choices [26]. The CFS consists of both "in-direct" services (IS) (food banking and rescue organisations who collect, bank and/or distribute unsaleable food) and 'direct' services (DS) who provide the food to those in need.

The non-profit (NP) sector's ability to effectively address problems such as food insecurity has also been questioned in the academic literature, which has been critical of food banks based on users' experiences such as shame, stigma and eligibility criteria in high-income countries [20,27]. Salamon's theory of voluntary failure was developed in 1987 to explain the effectiveness of the voluntary response to issues such as food insecurity [28]. His theory described market failure, voluntary failure, and third-party government failure in delivering effective welfare-government relationships in the United States. The CFS NP voluntary response in Australia has arisen as a result of both a market and a third-party government failure in delivering the "collective good" of providing a welfare safety net to prevent food insecurity. The Commonwealth Department of Social Services acknowledges the existence of Emergency Relief as "services delivered by community organisations".

Salamon's four types of voluntary failure include (i) philanthropic insufficiency, the "inability to generate resources on a scale that is both adequate enough and reliable enough to cope with the human-service problems" [28] (p. 39); (ii) philanthropic particularism, which occurs when "some subgroups of the community may not be adequately represented in the structure of voluntary organizations" [28] (p. 40) where the focus is on treating "the more 'deserving' of the poor" leaving serious service gaps or duplicating services and wasting resources; (iii) philanthropic paternalism, which refers to the notion that "those with the greatest resources have influence over the definition of community need" [28] (p. 41); and (iv) philanthropic amateurism, described as "amateur approaches to coping with human problems" [28] (p. 42). A current assessment of CFS in Perth shows evidence of one type of voluntary failure, namely philanthropic insufficiency [24].

There has been limited exploration of the scope and organisational capacity of the Australian CFS [12,29] and none in Western Australia. In 2014, due to increasing demand, food relief organisations expressed a need to understand the current and future capacity of the CFS in inner-city Perth to meet their clients' needs [25]. Understanding the practical organisational issues facing the CFS is important when considering options for change to improve end-user services [30]. The aim of this paper is to document the scope, nature and organisational capacity of the CFS located in or serving inner-city Perth.

2. Methods

Between July and September 2015, an organisational capacity audit was undertaken of the CFS located in or serving inner-city Perth. The audit identified and mapped component organisations, their values, human and financial resources, their networks, nutrition policies, and food service operations.

A research advisory group comprising the research team and five representatives from key organisations working with homelessness, social disadvantage and relief services identified the CFS organisations located in or serving inner-city Perth. They provided initial contact details which were confirmed via telephone or web search. A nomenclature for the types of food service models and their inter-relationships was agreed, for example IS and DS.

Two semi-structured interview schedules were developed for the IS and DS. The assessment of organisational capacity was guided by the approach used to improve nutrition for vulnerable groups, children in childcare in Australia [31] and food bank users in the United States [15]. The instrument was adapted from the Research Tools for Use in Studying Nutrition Policies and Practices in the Emergency Food Bank Network [15] and Food Service Planning in Child Care in Western Australia [32] surveys, which assessed organisational capacity for a safe, nutritious and appropriate food service. Table 1 provides an overview of the interview schedule.

Table 1. Semi-structured interview schedule.

Topics Covered	Indirect Services	Direct Services
Organisational values, length of operation, funding sources	Asked	Asked
Food service models/types, location, timing, description of recipients	Asked	Asked
Workforce profile including volunteers and training	Asked	Asked
Food storage capacity	Asked	Asked
Nutrition and food safety training, policy and practices	Asked	Asked
Sources of foods	Asked	Asked
Food transport (for food received and distributed)	Asked	Asked
Perception of donors influence on charitable food services (CFS)	Asked	Asked
Impact of government actions on CFS	Asked	Asked
Preferences for specific foods	Asked	Asked
Challenges and opportunities to increasing nutritious food	Asked	Asked
Agencies receiving food, quantities and recipients	Asked	Not asked

The surveys were trialled with senior managers from two CFS organisations, with changes made to the order and phrasing of questions post-pilot to ensure clarity. Background information was obtained from organisational websites, and interviewees were asked to provide written documentation such as annual reports or service brochures.

Two researchers (Bruce Mackintosh and Cathy Campbell) with extensive experience in food relief and public health nutrition conducted the interviews. Thirty DS and five IS were telephoned to screen for interview suitability. If the organisation played a role in food service delivery in inner-city Perth, the chief executive officer, director or manager, or a nominated proxy was invited for face-to-face interview. Twelve face-to-face interviews were conducted (nine DS and three IS). Eight telephone interviews were conducted with DS offering limited food relief; for example, only supermarket vouchers or one-off cash payments to their clients. Both researchers attended each interview, filled in the written questionnaire and took additional notes. The three lots of data—the audit of the websites, interviewee responses to the survey instrument and interviewer notes—were collated, reported in tables where appropriate, and general findings were summarised by the interviewers. The study was conducted according to guidelines in the Declaration of Helsinki and all procedures involving human subjects were approved by the Curtin University Human Research Ethics Committee (HR183/2015). Written informed consent was obtained from all subjects.

3. Results

This study is the first to describe the organisational capacity of the CFS located in or servicing a capital city in Australia. The inner-city Perth CFS comprised three indirect services (IS) who sourced, banked and/or distributed food to 15 direct services (DS), who in turn provided food to recipients. DS offered 30 different food services at 34 locations feeding over 5670 people/week via 16 models including mobile and seated meals, food parcels, supermarket vouchers, and food pantries: see Table 1.

The CFS organisational capacity is described in terms of purpose; years of operation; funding sources and workforce structure; food supply and food service models offered; commitment to and structures to support the provision of nutritious food; the influence/impact of government regulation or legislation. The organisational overview of the CFS serving inner-City Perth is shown in Figure 1, and the audit results described for IS and then for DS followed by the barriers to improvement and interviewee recommendations.

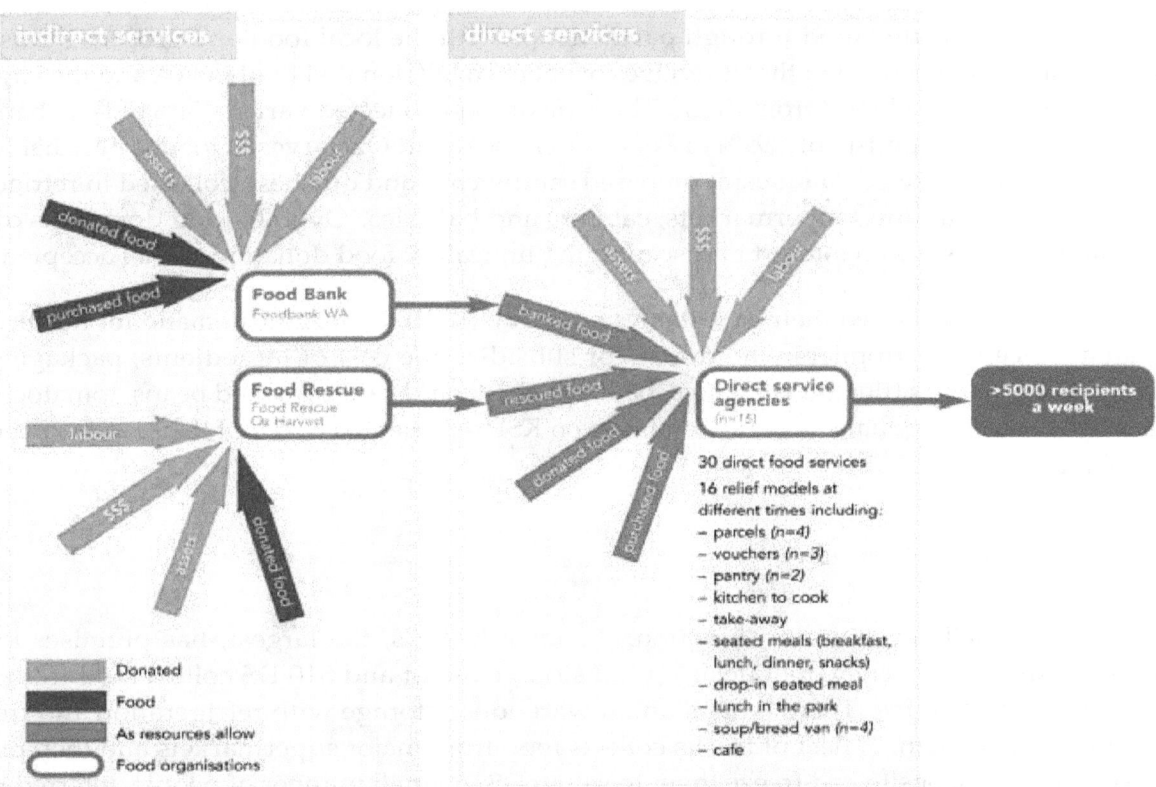

Figure 1. Model of the charitable food sector in inner-city Perth.

3.1. Indirect Services

Three IS were either located in or serviced inner-city Perth at the time of the research who procured food and either banked, sorted or directly distributed it to DS; Supplementary Table S1 shows the characteristics of the IS.

3.1.1. Organisational Intent, Funding and Workforce

Foodbank WA (Perth Western Australia), had operated for 21 years in, compared to 2 and 5 years for OzHarvest and Food Rescue WA, respectively. All three IS aimed to rescue surplus food and reduce food waste to provide for people in need, either via DS or directly. Foodbank WA and Food Rescue WA included reducing hunger with nutritious food and Foodbank WA and OzHarvest mentioned quality food. Food Rescue WA merged with Uniting Care West, a community services agency of the Uniting Church in Australia Synod of WA in 2013.

IS managers said their funding was ad hoc, unreliable, and from different sources including corporate and private donations, sponsorships and government grants. Foodbank WA also charged DS a per-kilogram handling fee to cover operating costs which generated AUD$3.78 million in 2017 [33]. OzHarvest and Food Rescue WA relied entirely on donations.

The workforce varied with organisational size: the number of paid full-time equivalent (FTE) staff ranged from two to 50 (Food Rescue WA and Foodbank WA respectively). Foodbank and OzHarvest employed nutritionists/dietitians (10 FTE and 1 casual respectively), one chef (1 FTE and 1 casual respectively) and hosted student placements. All three IS relied heavily on volunteers: Food Rescue WA had 2 paid staff and 100 volunteers (1:50), Foodbank WA has 1:45 and OzHarvest 1:25.

3.1.2. Food Types, Sources, Collection and Distribution

All IS sourced donated food through partnerships with the local food and grocery industry or retailers. Foodbank WA estimated that it receives over 80% of all donated food in WA and the larger DS in inner-city Perth sourced food from them. The type of food collected varied: 74% of Foodbank WA food was packaged non-perishable; 99% of Food Rescue WA and OzHarvest's food is perishable (e.g., fruit and vegetables, frozen meals, sushi, prepared sandwiches and quiches), collected in refrigerated vans from cafes, restaurants, supermarkets, caterers and bakeries. Overall, food donations did not meet demand and, despite an interest in discouraging unhealthy food donations, IS all accepted them.

Foodbank WA established their 'key staples program' (KSP) to meet the demand for healthy food. KSP is an alliance with suppliers who donate or subsidize the cost of ingredients, packaging and delivery of nine products (flour, pasta sauce, oats, spaghetti, and canned baked beans, tomatoes, fruit, vegetables and soup). Foodbank WA's expenditure on KSP represented 8.95% of their total expenditure in 2017 [33].

3.1.3. Facilities, Size and Function

IS varied in facilities, size and function. Foodbank WA's, the largest, has premises located 27 kilometres from CBD. They operate as a food storage depot and 510 DS collect food from them, paying a small handing fee. There is substantial warehouse storage with refrigeration and freezers and a commercial kitchen. A fleet of trucks collects food from major supermarkets and they prepare 2000 meals each week onsite and freeze them to sell to DS. A small number of people, referred by DS, can purchase food from directly as well.

Food Rescue WA has premises 10 km from the CBD with refrigerated and freezer storage space where they sort and repack the food they collect in two refrigerated trucks from supermarkets, then deliver to DS. They also use 'cargo carts' to collect and redistribute sandwiches and wraps from cafes in the CBD each day. OzHarvest distributes the food to DS immediately.

In 2016, Foodbank WA rescued 2.8 million kg of food, OzHarvest rescued 348,627 kg and distributed it to 84 DS [34] and Food Rescue WA distributed 478,000 kg of food [33]. Most (75%) of OzHarvest's food is rescued from supermarkets.

Overall, despite rescuing and redistributing significant quantities of food, the IS said they were unable to meet the demand and provide a sustainable, consistent supply of nutritious food to DS agencies who consequently had to make daily modifications to their services.

3.1.4. Nutrition Policy and Capacity

No IS had a formal nutrition policy to specify the types of foods procured. The Foodbank WA interviewee said that the presence of the nutrition staff encouraged a preference for nutritionally preferable KSP and the amount of sugar-sweetened beverages and potato crisps they distributed had declined. Food Rescue WA mainly focused their effort on the procurement of fresh fruit and vegetables.

All paid food preparation staff at Foodbank WA were food safety trained and premises were regularly inspected by local government officers. The two food rescue organisations said they did not accept unsafe food so did not train staff in food safety. OzHarvest offered two sessions of their Nutrition Education Sustenance Training (NEST) nutrition education program for staff, volunteers and service recipients.

3.1.5. Organisational Relationships

Some DS were not aware of the extent and nature of Foodbank WA's services and capacity to supply, at no or a very small cost, many of the items they were purchasing at full price from supermarkets. Some of those who were aware did not use Foodbank WA because they lacked regular transport and the distance from the CBD was a barrier. Others who accessed Foodbank WA purchased energy dense-nutrient poor foods such as potato crisps because they were cheaper by weight than heavier nutritious foods.

3.2. Direct Services

3.2.1. Organisational Intent, Funding and Workforce

The DS had provided food charity in inner-city Perth for many years: for example, the Salvation Army has provided food relief for 125 years while others have done so for 35 to 60 years. Ten of the 15 organisations had faith-based origins. Humanitarian values with a commitment to human dignity and a finding pathway out of food security guided most, typified by one interviewee's comment: "We believe that by nourishing the homeless and the vulnerable in a non-judgmental and compassionate way, we give hope, raise awareness about poverty and provide better outcomes for the wider community".

Funding sources were described as diverse and difficult to quantify. Three of the 15 DS received government funding (e.g., grants from State Government (Departments of Health or Child Protection and Family Support) or the Commonwealth Department of Social Services via their Emergency Relief Fund). Faith-based DS relied on parent organisations such as their church as well as corporate or public donations. Non-faith-based DS relied on philanthropic donations, fundraising activities, and community grants from funders such as Lotterywest, the official State lottery for WA. Specific information on corporate donors was not provided for confidentiality reasons.

The DS workforce structure is summarized in Table 2. The reliance on volunteers was high at a paid staff to volunteer ratio of 1:37. Although many interviewees said that they would value input from a nutritionist or dietitian, only two DS had access to formally trained nutrition personnel. One had employed a full-time dietitian but terminated the position in December 2015 due to lack of funds and the other dietitian was only employed on a casual basis to plan menus.

Table 2. Snapshot of the types and extent of direct food service in inner-city Perth, January 2015.

Funding	Food Source	Food Model	Days of Operation							Serve	Staff	
			M	T	W	T	F	S	Su	/wk	Paid	Vol
G (CP)	D	S, S/W (MS)	√	√	√	√	√	√	√	500	4	565
CH	D	Parcels		√			√			-		
CH	D	BBQ Monthly								-		
G (CP, H)	P	Kitchen	√	√	√	√	√	√	√	-		
D	D (f&P), B, R	TA noon	√	√	√	√	√	√		1250	5	200
CH	D (f&P)	BF (SM)	√	√	√					30–45		
CH	D (f&P)	Lunch (SM)	√	√	√		√			30–45		
CH	D (f&P)	D (SM)				√	√	√		120		
D, CH	D (f&P), B, R	BF (SM)	√	√	√	√				150	6	
D, CH	D (f&P), B, R	Food Any	√	√	√	√	√			-		
D, CH	D (f&P), B, R	Lunch					√			-		
D, CH	D (f&P), B, R	Parcel	√	√	√	√	√			-		
D, CH	D (f&$), B, R	Voucher	√	√	√	√	√			-		
Lottery	D	Parcel	√	√	√	√	√			5		
Lottery	D	Voucher	√	√	√	√	√			-		
G (CP)	D, R	MT	√	√	√	√	√			650	4	40
CH	D (f&$)	S Kitchen						√		20–50		
G (CP, H)	B, R	All meals	√	√	√	√	√	√	√	144	4	6
Lottery	D	S/W	√	√	√	√	√			5		
CH	D	Pantry	√	√	√	√	√			75		
CH	D (f&P), B, R	Café	√	√	√	√	√			-	2	153
CH	D (f&P), B, R	Parcel/Pantry	√	√	√	√	√			250		
CH	D (f&P), B, R	Voucher $20	√	√	√	√	√			150		
CH	D (f&P), B, R	S, S/W (Van)	√	√	√	√	√	√	√	350		
CH	D (f&P), B, R	S, S/W (Van)					√	√	√	150		
CH	D (f&P), B, R	All meals	√	√	√	√	√	√	√	600	4	20
CH, G CP	D (f&P), B, R	Drop-in (SM)	√	√	√	√	√			500	1	1
Total										5029	30	985

√: yes; &: and; G: government; CP: Department of Child Protection; CH: church; H: Department of Health; TA: take-away, P: purchased; D: donated; f: food; $: money; B: bank; R: rescue; SM: seated meal; UCW: Uniting Care West; BF: breakfast; MT: morning tea; L: lunch; D: dinner; S: soup; S/W: sandwich; M: Monday; T: Tuesday; W: Wednesday; T: Thursday; F: Friday; S: Saturday; Su: Sunday; wk: week; Fed: Federal; Vol: volunteers.

3.2.2. Food Service Models, Number and Facilities

Table 2 outlines the types of food service models and number of facilities (4 mobile services, 7 with premises, 2 shelters and 4 for specific client groups, e.g., people at risk of HIV/AIDS). There were 16 food service models offered at different locations on various days in the week: mobile and seated meals food parcels and pantries, and vouchers. Most DS recipients were homeless men, with a high proportion of Aboriginal and/or Torres Strait Islander people. Weekend coverage was limited. Four vans distributed prepared food in parks: one offered a three-course lunchtime meal 5-days/week, one offered soup, pies, sandwiches, tea and coffee each morning, another soup and bread each evening, and the fourth offered sandwiches to young people on the street 5 days/week.

Seven DS with premises had food preparation and serving areas and offered seated meals, usually on weekdays in one large room. Based on an eligibility assessment of need, five provided food parcels and pantry (a small storeroom with mostly non-perishable food items arranged on shelves) visits. A staff member accompanied eligible recipients to the pantry where they choose a set number of free food items or a food parcel, deemed sufficient for 1–2 days to enable a single person or a family to "get back on their feet". Pantry visits are restricted to once or twice a year.

Two DS only provided vouchers or "gift cards" to purchase food from supermarkets with eligibility based on DS-assessed need. Vouchers can be redeemed for food and/or any supermarket items other than cigarettes and alcohol. Recipients often purchase non-food items: for example, toiletries or dog food. Several DS provided school breakfasts or delivered frozen meals to other agencies.

3.2.3. Food Sources

Figure 1 shows DS food sources. Most DS use more than one source of food (either from IS or from direct food donations or purchased directly from supermarkets using donated money) and quantities varied from week to week. Some went to Foodbank WA for free food but chose lighter food by weight due to the handling fee while others relied on food rescue delivered daily. Church groups and philanthropic supporters intermittently offered food to DS. Most of the DS food supply was non-perishable and shelf-stable such as pasta or canned tuna, with the exception of daily rescued food. Interviewees said they needed more donations of perishable whole foods, particularly fruit and vegetables, meat, fish and dairy products.

3.2.4. Nutrition Policy and Capacity

Interviewees said that DS were generally wanting to improve nutrition standards but none had a formal nutrition policy and only one listed nutrition and food safety as program priorities. Interviewees did not believe that their reliance on donated food would influence nutrition policy actions they might choose to implement, but also said that they were unwilling to refuse donations of poor nutrition quality. The increasing and unmet demand for food, uncertain and unreliable food supply, and the salience of nutrition messages among volunteers and recipients were listed as barriers to improving the healthfulness of the food DS provided. The interviewers noted the poor nutrition knowledge of interviewees.

Interviewees were aware of the importance of nutrition and the relationship between the food provided and recipients' health. They said that some recipients had special dietary needs due to diabetes, heart disease, poor oral health, excessive body weight, or drug or alcohol dependency.

Food handling and safety training was rare for staff and not available for volunteers. The exception was DS with premises, such as the aged care nursing home, whose license required that all staff be trained to meet Australian food safety standards. Although no DS received government funding to deliver nutrition education, four had nutrition programs adapted from the FOODCents© budgeting, purchasing, and cooking skills development program [35,36] and several expressed interest in nutrition and budgeting training.

3.2.5. Influence of Government Policies or Legislation

DS interviewees said that state or federal government food-related policies were limited and had little or no day to day influence on the operations of DS. However, local government parking and public nuisance by-laws negatively impacted mobile services by limiting the locations where they could operate. DS referred to "Good Samaritan" legislation that protected them from liability for any unintended consequences of their activity and they were aware that food safety regulations did not currently apply to them as they did not sell food.

When asked about what was needed to improve DS, they wanted more meat, fish and dairy, fresh fruit and vegetables, sliced bread, facilities and equipment (larger kitchen, more vans, refrigerators, commercial bread slicers), the capacity to extend their weekend outreach services, including a bus with more refrigeration and a barbecue onboard, and the resources and capacity to serve a three-course seated meal.

3.2.6. Overall Barriers to CFS Meeting Demand for Nutritious Food

There is no overarching system or policies directing the CFS in inner-city Perth. Many interviewees did not know or communicate with other services. Even though IS said they preferred to supply nutritious foods to DS, they all received and passed-on donated food (for example, cakes, pastries, soft drinks and other unhealthy foods and drinks, particularly those from bakeries and supermarkets). IS said that their reliance on donated food was the main influence on the food they supplied to DS; they cannot predict their food inventory and are often not able to meet DS needs. Foodbank WA and Food

Rescue WA had more consistent donations, but OzHarvest said that donations were unreliable in the type and quantity of food and that they never know what they will get from donors and remarked on the challenges this presents. The IS recommended that food donors be educated regarding the importance of healthy food.

While one DS said they preferred to provide fruit juice and not carbonated sugar-sweetened beverages, another said that "food is food" and they did not hesitate to provide any food. Mobile services purchased and distributed meat pies because they were convenient, easy to prepare and recipients preferred them. One DS interviewee said it was important to give people the occasional "treat" food.

4. Discussion

The findings of this study need to be considered in the context of neo-liberal market economies, where a decline in social welfare creates conditions for individual insecurity and stress [37]. Efforts to reduce pressure on government spending has seen a rise in third sector or voluntary organisations involved in efforts to address complex human problems such as food insecurity [38,39]. The study findings show the CFS in inner-city Perth is complex, with disparate organisations working in an uncoordinated way in difficult conditions. A significant number of operational challenges face both IS and DS, limiting their ability to deliver nutritious or appropriate food relief to recipients. These include the increasing demand and long-term nature of food insecurity (with some models consisting of 1–2 days of emergency relief); their human resource capacity being heavily reliant on volunteers; declining and/or unreliable financial support; an unreliable and inconsistent food supply based primarily on donated or rescued waste food; no food safety or nutrition policy or regulatory framework; and limited nutrition capacity and expertise. No organisation has a standalone ratified nutrition policy supporting the regular acquisition of a nutrition-focused food supply. Disconnected and incoherent policy making is a key challenge in global food systems [40] but equally applies to charitable food systems. In CFS, the policy disconnect and incoherence occurs because decisions are being made in different spaces by diverse policy actors, e.g., government departments, IS, DS, food donors and referring social welfare agencies, which serve diverse interests. Good policy requires a clear understanding of what we want to achieve; so, in this example, is it reducing food waste or reducing food poverty?

DS have offered food relief for up to 125 years demonstrating both the long-term nature of food insecurity and their commitment to providing food to people in need. IS, a more recent addition to the CFS, bring a sophisticated business proposition to food rescue, particularly Foodbank WA based on its organisational capacity. The intent of DS was that they were aspiring to achieve what Hamm and Bellows (2003) call community food security, "a situation in which all community residents obtain a safe, culturally acceptable, nutritionally adequate diet through a sustainable food system that maximizes community self-reliance, social justice, and democratic decision-making" (p. 37) [41,42], whereas IS focused on redistributing food waste without the emphasis on empowering people out of food security.

The inner-city Perth CFS exhibit all three failures (market, government and voluntary) of welfarism described 30 years ago by Lester Salamon [28]. The inability of some citizens to be able to afford to purchase sufficient food in a wealthy country such as Australia is evidence of market failure. The size, scope, expansion and longevity of the food relief sector is a marker of both Government social policy failure in terms of living and income standards and dignified food access [20]. It is also a government failure in terms of the Nation states obligation with respect to the right to food for all citizens—namely to respect, protect and fulfill. Evidence of the four voluntary failures of the non-profit sector includes the following.

4.1. Philanthropic Insufficiency

The increasing demand for food relief and the failure of the CFS to meet that demand is evidence of philanthropic insufficiency. The unreliable and inadequate funding, workforce, food and limited facilities undermine the capacity to support the provision of appropriate food relief. The length of CFS organisations' operation supports the findings of a 2012 review of the WA Emergency Relief secto, which concluded that it will always exist as a safety net, arguing that government should make it a program within a legitimate framework with a funding process [25]. The current findings suggest insufficient government policy, in particular, to assist the CFS to provide safe, reliable and nutritious food to recipients who represent a population sub-group vulnerable to poor health.

CFS relied heavily on corporate, philanthropic and individual donors in inner-city Perth and Victoria due to the limited and unreliable government funding [20]. Charities contribute a significant proportion of their income to CFS; for example, food accounted for 62% of the assistance provided by St Vincent de Paul Inc. in WA in 2017, an expenditure of AUD$1.15 million [43]. During the same period, the Victorian arm provided AUD$14.9 million in material aid, of which 71% was food-related (47% as food vouchers or gift cards) [44]. Getting food to recipients is the focus of effort, leaving little if any time for evaluation of activities for effectiveness or efficiencies. There is some concern that charitable donations have been declining in WA; for example, in 2014–2015 the Salvation Army's income was AUD$700,000 short of its donation target [45].

Interestingly the sentiment expressed by interviewees in this study was that there was enough food, but that it was not able to be distributed effectively, and that resources were wasted. As far back as the 1890s, there was a recommendation that charities in a local area should coordinate to achieve their common purpose and there is limited evidence of co-ordination in our study [28].

4.2. Philanthropic Particularism

DS who focused their donations towards particular subgroups—for example, only providing sandwiches for homeless young people on the street or food for people with HIV—were evident. Particularism also extended to local government, who prefer "pop-up" commercial food trucks catering for transient community events. As a consequence of this example, DS mobile vans and their recipients were regularly asked to move on.

4.3. Philanthropic Paternalism

There was a discord between DS organisations' intent to relieve hunger and promote pathways out of food insecurity and the current practice. The unreliable food supply and lack of nutrition policy meant DS were unlikely to refuse food or beverages of poor nutritional value. The lack of a nutrition policy in Australia is well known [12,26]. Yet, interviewees did not feel that complying with a nutrition policy would limit their food acquisition, consistent with previous research that has found no detriment to services with the establishment of nutrition policy that increases nutritious food acquisition and provision [13,14,46]. A more formal and professional approach is needed to ensure recipients of food relief needs are met.

4.4. Philanthropic Amateurism

Philanthropic amateurism was demonstrated by a lack of food service and/or nutrition training, in part due to the reliance on a "well-meaning but largely untrained workforce to deliver the service". As in other Australian cities, volunteers underpin the CFS workforce in inner-city Perth, suggesting a need for specific volunteer and staff training [20]. Volunteers were mainly retired older people, students, or from large corporate organisations who gift their workforce's time for community service. Although there are acknowledged benefits of reciprocity, there are also challenges relating to the health, financial resources and the preferred contribution of the workforce [47,48]. Complying with Australian standards for volunteering (matching roles to skills, supporting and developing the workforce, protecting their safety and wellbeing, recognizing contribution and continuously improving) [24] is difficult.

The lack of supportive government policy and legislation contributed to the CFS voluntary failure. Mobile food services were vulnerable to local government regulations who can withdraw permission to operate at their discretion. Interviewees described numerous examples of services being moved on due to construction, festivals, parking restrictions, or conflict. Locating DS indoors would alleviate these problems and provide dignified seated meal services and socialisation, critical for people who are socially isolated [24]. This would also facilitate contact with additional services (e.g., health, accommodation, or supports for employment readiness). The FreshPlace model is an example of this type of integrated service which provides both food and assists pathways out of food insecurity [49].

Maintaining food safety along the logistics supply chain is likely to be difficult in the current CFS given the reliance on rescuing perishable waste food that may be past or close to expiry, and untrained volunteers handling food. Ensuring food handling and safety practices could protect this high-risk population sub-group against foodborne illness. Food safety legislation was designed to reduce the public health risk to the individual, yet the Western Australian Civil Liabilities Act 2002 Volunteers and Food and other Donors Act "protects persons who donate food or grocery products from incurring civil liability for personal injury resulting from the consumption of that food or the use of those grocery products, and for related purposes." [50] (p. 1).

CFS-focussed hospitality training would build the confidence and efficiency of the workforce in food service management, food procurement, menu planning, food preparation, occupational health and safety, food safety, and nutrition.

4.5. Equity, Effectiveness and Efficiency

This current study also provides evidence of inadequacy and the corresponding need for action to address all three areas of the 'iron triangle of hunger relief' described by Sengul Orgut et al. (2017) [51]. The three areas are equity (serving the needs of the recipient fairly in regard to both the quantity and quality or type of food received), effectiveness (the ability to meet the needs of the food insecure recipient), and efficiency (cost of resources needed to collect, manage, store and distribute donated food). Each dimension is in turn affected by supply (uncertain monetary supply, donations, and perishability), distribution (uncertain demand) and capacity factors (physical storage, transportation, workforce, and budget). Inefficient food redistribution is exacerbated by a lack of communication between CFS organisations and concerns were raised about overlapping or even competing services, and apparent lack of coordination.

4.6. Strategic Partnerships—The Way Forward

Based on the findings of this organisational audit, there are seven recommendations to guide action to improve the capacity of the CFS to provide a food service that meet the needs of its recipients. The recommendations are ranked in order of priority and given the similarities of the CFS in other Australian States and Territories, we believe they have national applicability.

1. Government-led framework with strategic coordinated partnerships with policy, licensing and funding supports

Streamlining the coordination and collaboration to reduce duplication and provide a better-quality service is recommended. The voluntary sector's weaknesses correspond to government strengths, and vice versa. In the case of the CFS, all levels of government (national, state and local) could partner with the DS and IS. Each level of government has a different imperative; for example, local area health plans are required to address significant health needs of the community, statewide departments act as system managers to set policy priority and conduct monitoring and surveillance activities, and the Federal government sets national standards, develops quality improvement schemes and is responsible for emergency response and social welfare decision making. Funding opportunities and decisions could then occur across all three levels of government and with all partners. Special care would need to be taken to ensure this is achieved without the loss of autonomy or flexibility for the CFS to meet recipient's needs.

2. Refocus, resource and prioritise the requirements for a nutrition-focussed CFS.

Planned menus are integral to the provision of a safe, nutritious and appropriate food service, and a reliable food supply is essential. The scope and nature of the IS suggest that the timing is right for them to focus on nutritious food acquisition with a formalized policy, such as that achieved with nutrition-focussed food banking [13]. Government can support the policy development and implementation through appropriate licensing and/or regulation to address any food safety or nutrition risk and sustain the change with additional resources.

3. Establish CFS principles and standards for appropriate food service needs.

The duty of care is described and controls (policy, licensing, legislation, accreditation and/or training) are implemented in other areas where foodservices are offered to vulnerable population sub-groups; for example, for children (in childcare centers, schools, or day care [31,32]) or people in custodial facilities, aged care facilities, or hospitals where recipients are reliant of the food provided to meet their welfare needs. At a local government level, compliance with food safety regulations for events such as festivals, music concerts are tightly controlled but do not apply for CFS.

Local government is currently considering licensing mobile CFS, including standards that translate nutrition needs across the continuum of care into the types and amounts of foods that should be acquired and supplied to meet CFS recipients' needs in a timely, cost-effective way to improve CFS. Work needs to be undertaken to determine both the content and 'format' (how the food is distributed, utilised and mechanisms for social inclusion) as was undertaken in Belgium [52]. A realistic individual assessment of the length of time the DS is needed should be included in the assessment.

Food safety training should be a mandatory requirement for all CFS workers handling food. As with retail food business, measures should be taken to ensure food safety. The large and changeable volunteer workforce and limited funding may hamper training opportunities; however, given the types of perishable foods distributed, particularly eggs, meat, prepared meals, sushi, there is likely an increased the risk of food poisoning in a system without a food safety and handling framework.

4. Explore options to increase the sufficiency and efficiency of the food supply

Efficiencies are needed in both the distribution of food from IS to DS to recipients and its transformation into appropriate forms suitable for different food service models. With coordination, many options are available to improve food supply logistics and efficiencies. Technology-based online inventories of donated food used to improve food distribution efficiencies in other developed countries [53–55] are not used in Perth. These systems could improve efficiencies by signposting food availability earlier based on "use-by" or "best-by" dates; increasing donations of perishable items; assisting small CFS with limited food storage and with disaster relief emergency responses for food at short notice and in large quantities.

For a sustainable CFS system, government and the commercial and voluntary sector should consider the following: what are the cost benefits of redistributing food waste from the retail sector? Who pays, and what are the costs at each stage of the supply chain, including the food service end? Are there other preferred options? Improving efficiencies may also lead to resources being freed up to re-direct to other priorities; for example, providing meal services on weekends and during holiday periods where they are currently not provided.

5. Training and development of the CFS workforce is needed

Develop and provide CFS workforce training to enable delivery of services to meet their organisational intent and recipient's needs, framed as providing community food security. Cost-effective options should be investigated such as using the massive open online course (MOOC) platform, which enables flexible participation and uses a contemporary educational design to show case studies and provide opportunities for interactive learning and has been shown to be effective [56,57]. The "Developing Food Bank Nutrition Policy to Procure Healthful Foods" (Canvas.net) MOOC for food banks provides a precedent [58]. Local government, peak volunteering bodies, or hospitality training colleges or universities could consider offering gratis training for CFS staff and volunteers.

6. Develop a CFS measurement system monitoring demand, distribution, impact and economic benefit

The CFS works to provide community food security, yet currently measures their impact in terms of kilograms of food rescued or meals provided. Consistent system-wide measures would enable all players in the CFS to articulate its value in terms of achieving community food security. Specific cross-discipline higher degree research should be a university research and government funding priority.

7. Reorient the CFS to create pathways to build sustained food insecurity for recipients

The values of DS organisations suggest that the aim of the CFS approach should be to ensure "community food security" which focusses on local sustainable solutions to ensure ongoing food security rather than just providing short-term food relief. Inherent in any CFS response is the need for higher degrees of citizen empowerment and food democracy, not evident in Perth CFS recipient views [24]. Reducing food insecurity is also an internationally acknowledged government public health priority. Placing people's lived experiences at the centre of decision delivers better integrated policy solutions and effective pathways out of food insecurity [40]. The lack of uptake of innovative social enterprises as a response to food insecurity in Australia has been attributed to the resistance from dominant commercial players and restrictive government legislation [20]. There is a need to work with these actors to support the development and trialing of alternative models to address the market, government and voluntary failures that exist in the current CFS.

4.7. Strengths, Limitations and Further Research

This study is the first comprehensive examination of the scope and operational capacity of the charitable food sector in inner-city Perth and provides a detailed picture of the workings of the sector in an Australian capital city. Specific information on corporate donors and funding was not provided due to confidentiality; however, additional information was sought from financial reports. Service delivery achievements and shortfalls were inconsistently expressed across organisations; for example, millions of meals served versus tonnes of food waste diverted from landfill and numbers of people provided meals. Turn away rates due to short falls in food supply were not available but would assist in the assessment of the effectiveness of the CFS. The findings of this study are limited to the CFS provided in inner-city Perth and provide only a snapshot at a point in time; however, they are likely to be relevant to other the inner-city precincts of Australian and international capital cities with a welfare safety net.

Further research is needed to quantify the types, amount and form of food supplied and the environment in which it is delivered. This will help to determine the suitability and capacity of CFS to meet of the needs of their recipients in terms of food security, nutrition status, and social inclusion. Current decision-making is divorced from lived experience. Decision makers are crafting solutions devoid of an understanding of those who are affected by the problem. Further research validating people lived experience of food insecurity and trialing new responses which offer pathways out is a priority.

Further research recommendations include an economic cost-benefit analysis of the efficiencies of the CFS; further exploration of the government (federal, state and local) and private sector roles in the CFS; and the development and piloting of other models of food relief with an emphasis on social inclusion and pathways out of food insecurity.

5. Conclusions

This research is a timely contribution that shines a light on the NP sector as it struggles to cope with the chronicity of embedded food insecurity, the ad hoc nature of donated food, declining funding and resource constraints. The lack of formalised nutrition policy and training is likely to hinder the acquisition and provision of nutritious and appropriate food relief for people vulnerable to food insecurity. Coordination, reliable funding and food acquisition, food handling and nutrition policy and training and volunteer support is needed to build the capacity of the sector. The findings suggest a CFS at breaking point and highlight the urgent need for debate and investigation of other models to better address food insecurity.

Author Contributions: C.M.P., S.B., A.B., D.K., J.B., B.M., M.C. and J.J. conceived the study design and research objectives, all authors and the research advisory team developed the research questions and interview guide; B.M. and C.C. conducted the interviews; B.M., C.C., C.M.P., and S.B. analyzed the data; B.M., C.C., C.M.P., and S.B. wrote the paper; all authors reviewed and edited the manuscript.

Acknowledgments: This work was funded by Healthway, the Western Australian Health Promotion Foundation, who funded Curtin University to undertake this Special Research Initiative entitled "Charitable Food Services and the Needs of Homeless and Disadvantaged People" (Grant number 24266). Healthway had no role in the design, analysis or writing of this article. We wish to acknowledge the partner organisations (The Salvation Army, United Care West, Noongar Patrol Services, Australian Red Cross, Foodbank, Western Australian Council of Social Services WACOSS—Emergency Relief Forum, Vincentcare, Perth City Council) who formed the research advisory group. We would like to thank members of the research team who have contributed to the work of the project particularly Lieutenant Kris Halliday from The Salvation Army's Doorways Community Programs and Bernie Fisher from WACOSS, Rex Milligan from Foodbank WA as well as the interviewees who willingly gave their time and shared their insights and experience with the ambition of creating a better CFS.

References

1.   Seligman, H.K.; Laraia, B.A.; Kushel, M.B. Food insecurity is associated with chronic disease among low-income NHANES participants. *J. Nutr.* **2010**, *140*, 304–310. [CrossRef] [PubMed]

2.   Marmot, M. Inclusion health: Addressing the causes of the causes. *Lancet* **2017**, *10117*, 186–188. [CrossRef]

3.   McKee, M.; Reeves, A.; Clair, A.; Stuckler, D. Living on the edge: Precariousness and why it matters for health. *Arch. Public Health* **2017**, *75*, 13. [CrossRef] [PubMed]

4.   Fazel, S.; Geddes, J.R.; Kushel, M. The health of homeless people in high-income countries: Descriptive epidemiology, health consequences, and clinical and policy recommendations. *Lancet* **2014**, *384*, 1529–1540. [CrossRef]

5.   Baggett, T.P.; Singer, D.E.; Rao, S.R.; O'Connell, J.J.; Bharel, M.; Rigotti, N.A. Food insufficiency and health services utilization in a national sample of homeless adults. *J. Gen. Intern. Med.* **2011**, *26*, 627–634. [CrossRef] [PubMed]

6.   Cook, J.T.; Black, M.; Chilton, M.; Cutts, D.; Ettinger de Cuba, S.; Heeren, T.C.; Rose-Jacobs, R.; Sandel, M.; Casey, P.H.; Coleman, S. Are food insecurity's health impacts underestimated in the U.S. population? Marginal food security also predicts adverse health outcomes in young us children and mothers. *Adv. Nutr.* **2013**, *4*, 51–61. [CrossRef] [PubMed]

7.   Hamelin, A.-M.; Hamel, D. Food insufficiency in currently or formerly homeless persons is associated with poorer health. *Can. J. Urban Res.* **2009**, *18*, 1.

8.   Quine, S.; Kendig, H.; Russell, C.; Touchard, D. Health promotion for socially disadvantaged groups: The case of homeless older men in Australia. *Health Promot. Int.* **2004**, *19*, 157–165. [CrossRef] [PubMed]

9.   Lee, B.A.; Greif, M.J. Homelessness and hunger. *J. Health Soc. Behav.* **2008**, *49*, 3–19. [CrossRef] [PubMed]

10. Crawford, B.; Yamazaki, R.; Franke, E.; Amanatidis, S.; Ravulo, J.; Steinbeck, K.; Ritchie, J.; Torvaldsen, S.
     Sustaining dignity? Food insecurity in homeless young people in urban Australia. *Health Promot. J. Austr.*
     2014, *25*, 71–78. [CrossRef] [PubMed]

11. Ruah. *Ruah Community Service*; Registry Week 2016 Report; Ruah: Perth, Australia, 2016.

12. Lindberg, R.; Whelan, J.; Lawrence, M.; Gold, L.; Friel, S. Still serving hot soup? Two hundred years of
     a charitable food sector in Australia: A narrative review. *Aust. N. Z. J. Public Health* **2015**, *39*, 358–365.
     [CrossRef] [PubMed]

13. Simmet, A.; Depa, J.; Tinnemann, P.; Stroebele-Benschop, N. The nutritional quality of food provided from
     food pantries: A systematic review of existing literature. *J. Acad. Nutr. Diet.* **2017**, *117*, 577–588. [CrossRef]
     [PubMed]

14. Campbell, E.; Webb, K.; Michelle, R.; Crawford, P.; Hudson, H.; Hecht, K. *Nutrition-Focused Food Banking*;
     Institute of Medicine: Washington, DC, USA, 2015.

15. Campbell, E.C.; Ross, M.; Webb, K.L. Improving the nutritional quality of emergency food: A study of food
     bank organizational culture, capacity, and practices. *J. Hunger Environ. Nutr.* **2013**, *8*, 261–280. [CrossRef]

16. Pollard, C.; Begley, A.; Landrigan, T. The rise of food inequality in Australia. In *Food Poverty and Insecurity:
     International Food Inequalities*; Caraher, M., Coveney, J., Eds.; Springer International Publishing Switzerland:
     Basel, Switzerland, 2016; pp. 89–103.

17. Australian Government Department of Human Services. Age Pension. Available online: https://www.
     humanservices.gov.au/individuals/services/centrelink/age-pension (accessed on 18 April 2018).

18. Australian Government Department of Human Services. Families. Available online: https://www.
     humanservices.gov.au/individuals/families (accessed on 18 April 2018).

19. Australian Government Department of Human Services. Newstart Allowance. Available online:
     https://www.humanservices.gov.au/individuals/services/centrelink/newstart-allowance (accessed on
     18 April 2018).

20. Wills, B. Eating at the limits: Barriers to the emergence of social enterprise initiatives in the australian
     emergency food relief sector. *Food Policy* **2017**, *70*, 62–70. [CrossRef]

21. Foodbank Hunger Report 2016. Available online: https://www.foodbank.org.au/wp-content/uploads/
     2016/05/Foodbank-Hunger-Report-2016.pdf (accessed on 1 December 2017).

22. Wingrove, K.; Barbour, L.; Palermo, C. Exploring nutrition capacity in australia's charitable food sector.
     Nutr. Diet. **2016**, *74*, 495–501. [CrossRef] [PubMed]

23. Wicks, R.; Trevena, L.J.; Quine, S. Experiences of food insecurity among urban soup kitchen consumers:
     Insights for improving nutrition and well-being. *J. Acad. Nutr. Diet.* **2006**, *106*, 921–924. [CrossRef] [PubMed]

24. Booth, S.; Begely, A.; Mackntosh, K.A.; Jancy, J.; Caraher, M.; Whelan, J.; Pollard, C.M. Gratitude, resignation,
     and the desire for dignity: Lived experience of food charity recipients and their recommendations for
     improvement, Perth, Western Australia. *Public Health Nutr.* **2018**. accepted for publication.

25. Western Australian Council of Social Service. *Giving Shape to the Emergency Relief Sector*; Western Australian
     Council of Social Service: West Perth, Australia, 2012.

26. Middleton, G.; Mehta, K.; McNaughton, D.; Booth, S. The experiences and perceptions of food banks amongst
     users in high-income countries: An international scoping review. *Appetite* **2018**, *120*, 698–708. [CrossRef]
     [PubMed]

27. Booth, S.; Whelan, J. Hungry for change: The food banking industry in Australia. *Br. Food J.* **2014**,
     116, 1392–1404. [CrossRef]

28. Salamon, L.M. Of market failure, voluntary failure, and third-party government: Toward a theory of
     government-nonprofit relations in the modern welfare state. *Nonprofit Volunt. Sect. Q.* **1987**, *16*, 29–49.
     [CrossRef]

29. McKay, F.H.; McKenzie, H. Food aid provision in metropolitan Melbourne: A mixed methods study. *J. Hunger
     Environ. Nutr.* **2017**, *12*, 11–25. [CrossRef]

30. Harris, E.; Wise, M.; Hawe, P.; Finlay, P.; Nutbeam, D. *Working Together: Intersectoral Action for Health*;
     Australian Government Publishing Service: Canberra, Australia, 1995.

31. Pollard, C.; Lewis, J.; Miller, M. Start right–eat right award scheme: Implementing food and nutrition policy
     in child care centers. *Health Educ. Behav.* **2001**, *28*, 320–330. [CrossRef] [PubMed]

32. Pollard, C.M.; Lewis, J.M.; Miller, M.R. Food service in long day care centres—An opportunity for public
     health intervention. *Aust. N. Z. J. Public Health* **1999**, *23*, 606–610. [CrossRef] [PubMed]

33. Foodbank Western Australia Annual Report 2017. Available online: https://www.foodbankwa.org.au/wp-content/blogs.dir/5/files/2017/10/FB-AR-17_online.pdf (accessed on 12 April 2018).

34. The Ozharvest Effect 2016. Available online: https://www.ozharvest.org/wp-content/uploads/2014/04/OZHF0034F_OzHarvest_AnnualReport_Book2_FA3_LR41.pdf (accessed on 12 April 2018).

35. Foley, R.M.; Pollard, C.M. Food cent $—Implementing and evaluating a nutrition education project focusing on value for money. *Aust. N. Z. J. Public Health* **1998**, *22*, 494–501. [CrossRef] [PubMed]

36. Pettigrew, S.; Moore, S.; Pratt, I.S.; Jongenelis, M. Evaluation outcomes of a long-running adult nutrition education programme. *Public Health Nutr.* **2016**, *19*, 743–752. [CrossRef] [PubMed]

37. Offer, A.; Pechey, R.; Ulijaszek, S. Obesity under affluence varies by welfare regimes: The effect of fast food, insecurity, and inequality. *Econ. Hum. Biol.* **2010**, *8*, 297–308. [CrossRef] [PubMed]

38. Enjolras, B.; Salamon, L.M.; Sivesind, K.H.; Zimmer, A. *The Third Sector as a Renewable Resource for Europe: Concepts, Impacts, Challenges and Opportunities*; Springer: Berlin/Hamburg, Germany, 2018.

39. Casey, J. *The Nonprofit World: Civil Society and the Rise of the Nonprofit Sector*; Kumarian Press: Sterling, VA, USA, 2016.

40. Hawkes, C. The role of law, regulation, and policy in meeting 21st century challenges to the food supply. In *Food Governance Conference*; Sydney University: Sydney, Australia, 2016.

41. Bellows, A.C.; Hamm, M.W. U.S.-based community food security: Influences, practice, debate. *J. Study Food Soc.* **2002**, *6*, 31–44. [CrossRef]

42. Hamm, M.W.; Bellows, A.C. Community food security and nutrition educators. *J. Nutr. Educ. Behav.* **2003**, *35*, 37–43. [CrossRef]

43. St Vincent de Paul Society (WA) Inc. Annual Review 2017: Restoring Hope. Available online: https://www.vinnies.org.au/icms_docs/276248_Vinnies_WA_2017_Annual_Report.pdf (accessed on 12 April 2018).

44. St Vincent de Paul Society (Victoria) Inc. 2016–2017 Annual Review Face to Face Side by Side Walking together. Available online: https://www.vinnies.org.au/icms_docs/276542_2016-2017_Annual_Report.pdf (accessed on 12 April 2018).

45. Claire, D. *Salvation Army May Cut Services in WA as Donations Decline for Third Year in a Row*; ABC New 2015; Australian Broadcasting Commission: Perth, Australia, 2015.

46. Simmet, A.; Depa, J.; Tinnemann, P.; Stroebele-Benschop, N. The dietary quality of food pantry users: A systematic review of existing literature. *J. Acad. Nutr. Diet.* **2017**, *117*, 563–576. [CrossRef] [PubMed]

47. Stephens, C.; Breheny, M.; Mansvelt, J. Volunteering as reciprocity: Beneficial and harmful effects of social policies to encourage contribution in older age. *J. Aging Stud.* **2015**, *33*, 22–27. [CrossRef] [PubMed]

48. Wheeler, J.A.; Gorey, K.M.; Greenblatt, B. The beneficial effects of volunteering for older volunteers and the people they serve: A meta-analysis. *Int. J. Aging Hum. Dev.* **1998**, *47*, 69–79. [CrossRef] [PubMed]

49. Martin, K.S.; Colantonio, A.G.; Picho, K.; Boyle, K.E. Self-efficacy is associated with increased food security in novel food pantry program. *SSM-Popul. Health* **2016**, *2*, 62–67. [CrossRef] [PubMed]

50. Government of Western Australia; Department of Communities. *Volunteers and Food and Other Donors (Protection from Liability) Act 2002*; Government of Western Australia; Department of Communities: Perth Western, Australia, 2016; Volume 32.

51. Orgut, I.S.; Brock, L.G., III; Davis, L.B.; Ivy, J.S.; Jiang, S.; Morgan, S.D.; Uzsoy, R.; Hale, C.; Middleton, E. Achieving equity, effectiveness, and efficiency in food bank operations: Strategies for feeding America with implications for global hunger relief. In *Advances in Managing Humanitarian Operations*; Springer: Berlin/Hamburg, Germany, 2016; pp. 229–256.

52. Stepman, E.; Uyttendaele, M.; De Boeck, E.; Jacxsens, L. Needs of beneficiaries related to the format and content of food parcels in Ghent, Belgium. *Br. Food J.* **2018**, *120*, 578–587. [CrossRef]

53. Bazerghi, C.; McKay, F.H.; Dunn, M. The role of food banks in addressing food insecurity: A systematic review. *J. Community Health* **2016**, *41*, 732–740. [CrossRef] [PubMed]

54. Chow Match. *Food Sharing Database*; Chow Match: San Francisco, CA, USA, 2015.

55. Corbo, C.; Fraticelli, F. The use of web-based technology as an emerging option for food waste reduction. In *Envisioning a Future Without Food Waste and Food Poverty: Societal Challenges*; San-Epifanio, L.E., Scheifler, M.D.R., Eds.; Wageningen Academic Publishers: Wageningen, The Netherlands, 2015; pp. 1–2.

56. Bozkurt, A.; Akgun-Ozbek, E.; Yilmazel, S.; Erdogdu, E.; Ucar, H.; Guler, E.; Sezgin, S.; Karadeniz, A.; Sen-Ersoy, N.; Goksel-Canbek, N. Trends in distance education research: A content analysis of journals 2009–2013. *Int. Rev. Res. Open Distrib. Learn.* **2015**. [CrossRef]

57.   Adam, M.; Young-Wolff, K.C.; Konar, E.; Winkleby, M. Massive open online nutrition and cooking course for improved eating behaviors and meal composition. *Int. J. Behav. Nutr. Phys. Act.* **2015**, *12*, 143. [CrossRef] [PubMed]

58.   Webb, K.; Campbell, E.M.R. Developing Food Bank Nutrition Policy to Procure Healthful Foods (Canvas.Net). Available online: https://www.canvas.net/browse/cwh/courses/food-bank-nutrition-policy (accessed on 12 April 2018).

Permissions

The contributors of this book come from diverse backgrounds, making this book a truly international effort. This book will bring forth new frontiers with its revolutionizing research information and detailed analysis of the nascent developments around the world.

We would like to thank all the contributing authors for lending their expertise to make the book truly unique. They have played a crucial role in the development of this book. Without their invaluable contributions this book wouldn't have been possible. They have made vital efforts to compile up to date information on the varied aspects of this subject to make this book a valuable addition to the collection of many professionals and students.

This book was conceptualized with the vision of imparting up-to-date information and advanced data in this field. To ensure the same, a matchless editorial board was set up. Every individual on the board went through rigorous rounds of assessment to prove their worth. After which they invested a large part of their time researching and compiling the most relevant data for our readers.

The editorial board has been involved in producing this book since its inception. They have spent rigorous hours researching and exploring the diverse topics which have resulted in the successful publishing of this book. They have passed on their knowledge of decades through this book. To expedite this challenging task, the publisher supported the team at every step. A small team of assistant editors was also appointed to further simplify the editing procedure and attain best results for the readers.

Apart from the editorial board, the designing team has also invested a significant amount of their time in understanding the subject and creating the most relevant covers. They scrutinized every image to scout for the most suitable representation of the subject and create an appropriate cover for the book.

The publishing team has been an ardent support to the editorial, designing and production team. Their endless efforts to recruit the best for this project, has resulted in the accomplishment of this book. They are a veteran in the field of academics and their pool of knowledge is as vast as their experience in printing. Their expertise and guidance has proved useful at every step. Their uncompromising quality standards have made this book an exceptional effort. Their encouragement from time to time has been an inspiration for everyone.

The publisher and the editorial board hope that this book will prove to be a valuable piece of knowledge for researchers, students, practitioners and scholars across the globe.

List of Contributors

Raissa Sorgho
Heidelberg Research to Practice Group, Heidelberg Institute of Global Health (HIGH), Heidelberg University Hospital, Heidelberg University, Im Neuenheimer Feld 365, 69120 Heidelberg, Germany
Working Group on Climate Change, Nutrition & Health, Heidelberg Institute of Global Health (HIGH), Heidelberg University Hospital, Heidelberg University, Im Neuenheimer Feld 324, 69120 Heidelberg, Germany

Carlos A. Montenegro Quiñonez, Valérie R. Louis, Volker Winkler, Peter Dambach and Olaf Horstick
Heidelberg Research to Practice Group, Heidelberg Institute of Global Health (HIGH), Heidelberg University Hospital, Heidelberg University, Im Neuenheimer Feld 365, 69120 Heidelberg, Germany

Rainer Sauerborn
Working Group on Climate Change, Nutrition & Health, Heidelberg Institute of Global Health (HIGH), Heidelberg University Hospital, Heidelberg University, Im Neuenheimer Feld 324, 69120 Heidelberg, Germany

Jiuliang Xu, Fusuo Zhang and Xuexian Li
Department of Plant Nutrition, The Key Plant-Soil Interaction Laboratory, Ministry of Education, China Agricultural University, Beijing 100193, China
National Academy of Agriculture Green Development, China Agricultural University, Beijing 100193, China
Chinese Academy of Green Food Development, Beijing 100193, China

Muhammad Ishfaq and Jiahui Zhong
Department of Plant Nutrition, The Key Plant-Soil Interaction Laboratory, Ministry of Education, China Agricultural University, Beijing 100193, China

Zhihua Zhang and Xian Zhang
China Green Food Development Center, Beijing 100081, China

Wei Li
Fujian Key Laboratory of Agro-Product Quality and Safety, Fuzhou 350003, China

Jeromey B. Temple
Demography and Ageing Unit, Melbourne School of Population and Global Health, University of Melbourne, Melbourne 3010, Australia

Flora Douglas
School of Nursing and Midwifery, Robert Gordon University, Aberdeen AB10 7QG, Scotland
Rowett Institute, University of Aberdeen, Aberdeen AB25 2ZD, UK

Fiona MacKenzie
Institute of Applied Health Sciences, University of Aberdeen, Aberdeen AB25 2ZD, Scotland

Lynda McKenzie, Anne Ludbrook and Ourega-Zoé Ejebu
Health Economics Research Unit, University of Aberdeen, Aberdeen AB25 2ZD, Scotland

Stephen Whybrow
The Rowett Institute, University of Aberdeen, Aberdeen AB25 2ZD, Scotland

Ada L. Garcia
Human Nutrition, School of Medicine, Dentistry and Nursing, College of Medical, Veterinary and Life Sciences, University of Glasgow, Glasgow G31 2ER, Scotland

Elizabeth Dowler
Emeritus Professor of Food & Social Policy, Department Sociology, University of Warwick, Coventry CV4 7AL, UK

Anna Sofia Salonen and Tuomo Laihiala
Faculty of Social Sciences, University of Tampere, 33014 Tampere, Finland

Maria Ohisalo
Y-Foundation, 00531 Helsinki, Finland

Megan Ferguson
School of Public Health, The University of Queensland, Brisbane 4072, Australia
Wellbeing and Preventable Chronic Diseases, Menzies School of Health Research, Darwin 0811, Australia

Kerin O'Dea
Division of Health Sciences, University of South Australia, Adelaide 5001, Australia

Jon Altman
Alfred Deakin Institute for Citizenship and Globalisation, Deakin University, Burwood 3125, Australia

Marjory Moodie
Deakin Health Economics, Centre for Population Health Research, Deakin University, Geelong 3220, Australia

Julie Brimblecombe
Wellbeing and Preventable Chronic Diseases, Menzies School of Health Research, Darwin 0811, Australia
Faculty of Medicine, Nursing and Health Sciences, Monash University, Melbourne 3168, Australia
Department of Nutrition, Dietetics and Food, Monash University, 3168 Melbourne, Australia

Sue Booth
College of Medicine & Public Health, Flinders University, Adelaide 5000, Australia

Mia A. Papas
Christiana Care Health System, Value Institute, Wilmington, DE 19899, USA

Kimberly B. Gill
Disaster Research Center, University of Delaware, Newark, DE 19716, USA

David M. Abramson
College of Global Public Health, New York University, New York, NY 10012, USA

Lauren A. Clay
Health Services Administration, D'Youville College, Buffalo, NY 14201, USA
Disaster Research Center, University of Delaware, Newark, DE 19716, USA
College of Global Public Health, New York University, New York, NY 10012, USA

Timothy J. Landrigan, Satvinder S. Dhaliwal, Alison Daly, Christina M. Pollard, Deborah A. Kerr, Colin W. Binns, Cathy Campbell, Deborah Kerr, Andrea Begley and Jonine Jancey
Faculty of Health Science, School of Public Health, Curtin University, Perth 6845, Western Australia, Australia

Jill Whelan and Colin Bell
School of Medicine, Global Obesity Centre, Deakin University, Geelong 3220, Australia

Lynne Millar
Australian Health Policy Collaboration, Victoria University, Melbourne 3000, Australia
Australian Institute for Musculoskeletal Science (AIMSS), The University of Melbourne and Western Health, St Albans 3021, Australia

Felicity Grainger
School of Exercise and Nutrition Sciences, Deakin University, Geelong 3220, Australia

Steven Allender
School of Health and Social Development, Global Obesity Centre, Deakin University, Geelong 3220, Australia

Penelope Love
School of Exercise and Nutrition Sciences, Deakin University, Geelong 3220, Australia
Institute for Physical Activity and Nutrition (IPAN), Deakin University, Geelong 3220, Australia

Clare Brown, Cara Laws, Lea Merone, Melinda Hammond and Kani Thompson
Apunipima Cape York Health Council, 4870 Cairns, Australia

Dympna Leonard
Australian Institute of Tropical Health and Medicine, College of Public Health Medical and Veterinary Sciences, James Cook University, 4870 Cairns, Australia

Sandy Campbell
Centre for Indigenous Health Equity Research, Central Queensland University, 4870 Cairns, Australia

Karla Canuto
Apunipima Cape York Health Council, 4870 Cairns, Australia
Wardliparingga Aboriginal Health, South Australian Health and Medical Research Institute, 5001 Adelaide, Australia

Geneviève Jessiman-Perreault and Lynn McIntyre
Department of Community Health Sciences, Cumming School of Medicine, University of Calgary, Calgary, AB T2N 1N4, Canada

Martin Caraher
Centre for Food Policy, City University of London, Northampton Square, London EC1V 0HB, UK

Michael Phillips
Harry Perkins Institute for Medical Research, University of Western Australia, Perth 6009, Western Australia, Australia

Ada L Garcia
Human Nutrition, University of Glasgow, Glasgow G31 2ER, UK

Karen Louise Barton
Division of Food and Drink, Abertay University, Dundee DD1 1HG, UK

Wendy Louise Wrieden
Human Nutrition Research Centre and Institute of Health & Society, Newcastle University, Newcastle upon Tyne NE2 4HH, UK

Penelope Love and Cherie Russell
Institute for Physical Activity and Nutrition (IPAN), Deakin University, Geelong 3220, Australia
School of Exercise and Nutrition Sciences, Deakin University, Geelong 3220, Australia

Meron Lewis
The Australian Prevention Partnership Centre (TAPPC), Sax Institute, Sydney 2007, Australia

Amanda Lee
The Australian Prevention Partnership Centre (TAPPC), Sax Institute, Sydney 2007, Australia
School of Public Health, University of Queensland, Herston QLD 4006, Australia

Bruce Mackintosh
School of Agriculture and Environment, The University of Western Australia, 35 Stirling Highway, Crawley, Perth 6009, Australia

Joel Berg
Hunger Free America, 50 Broad Street, Suite 1103, New York 10004, NY, USA

Index

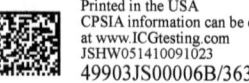

Printed in the USA
CPSIA information can be obtained
at www.ICGtesting.com
JSHW051410091023
49903JS00006B/363

9 781639 897216